In Vitro Fertilization

The A.R.T. of Making Babies

(Assisted Reproductive Technology)

Fourth Edition

Geoffrey Sher, MD
Virginia Marriage Davis, RN, MN
Jean Stoess, MA

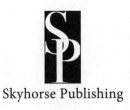

Skyhorse Publishing

Skyhorse Publishing books may be purchased in bulk at special discounts for sales promotion, corporate gifts, fund-raising, or educational purposes. Special editions can also be created to specifications. For details, contact the Special Sales Department, Skyhorse Publishing, 307 West 36th Street, 11th Floor, New York, NY 10018 or info@skyhorsepublishing.com.

Skyhorse® and Skyhorse Publishing® are registered trademarks of Skyhorse Publishing, Inc.®, a Delaware corporation.

Visit our website at www.skyhorsepublishing.com.

10 9 8 7 6 5 4 3 2

Library of Congress Cataloging-in-Publication Data on file

ISBN: 978-1-62087-606-0

Text design adapted by James Scotto-Lavino
Cover design by Owen Corrigan
Illustrations by Marc Greene and Dale Williams
Printed in the United States of America

This book is dedicated to all of the brave, strong

couples who, despite enduring difficult struggles, still believe

in the possibility of parenthood.

TABLE OF CONTENTS

Chapter 10: Is IVF the Most Appropriate Option? 206

Chapter 11: Shaping Realistic Expectations about IVF 225

Chapter 12: How to Find the Right IVF Program 242

Chapter 13: IUI, GIFT, and Other Alternatives to IVF 255

FOREWORD BY BRIAN COHEN, MD

It is my privilege to write a few words and introduce the 4th edition of *In Vitro Fertilization: The A.R.T of Making Babies* by Dr. Geoffrey Sher.

I have known Dr. Sher the past forty-five years. He has always had a particular interest and commitment to the diagnosis and treatment of infertility.

Early on, Dr. Sher had extensive experience with the use of human menopausal gonadotropin therapy. It is thus no surprise that the advent of in vitro fertilization was accompanied by Dr. Sher being amongst those with the highest success rates in the United States.

When the work of Dr. Patrick Steptoe and Dr. Robert Edward resulted in the first pregnancy due to in vitro fertilization, Dr. Sher, accompanied by two highly experienced cellular biologists, went to learn firsthand the basic laboratory techniques and the clinical management of this process.

From the beginning Dr. Sher has always been committed to ensuring scientific quality and accountability in the field of in vitro fertilization. If considered controversial, it is because he has always chosen to seek the scientific truth in the interests of benefiting the patient. He has consistently chosen science over politics. His attitude is refreshing, for when politics trumps science in medicine, the only one who suffers is the patient.

This book provides insight for those who seek and need in vitro fertilization. It illustrates step-by-step information and a detailed account of what to expect in the process of in vitro fertilization.

Chapters on preimplantation genetic diagnosis to ensure the highest quality of embryos and the description of cutting-edge methods for egg/embryo genetic analysis and freezing are illuminating.

Particular attention should be paid to the section on Reproductive Immunology. It remains an area of controversy where general medical politics has trumped the science at this time. This is particularly important for the patient who has had two or three failures at in vitro fertilization despite the presence of healthy embryos. Measuring the scientific parameters of immunological causes enables us to achieve a diagnosis and to treat it appropriately.

I have no hesitation in recommending this book for patients who seek knowledge in the field of in vitro fertilization. I am sure it will provide much positive detailed information empowering the patient to ask the correct questions and to ensure that they find the right program to optimize their treatment.

Such knowledge should facilitate patients getting the most up-to-date and adequate care and hopefully a positive result…the child they so earnestly desire.

Brian M. Cohen, MBChB, MD (Post Doctoral)
Clinical Professor, University of Texas Southwestern Medical Center at Dallas, Dallas, TX
Director, Cohen Center, P.A., Dallas, TX

FOREWORD BY NANCY HEMENWAY

D esigner egg auctions, cloning, and "test-tube babies" are all "hot topics" used by the media to fuel the controversial fires surrounding infertility treatment options. More than 5 million couples are faced with the prospect of navigating and filtering a colossal maze of information and misinformation in order to successfully build their families. This winding road to family can be extremely lonely, physically demanding, and emotionally draining. Dr. Geoffrey Sher is a cool oasis and a breath of fresh air for couples embarking on this exhausting journey.

Dr. Geoffrey Sher, executive medical director of Sher Institutes for Reproductive Medicine, practicing in Las Vegas, Nevada, and St. Louis, Missouri, is one of a kind. He is entrepreneurial, energetic, passionate, and compassionate in his approach to both the science and medical aspects of reproductive medicine. Dr. Sher's book, *In Vitro Fertilization: The A.R.T. of Making Babies*, is a beacon and road map for those plotting their treatment course.

In Vitro Fertilization: The A.R.T. of Making Babies empowers the individual with reliable information, in down-to-earth language. Sher's forward-thinking and frank dialogue tackles difficult and controversial topics with honesty and integrity. Together the authors further the idea that working in tandem with one's physician to build a family should be the rule—not the exception.

Over the last 20 years, I have been an advocate, educator, a patient, a consumer, and, finally, after years of navigating the infertility labyrinth, a parent twice blessed. I am a survivor of many infertility battles and the cofounder and executive director of the InterNational Council on Infertility Information Dissemination, Inc. (INCIID—pronounced "inside"), the world's largest infertility advocacy organization. I've worked alongside some of the leading names in the field of reproductive medicine. Yet there is none I am more honored to call friend and colleague than Geoffrey Sher, MD; a man of many talents, who has a clear vision for the future.

Nancy Hemenway
Executive Director
International Council on Infertility Information Dissemination (INCIID)
www.INCIID.org

PREFACE

"Innovators are rarely received with joy, and established authorities launch into condemnation of newer truths; for at every crossroad to the future are a thousand self-appointed guardians of the past."

—Betty MacQuitty, Victory Over Pain: Morton's
Discovery of Anesthesia

In vitro fertilization (IVF) has come a long way since 1978, when Louise Brown, christened "the world's first test-tube baby" by the press, was born in England. The first in vitro fertilization program in the United States was introduced at the Eastern Virginia Medical School at Norfolk in the late 1970s. Now, more than 400 clinics throughout the United States offer IVF, with varying degrees of reported success.

In vitro fertilization literally means "fertilization in glass." Traditionally known as in vitro fertilization and embryo transfer (IVF/ET), the procedure is more commonly referred to simply as in vitro fertilization, or IVF. (The term *IVF* will be used throughout this book instead of the more cumbersome *IVF/ET*.)

IVF is composed of several basic steps. First, the woman is given fertility drugs that stimulate her ovaries to produce as many mature eggs possible. Then, when the ovaries have been properly stimulated, the eggs are retrieved by suction through a needle inserted into her ovaries. The harvested eggs are then fertilized in a petri dish in the laboratory with her partner's or a donor's sperm. Several days later, the fertilized egg(s)—now known as embryo(s)—are transferred by a thin catheter through the woman's vagina into her uterus, where it is hoped they will grow into one or more healthy babies.

It is essential that the infertile couple and their physician identify the cause of the infertility in order to determine the most appropriate form of treatment. This does not mean that IVF should be regarded as a treatment of last resort. It may well be that IVF offers the best hope for a healthy pregnancy. At most reputable IVF centers, the chance of a woman becoming pregnant with IVF is much greater than that of a fertile woman conceiving (without treatment) in any given month of trying. Nevertheless, the couple should understand that IVF is not everything to everyone and that some women never get pregnant through IVF, no matter how many times they try.

Many infertile couples who have experienced repeated disappointments over the years in their attempts to conceive have become desperate. Most have previously tried a variety of unsuccessful procedures: fertility drugs for the woman and/or man, medications to treat various hormonal problems, nonsurgical alternatives such as artificial insemination, and pelvic surgery to repair anatomical defects. These couples look to IVF as a promising procedure that might help them conceive after all of their other attempts have failed.

Yet, of the more than 2 million couples in the United States for whom IVF offers the best option for pregnancy, less than 200,000 undergo the procedure annually. Clearly, eligible infertile couples in the United States are not even coming close to tapping into the potential of IVF. Why is this so?

One reason is that some people still consider IVF to be experimental. However, the evidence proves otherwise—about 350,000 IVF babies have already been born in the United States. Yet the public, in company with many members of the medical profession, still knows relatively little about IVF beyond the way it is characterized by the media.

People get a distorted idea about IVF when they turn on the television and see a slide of a test tube with a baby inside. By no means are either test tubes or babies involved at that point. There are just a momentary couple of days when fertilization takes place outside the body, and then the embryo(s) is placed in the woman's uterus and begins to grow there. The phrase *test-tube baby* is a convenient handle for the media, but it misleadingly implies that the whole process occurs outside the body, which is not true.

Unfortunately, consumers find it difficult to get much in-depth information about this exciting procedure. (The term *consumers* is used here to mean both infertile couples and physicians who refer their patients to a particular program.) Currently, no credible source provides prospectively audited, verifiable information about success rates obtained from IVF programs in the United States. As a result, people trying to learn about IVF often feel as though they are stumbling in the dark.

Several national organizations, including the Society for Assisted Reproductive Technology (SART), an affiliated society of the American Society for Reproductive Medicine (ASRM), and a number of support groups for infertile couples provide limited information about IVF and related procedures. SART was formed in 1988 under the umbrella of the ASRM, which is primarily made up of physicians but also includes laboratory personnel, psychologists, nurses, and other paramedical personnel interested in infertility.

SART provides a list of IVF programs in the United States, but it does not recommend or endorse any specific programs. Instead, SART encourages consumers to contact IVF programs individually for more information.

Aside from the problem of insufficient information, another obstacle to widespread acceptance of IVF is its high cost. IVF is relatively expensive—$10,000 to $20,000 per procedure, depending on the program and the type of IVF procedure performed.

Many couples pass up IVF because of the financial burden, although it may be the most appropriate treatment for them. They simply can't afford it. Some states have passed laws requiring insurance companies to reimburse in total for IVF, and several others are considering similar legislation. Nevertheless, we must inform consumers that a new form of payment for IVF services known as Financial Risk Sharing (FRS) promises to make IVF services more affordable. More than 100 IVF programs in the United States currently offer FRS in one form or another and the number is growing. (See Chapter 18 for a discussion about FRS that is offered by the Sher Institutes for Reproductive Medicine (SIRM) as well as the need for insurance reimbursement for IVF.)

Yet we must also warn consumers that the outlook on IVF-related issues is not likely to improve for some time. IVF will remain an expensive procedure. But by researching the IVF situation for themselves, couples will be able to answer these fundamental questions: (1) Are we eligible for IVF and, (2) How do we select the program that will give us the best results?

This book is designed to help answer these critical questions. It describes IVF and some other assisted reproductive technology (A.R.T.) procedures; outlines a variety of emotional, physical, financial, and moral/religious issues; and highlights points that should be considered when deciding whether IVF or another high-tech procedure is indeed the most appropriate option. We do not offer any judgments relating to ethics, religion, or morality. These kinds of decisions are private matters that must be resolved by each couple in their own way. We do not intend to imply that our approach is the only acceptable way and/or should be rigidly followed. Our function is to recommend, to inform, to educate, and to serve—but never to dictate.

We are particularly cognizant of the fact that many women who do conceive following IVF may have pregnancies that are at risk. Going from infertility to family can be extremely traumatic from an emotional, psychological, and physical point of view. One of the ways we prepare couples is by providing them with as much information about infertility, as well as IVF and related procedures, as they need. We believe that being as knowledgeable as possible helps them cope with the roller-coaster experience they will undergo.

Infertility is a condition that often disempowers those so affected. The only way to be re-impowered is through information. A very easy way to access such information is by going online to my blog at www. IVFauthority.com where you will see numerous articles (which I post, almost on a weekly basis). There you will find current information on a whole host of topics, all of which are directly and indirectly related to ART. Another very accessible source of information can be found on the SIRM website, www.haveababy.com, which also houses a very popular and active "discussion board." Thousands of individuals post questions and make comments with the full expectation of a very prompt response by an SIRM fertility specialist. Interested parties can also   call (800) 780-7437 to obtain additional information and schedule an in-person or Skype consultation (often at no cost). Those interested can also visit

SIRM on Facebook (http://www.facebook.com/HaveABaby) where one can post and read comments, learn about upcoming SIRM events and about what is new in our setting. There (as on the SIRM-website) one can also communicate with others as well as with an SIRM physician. Finally, this book, *In Vitro Fertilization: The A.R.T. of Making Babies* may also be purchased from most bookstores or can be obtained online at www. amazon.com.

This book was written to help consumers become better informed so as to enable them to develop and maintain realistic expectations about IVF. Realistic expectations revolve around the best and the worst possible scenarios, but all infertile couples should prepare themselves for the worst, just in case. However, by planning an effective strategy, asking the right questions, and evaluating the answers properly, candidates can determine whether they are eligible for IVF and can find the most appropriate program. Based upon what this 35-year-old new mother told us, doing that homework does pay off:

"I must have spent at least three hours talking with my own physician, trying to find out where to go for IVF. It was so frustrating not being able to find anyone who could give me any real answers. Several times I was tempted to go to the IVF clinic nearest us just because it was so convenient. But, thank God, I did my homework as thoroughly as I knew how. I must have called up fifteen different programs. I asked a lot of questions about success rates and what it was like to go through their programs, and then I had to sort everything out. I finally found a great program—and now we have a beautiful little girl who is the joy of our lives. I can hardly remember what life had been like without her. It was worth all that effort."

—Geoffrey Sher, M.D.

UNITS OF MEASUREMENT

The following abbreviations for units of measurement are used throughout this book.

cc	cubic centimeter
cm	centimeter
mcg	microgram
mg	milligram
miu	milli-international unit
ml	milliliter
mm	millimeter
ng	nanogram
pg	picogram

CHAPTER

1

THE GROWING DILEMMA OF INFERTILITY

It is estimated that there are about 45 million couples of childbearing age living together in the United States today. Approximately 5 million of these couples are infertile.

This estimate is based on a series of nationwide surveys of married couples in which the women were between 15 and 44 years of age. It was found that one out of every 12 couples, or 8 percent, were involuntarily infertile.

Infertility can be defined as the inability to conceive after one full year of normal, regular heterosexual intercourse without the use of any contraception. The odds that a woman will get pregnant without medical assistance when she has failed to do so after a year or two of unprotected intercourse are extremely low.

Only couples who have experienced the problem of infertility can truly understand its devastating emotional and physical impacts. As one woman who had been trying unsuccessfully to become pregnant for many years explained:

> *It has been two years since I learned the reason I wasn't getting pregnant was because my fallopian tubes were blocked. It is incredible to think that I have had more physical interventions on my body*

in the last two years than in the rest of my thirty years combined. I underwent it voluntarily, too, because I wanted to correct the problem and have a child. Yet all the surgeries, the tests, and the medications seemed relatively minor compared to the emotional burden I put on myself.

After my first surgery, when my physician said it was okay to try to become pregnant, I don't think there was ever a day, or perhaps even an hour, that I didn't think about conceiving. It was always there—when I would see a child in the grocery store. When my friends would gripe about their kids. When I was on day 1, or day 14, and every other day of my menstrual cycle. Whenever my husband and I made love. Was I ever going to get pregnant? I had conflicting fantasies of what I would be like as a 60-year-old woman who had never had children. I could never get it out of my mind.

One study of infertile couples illustrates the pervasive impact of infertility. When asked what they considered to be the primary problem in their lives, almost 80 percent of the couples replied that it was their inability to conceive. Most of the remaining 20 percent ranked infertility as their second most perplexing problem, after financial difficulties. The remaining fraction of respondents rated infertility a close third after financial problems and marital strife.

A newly pregnant woman, who had just completed her second IVF treatment cycle, summed up the emotional impact of infertility in this way:

You really can't understand what it's like to be infertile unless you are infertile yourself and have experienced what we've gone through. You can sympathize, but you can't empathize with us.

The traditional options available to infertile couples who want a baby have included counseling, surgery to repair anatomical damage, the use of fertility drugs to enhance ovulation and sperm function, and insemination of the woman with her partner's or a donor's sperm. Most authorities would agree that these methods are effective for approximately 50 percent of all infertile couples. For the about 5 million infertile couples in the United States, IVF is the only recourse; yet fewer than 250,000 procedures are being performed annually.

WHY THE NUMBER OF INFERTILE COUPLES IN THE UNITED STATES IS INCREASING EVERY YEAR

According to the National Center for Health Statistics, the rate of involuntary infertility has remained relatively constant at about 9 percent since 1965. This is an increase over the figures for the early 1950s through 1964, when it was thought that approximately 7–8 percent of all couples were unable to conceive. Although the rate of infertility has not changed since the mid-1960s, the number of infertile couples has increased every year in step with population growth. The following factors contribute to this trend.

Venereal Diseases Are Epidemic in the United States

Once considered largely under control because of the discovery and availability of proper medication, venereal diseases that damage the reproductive system are on the rise again. One of the major causes of this is the increased availability of effective birth control methods, which has undoubtedly contributed to a more open approach toward sexual activity. Consequently, both men and women often have relatively larger numbers of sexual partners. The unfortunate result has been a significant increase in sexually transmitted diseases.

Venereal disease such as gonorrhea is rampant in the United States. Gonorrhea lodges in the woman's fallopian tubes and often results in a severe illness. Unfortunately, in many cases gonorrhea causes so little physical discomfort that women frequently do not bother to seek treatment. But even a minor gonorrheal infection can damage the fallopian tubes, and many women find out they have had gonorrhea only when they investigate the cause of their infertility. In contrast, gonorrhea in men almost always produces sudden, painful symptoms that usually prompt an immediate visit to the doctor. For this reason, men are less likely to be infertile due to gonorrhea than are women.

The cure of sexually transmitted diseases is complicated by the emergence of new strains of gonorrhea and other venereal diseases that resist traditional treatment. These bacteria can be combated only by new and expensive antibiotics that often are not readily available.

Chlamydia, another infection that damages and blocks the fallopian tubes, is even more common today than gonorrhea. Chlamydia is relatively difficult to diagnose and culture and it responds well only to specific antibiotics. Past infection is diagnosed through a specific staining procedure of cervical secretions or by blood testing for anti-chlamydia antibodies. The symptoms of chlamydia are very similar to those of gonorrhea.

Syphilis, too, is again becoming widespread in the United States. Syphilis is easily cured in its early stages. In later stages its spread can be halted, but its effects cannot be reversed.

(See "Pelvic Inflammatory Diseases" in Chapter 9 for a discussion of the effect of sexually transmitted diseases on infertility.)

Medications and "Recreational Drugs" Are Taking Their Toll

Alcohol, nicotine, marijuana, cocaine, and other psychotropic drugs can significantly reduce both male and female fertility because they are capable of altering the genetic material of eggs and sperm. However, these substances can potentially have a far more severe and long-lasting effect on a woman than on a man. Because a woman is born with her lifetime quota of eggs already inside her ovaries, unwise use of medications and drugs can damage all the eggs her body will ever produce. In contrast, a man generates a completely new supply of sperm approximately every three months, so damaged sperm are replaced in a short time.

The Biological Clock Keeps on Ticking

Many women today choose to delay having a family in order to establish their careers, to be sure they and their partner can afford children because they married relatively late, or because they want to have a child with a new partner. However, there is a price to pay for having children later on. For example, some disorders that produce infertility tend to appear during the second half of a woman's reproductive life span. Thus, a woman who decides to have children after 35 might find she is infertile because of hormonal problems, a pelvic disease such as endometriosis, or the development of benign fibroid tumors of the uterus. In addition, the ability to ovulate healthy eggs and concurrently generate a hormonal environment that can adequately support a pregnancy becomes increasingly compromised as a woman gets older. Many women who plan to become pregnant later in their reproductive lives find themselves unable to do so.

Although the infertility rate has not increased, the aggregate number of couples whose last option for pregnancy is IVF is skyrocketing. Recent advances in the evolution of high-tech methods to evaluate and treat infertility offer the hope of pregnancy to couples who previously would have had no hope. Hundreds of thousands of very special miracles have been granted the gift of life through assisted reproductive technology (A.R.T) in the United States.

2

THE ANATOMY AND PHYSIOLOGY OF REPRODUCTION

In vitro fertilization can be viewed as an extension of the normal human reproductive process. It merely bypasses many of the anatomical or physiological causes of infertility by substituting IVF techniques for some of the processes that occur naturally in the body. In order to understand both natural conception and IVF, therefore, one must first be familiar with human reproductive anatomy and the process of reproduction.

THE FEMALE REPRODUCTIVE TRACT

The female reproductive tract consists of the vulva, vagina, cervix, uterus, fallopian tubes, and ovaries. The external portion of the female reproductive tract (see figure 2-1) is known as the *vulva*. The vulva includes the inner and outer lips, or *labia*. The hair-covered outer labia are called the *labia majora* (major lips). The *labia minora*, small inner lips partially hidden by the labia majora, are remnants of tissue whose embryologic counterpart in the male develops into the scrotum.

The *clitoris*, a small organ at the junction of the labia minora in the front of the vulva, is the embryologic counterpart of the male penis.

The clitoris undergoes erection during erotic stimulation and plays an important role in orgasm.

The area between the labia minora and the anus is called the *perineum*. It is formed by the outer portion of the fibromuscular wall and skin that separate the *anus* and *rectum* from the vagina and vulva.

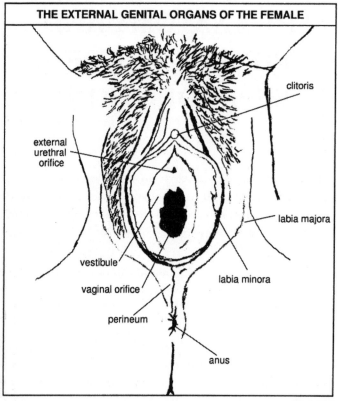

THE EXTERNAL GENITAL ORGANS OF THE FEMALE

clitoris

external urethral orifice

labia majora

vestibule

labia minora

vaginal orifice

perineum

anus

Figure 2-1

The *vagina*, a narrow passage about 3–4 inches long and about 1 inch wide, spans the area between the vulva and the cervix. It opens outward through the cleft between the labia minora, or *vestibule*. The vagina's elastic tissue, muscle, and skin have enormous ability to stretch so as to accommodate the penis during sex and the passage of a baby at birth.

The vagina is actually a potential space; it is a real space only when the penis enters it or during childbirth. At other times, the vaginal walls are collapsed against one another; a cross section of a relaxed vagina would resemble the letter H. In front of the vagina lie the *bladder* and the *urethra* (outlet from the bladder), and at the back is the rectum (see figure 2-2).

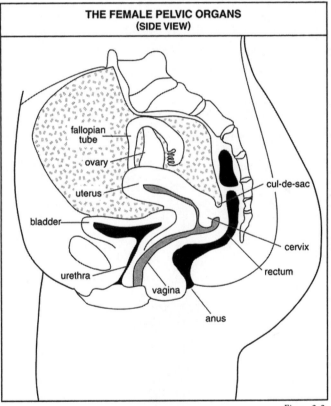

Figure 2-2

The cervix, which is the lowermost part of the uterus, protrudes like a bottleneck into the upper vagina. As figure 2-3 illustrates, a *fornix*, or deep recess, is created around the area where the cervix extends into the vagina. The area of the abdominal cavity behind the uterus is known as the *cul-de-sac*. The cervix opens into the uterus through a narrow canal, the lining of which contains glands that produce cervical mucus (the important role that cervical mucus plays in the reproductive process will be explained later in this chapter). The cervix is particularly vulnerable to infections and other diseases, such as cancer.

The *uterus*, which consists of strong muscle fibers, is able to stretch and grow from its normal size (when it resembles a pear) to accommodate a full-term pregnancy. The valve-like transition between the cervix and the uterine cavity enables a baby to grow within the uterus without prematurely dilating the cervix and thereby endangering the pregnancy through miscarriage or premature birth. The lining of the uterus, which nurtures and supports the developing embryo, is known as the *endometrium*.

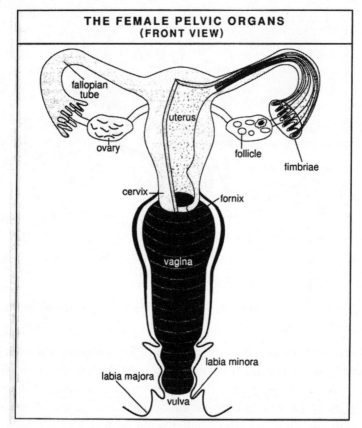

THE FEMALE PELVIC ORGANS
(FRONT VIEW)

Figure 2-3

The *fallopian tubes* are two narrow 4-inch-long structures that lead from either side of the uterus to the ovaries. At the end of the fallopian tubes are finger-like protrusions known as *fimbriae*.

The *ovaries* are two almond-sized structures attached to each side of the pelvis adjacent to the fimbriae. The ovaries both release eggs and discharge certain hormones into the bloodstream. The process of releasing the egg or eggs is called *ovulation*. Eggs are also known as *ova* or *oocytes*.

About the size of a grain of sand, eggs are the largest cells in the human body. A woman develops all the eggs she will ever have at the fetal age of 12 weeks. Although a female baby starts off with about 7 million eggs when she is inside her mother's womb, her ovaries contain only about 700,000 eggs by the time she reaches puberty. A woman uses about 300,000 of these eggs during the approximately 400 ovulations that occur during her reproductive life span.

Each month, the ovaries select a number of the woman's eggs for development and maturation. Eggs develop in blister-like structures, or *follicles*, that project from the surface of the ovaries. At ovulation, the egg is not simply expelled into the abdominal cavity. Instead, the fimbriae at the ends of the fallopian tubes gently vacuum the surface of the ovaries to retrieve the egg and direct it through the fallopian tubes for possible fertilization.

The human egg (see figure 2-4) is similar in structure to the eggs of many other species, including the chicken. In the center of the human egg is the nucleus, which bears the chromosomes. The surrounding *ooplasm* contains *micro-organelles*, which are cellular factories that produce energy for the egg. The ooplasm also contains nurturing material that supports the embryo during its early stages after fertilization, thus enabling it to grow before becoming attached to an external source of nourishment (the endometrium). Surrounding the ooplasm and nuclear material is the *perivitelline membrane*, which separates the internal matter from the *zona pellucida*. The zona pellucida is analogous to the shell of a chicken egg, and the perivitelline membrane corresponds to the membrane inside the eggshell.

The human egg, unlike the chicken egg, also contains a group of cells known as the *cumulus oophorus*, which are arranged in a starburst effect around the outside of the zona pellucida. (The critical role each of these structures plays in the fertilization process is explained later in this chapter under "How Fertilization Occurs.")

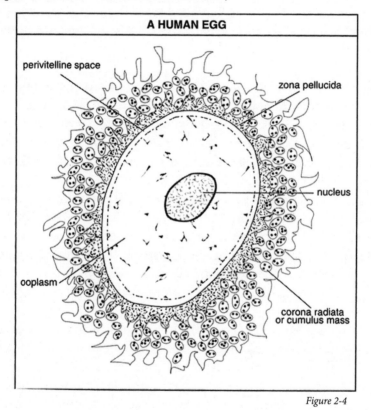

Figure 2-4

THE MALE REPRODUCTIVE TRACT

The male sex organs (see figure 2-5) comprise the *penis* and two *testicles*, or testes, which are located in a sac called the *scrotum*. The testicles (male counterparts of the woman's ovaries) produce *spermatozoa*, or *sperm* (the male equivalent of the woman's eggs).

In contrast to the woman, who is born with a lifetime quota of eggs, the man's testicles generate a new complement of sperm approximately every 100 days. The sperm begin to mature in the testicles and continue to develop as they travel through a long, thin, coiled tubular system in the scrotum called the *epididymis*. The epididymis is connected to a straight, thicker tube called the *vas deferens*. Just before the vas deferens enters the penis it joins the *urethra*, which originates in the bladder and allows the passage of urine from the bladder through the penis. Sperm are transported through this system by muscular contractions known as *peristalsis*.

Several glands, including the *seminal vesicles* and the *prostate gland*, are located along this tract. They release a large amount of milky secretions that nurture and promote the survival of the sperm. The combina-

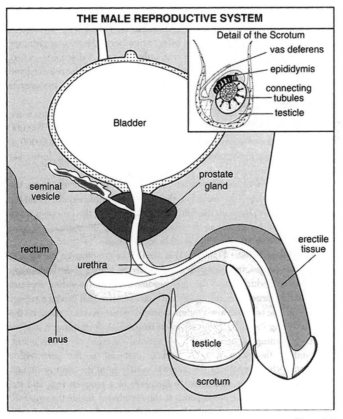

Figure 2-5

tion of sperm and milky fluid that is ejaculated during erotic experiences is known as *semen*. Semen and urine are not discharged simultaneously through the urethra. Urine is prevented from mixing with semen in the urethra because the bladder-urethra opening constricts during ejaculation. Similarly, closure of the vas deferens–urethra juncture prevents passage of semen during urination. In certain cases, removal of a diseased prostate gland may compromise this separation effect and cause the man to ejaculate backward into the bladder rather than outward through the penis, which is known as *retrograde ejaculation*. This condition may cause infertility, but it can be treated by inseminating the woman with sperm separated from urine the man would pass immediately following orgasm.

Sperm (see figure 2-6), in contrast to eggs, are the smallest cells in the body. They resemble microscopic tadpoles. Each sperm consists of a head, whose *nucleus* contains the genetic, or hereditary, material arrayed on chromosomes; a midsection that provides energy; and a tail that propels the sperm along the male reproductive system and through the woman's reproductive tract. The top of the head is covered by the *acrosome*, a protective structure containing enzymes that enable the sperm to penetrate the egg; and the surface of the acrosome is enveloped by the *plasma membrane*. (The function of the acrosome and plasma membrane will be explained under "How Fertilization Occurs" later in this chapter.)

Eggs and sperm are called *gametes* until fertilization. A fertilized egg is called a *zygote* until it begins to divide; from initial cell division through the first eight weeks of gestation it is known as an *embryo*, and from the ninth week of gestation until delivery it is called a *fetus*.

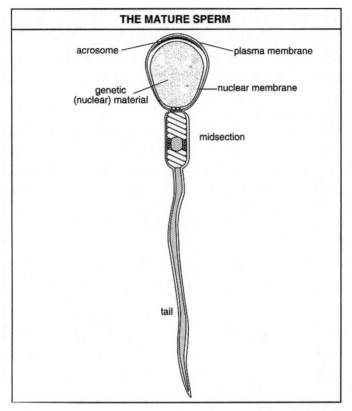

Figure 2-6

THE PROCESS OF FERTILIZATION

Fertilization is a complex process that must be accomplished within a strict time frame. Theoretically, a man is always fertile, but a woman's egg can only be fertilized within a specific 12- to 24-hour period shortly after ovulation. Therefore, there is a "window of opportunity" lasting only 24 to 48 hours each month when intercourse can be expected to result in fertilization. Timing is critical if the egg and sperm are to survive the journey through the woman's reproductive tract, unite, become fertilized, and result in the embryo implanting successfully into the uterine wall.

The man deposits between 100 million and 200 million sperm into the woman's vagina with each ejaculation of semen. During normal intercourse, or even after the woman has been artificially inseminated, much of the semen pools in the posterior fornix behind the protruding cervix. Because the cervix usually points partially backward into the posterior fornix, the cervix is usually immersed in the pool of ejaculated semen. This immersion helps direct the sperm through the cervix and into the reproductive tract.

The journey from the fornix to the fallopian tubes, which is about four inches, is hazardous and unbelievably taxing for the tiny sperm. For a cell the size of a sperm to travel this distance is equivalent to an adult human swimming the Pacific Ocean from Los Angeles to Tahiti. Only a small fraction of exceptionally strong, healthy sperm out of several million that were deposited in the fornix will survive that 24- to 48-hour

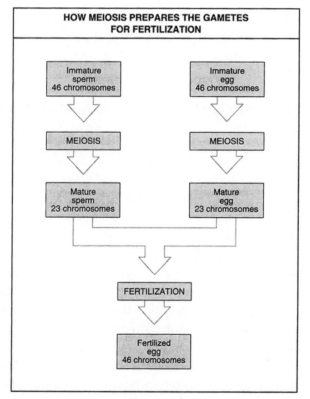

Figure 2-7

journey. Many are killed by the hostile environment in the vagina or cervix, and others simply do not survive the long swim. Peristaltic contractions in the fallopian tubes help the remaining sperm reach the egg, and the same contractions propel the fertilized egg or embryo back through the fallopian tube to the uterus. (The fertilization process occurs near the middle of the fallopian tube—not in the uterus.) Amazingly, out of the millions of sperm ejaculated into the vagina, only a few hundred to a few thousand successfully complete the journey to the waiting egg in the fallopian tube.

An egg presents a large target for the tiny sperm: about 1/180-inch as opposed to the sperm's 1/100,000-inch diameter. This means that the egg is about 550 times as wide as the sperm. The difference in size between the two gametes is due to the massive amount of cytoplasm within the egg that will nourish the newly formed embryo. Sperm, in contrast, consist almost entirely of genetic material with very little cytoplasm. They are little more than bags of chromosomes propelled by a tail.

IVF improves the odds that sperm can find and fertilize an egg. This is because the distance sperm have to swim to find the egg in a petri dish is considerably shorter than the "long-distance route to Tahiti" found in nature. The egg still lies passively within the dish, as it would in the fallopian tube; but in the significantly reduced volume of the petri dish, the sperm are far more likely to find the egg than they would be if they had to negotiate the entire distance from the fornix.

How Fertilization Occurs

The process whereby sperm are prepared to fertilize an egg, which is known as *capacitation*, takes place in two stages. First, as a sperm passes through the woman's reproductive tract, its acrosome fuses with its plasma membrane, slowly releasing the enzymes within the acrosome. Then, with its acrosome now exposed, the sperm attacks the cumulus granulosa and the zona pellucida (the shell-like covering) of the egg. The heads of a number of sperm fuse with the zona pellucida, and one successful sperm penetrates the egg. The process whereby a sperm fuses with the zona, the second state of capacitation, is called the *acrosome reaction*.

The sperm require from five to 10 hours of incubation in the fluids of the female reproductive tract to complete the acrosome reaction.

Capacitation takes place in the mucus secretions of the cervical canal, and continues in the uterus and fallopian tubes. It is believed that the passage of sperm through the cervical mucus around the time of ovulation promotes the necessary physical, chemical, and structural changes in the plasma membrane to facilitate release of acrosomal enzymes. (Because only sperm that have undergone capacitation are able to fertilize an egg, in IVF therapy the first stage of capacitation must be replicated in the laboratory prior to IVF if fertilization is to occur in the petri dish.)

After the acrosome reaction has taken place, the successful sperm completes the fertilization process by burrowing through the zona pellucida and ooplasm to the nuclear material. The sperm sheds its body and tail upon penetration, and only the head (containing the genetic material) actually enters the egg. Figure 2-8 illustrates the following steps in the capacitation-fertilization process:

- **Phase 1:** The plasma membrane fuses with the acrosome as the sperm pass into the reproductive tract to reach the egg, thus initiating capacitation.
- **Phase 2(a):** The acrosomal enzymes are released, and penetrate the cumulus mass cells of the egg.
- **Phase 2(b):** The acrosome fuses with the zona pellucida, thus completing capacitation.
- **Phase 3:** The sperm burrows through the zona pellucida into the ooplasm of the egg.

The moment a sperm penetrates the egg's zona pellucida, a reaction in the egg fuses the zona and the perivitelline membrane into an impermeable shield that prevents other sperm from entering.

When fertilization occurs, the egg starts dividing within the zona covering, drawing its metabolic supplies from the ooplasm within the egg. Propelled by contractions of the fallopian tube, the dividing embryo begins its three- or four-day journey to the uterus and continues to divide after reaching it.

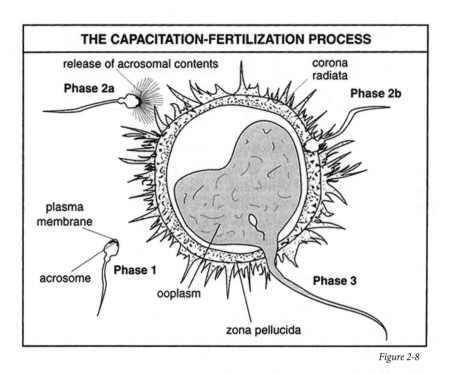

Figure 2-8

About two days after reaching the uterus, when the embryo has divided into more than 100 cells, it cracks open, and all the cells burst out through the fractured zona. This is known as *hatching*. These cells then try to burrow their way into the lining of the uterine wall. A portion of the growing embryo soon makes contact with the mother's circulatory system and becomes the earliest form of the *placenta*, from which the baby will receive its nourishment (see figure 2-9).

If an embryo implants anywhere but in the uterus, it is referred to as an *ectopic pregnancy*. In most cases, an ectopic pregnancy is due to embryonic implantation in the fallopian tube; this occurs about once in every 200 pregnancies. Isolated cases of implantation in the reproductive tract, such as on the ovary or elsewhere in the abdominal cavity, have been reported. In rare instances, such ectopic pregnancies have been known to develop to full term, but the baby invariably will not survive. (See Chapter 9 for more information on ectopic pregnancies.)

Figure 2-9 follows the progress of an egg as it is ovulated from the follicle, becomes fertilized in the fallopian tube, and implants into the endometrium of the uterus. The dotted line plots the days that normally elapse as:

1. Ovulation occurs (and meiosis takes place prior to and during fertilization)
2. The fertilized egg, which has not yet divided, is now called a zygote
3. The egg begins to divide and is now known as an embryo; at this point each *blastomere*, or cell, within the embryo is capable of developing into an identical embryo
4. The embryo develops into a mulberry-like structure known as a *morula*
5. A cavity develops within the embryo, which indicates the *blastocyst* stage
6. The process of *gastrulation* begins (cells are now dedicated to the development of specific embryonic layers that subsequently will form specific organs and structures; individual cells are no longer capable of developing into embryos)

At ovulation, the physical-chemical properties of the cervical mucus nurture the sperm as they pass through it, enhancing their quick passage and therefore capacitation as well. This is because hormonal changes around the time of ovulation ensure that the *microfibrilles*, or *myceles*, of the cervical mucus are arranged in a parallel manner. The sperm must then swim between the myceles in order to reach the uterus and, finally, the fallopian tubes. In addition, the cervical mucus becomes watery, and the amount produced (some of which may be discharged) increases significantly.

At another time during the menstrual cycle, the hormonal environment alters the arrangement of the myceles in the cervical mucus to form a barrier to the passage of sperm. During this time the mucus is thick, thus preventing the sperm from passing through the cervix.

The *Billings Method* of contraception is based on this phenomenon. A woman using the Billings Method predicts when she is likely to be

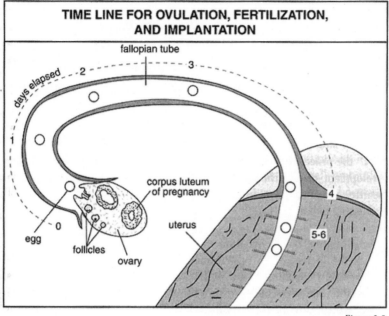

TIME LINE FOR OVULATION, FERTILIZATION, AND IMPLANTATION

Figure 2-9

ovulating by evaluating whether her cervical mucus is thick or watery. Because pregnancy can occur only around the time of ovulation, it is accordingly possible for her to identify the "safe period" when she is unlikely to conceive following unprotected intercourse.

HOW THE GENETIC BLUEPRINT IS DRAWN

After onset of the spontaneous LH surge or following controlled ovarian stimulation (COS) with fertility drugs where hCG is administered, the egg, which to this point has 23 pairs (46 total) of chromosomes, enters into a 38–42 hour process of maturation division known as meiosis. The objective is for the normal total number of 46 chromosomes to halve, so as to leave the mature egg with half the original number of chromosomes (i.e., 23). Such an egg is termed *euploid*. To achieve this, half the chromosomes of the immature egg are expelled from the egg substance in a membranous envelopment. This so-called *1st polar body* (PB-1) comes to lie in the *periviteline* space where within a day or two of fertilization it eventually degrades and disappears. The microscopic identification of PB-1 provides evidence that meiosis occurred and that the egg is "mature."

Each cell in a human being (except for the gametes) contains 46 chromosomes, which are bound together into 23 pairs. Chromosomes contain hundreds of thousands of genes, each of which transmits the hereditary messages of the man or woman.

If a *mature* sperm containing 46 chromosomes were to fertilize an egg that also contained 46 chromosomes, it is obvious that the two gametes would produce a zygote containing double the proper number of chromosomes. Therefore, nature has created a method through which the number of chromosomes in both the sperm and egg is reduced by half. The immature sperm (similar to the immature egg) contains 46 chromosomes.

As with the egg, each "immature" sperm also undergoes meiosis with the objective of dividing its 46 chromosomes in half. However, unlike the egg, which during meiosis halves its chromosomal component by discarding 23 chromosomes in the PB-1, each sperm divides into two (2) separate mature sperm each containing 23 chromosomes. When the mature egg and sperm, each with 23 chromosomes, fertilize, the resulting embryo will have 46 chromosomes. Such an embryo is *euploid* and has a maximum potential to develop into a healthy baby.

All this would be all be well and good were it not for the fact that in humans most *mature* eggs have an irregular chromosome component that is more than or less than 23 (*aneuploid*) and thus upon fertilization, will invariably develop into embryos that are likewise aneuploid (i.e., have more than or less than 46 chromosomes). It is important to bear in mind that with human reproduction, when it comes to the chromosomal integrity of the embryo, the egg plays a much more influential role than does the sperm. Moreover, in humans the rate of egg aneuploidy is higher than with any other mammal. In fact, more than 50% of mature eggs derived from women under 35 years of age are aneuploid and this incidence increases with advancing age, such that by the mid-40s more than 90% of a woman's eggs will be aneuploid. This growing incidence of egg aneuploidy explains the reciprocally high incidence of aneuploidy in human embryos. Aneuploid human embryos are "incompetent" (incapable of generating a normal pregnancy). Many such embryos will suffer developmental arrest, while those that continue to develop will either miscarry or result in aneuploid birth defect (e.g., Down syndrome). This serves to explain why infertility, miscarriages, and chromosomal birth defects increase with advancing age of the egg provider.

Immediately following fertilization of the egg by a sperm, the second polar body (PB-2) forms and is also extruded. Both polar bodies are located in the perivitelline space where they are readily detectable and are accessible to direct biopsy.

Once fertilized by sperm, the zygote starts to divide into cells (blastomeres). Now the blastomeres of this embryo divide repeatedly, replicating their chromosomal structure identically by a process called mitosis. The growth and development of all tissues—with the exception, of course, of the gametes—is done by mitosis. Mitotic cell division begins within 24–48 hours of fertilization occurring. Its rate of cleavage (division) is believed to be indicative of its "competency" to produce a viable embryo and its potential to implant into the uterine lining. Blastomeres which have all 46 chromosomes in place are referred to as being euploid, while those that have an irregular number of chromosomes (more, or less than 46) are termed "aneuploid." Embryos in which euploid blastomeres overwhelmingly predominate have a high potential to develop into a normal baby (i.e., "competent") while those with predominantly aneuploid blastomeres are "incompetent." Competent embryos usually develop in an orderly fashion, cleaving to the 5–9 cells (blastomeres) stage within 72 hours of fertilization. Thereupon, in the following 24 hours, they will divide so rapidly that the blastomeres "compact." Now it is referred to as a "morula" (mulberry). Over the ensuing 24–48 hours the cells begin to differentiate into a blastocyst, which has an inner fluid cavity, an outer layer known as the trophectoderm that subsequently develops into the root system (placenta) and membranes surrounding the baby, and an inner collection of cells known as the "inner cell mass," which ultimately develops into the baby itself.

Since the immature egg comprises two X chromosomes (XX), it follows that by halving in the process normal meiosis (reduction division), there will be only one X chromosome in the nucleus and one in the first polar body. In contrast, blastomeres comprise the chromosomes of both the egg and the sperm. Since the sex chromosome makeup of the immature sperm is X+Y, it follows that after dividing its chromosomes in half with meiosis, the mature will contain either an X or a Y chromosome. When a mature Y-carrying sperm fertilizes an egg, the resulting embryo will be male (XY), and if it contributes an X chromosome, the embryo will be female (XX). Thus it is the sperm rather than the egg that determines the sex of the offspring.

Thus the embryo is actually quite complex, for within the boundaries of each blastomere, placed strategically on each chromosome, are the genes that carry information for 100,000 chemical reactions and represent the genomic blueprint for a new individual. The set of instructions carried on the chromosomes is complete, and a virtual explosion of embryonic development is imminent.

HORMONES PREPARE THE BODY FOR CONCEPTION

Pregnancy, of course, begins with the fusion of the two gametes, but the preparations for conception begin long before fertilization occurs. The onset of puberty in both the man and the woman sets the stage for a biorhythmical hormonal orchestration that becomes more and more fine-tuned over the ensuing decade. It begins with the formation and release of hormones into the bloodstream, and the bodies of both sexes rely on a complex feedback mechanism to measure existing hormonal levels and determine when additional hormones should be released.

The *hypothalamus* (a small area in the midportion of the brain) and the *pituitary gland* (a small, grape-like structure that hangs from the base of the brain by a thin stalk) together regulate the formation and release of hormones. The hypothalamus, through its sensors, or *receptors*, constantly monitors female and male hormonal concentrations in the bloodstream and responds by regulating the release of small, protein-like "messenger hormones" to the pituitary gland. These messenger hormones are known as *gonadotropin-releasing hormones* or GnRH (see figure 2-10).

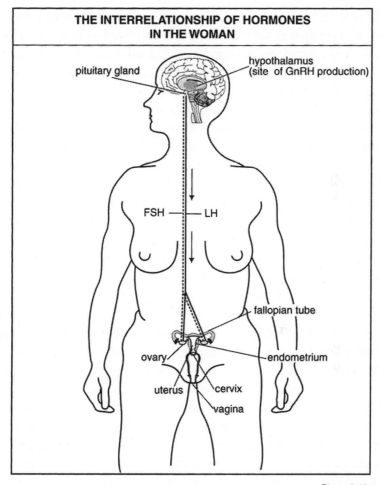

Figure 2-10

In response to the messenger hormones from the hypothalamus, the pituitary gland determines the exact amount of hormones that it in turn will release to stimulate the *gonads* (ovaries in the woman and testicles in the man). These hormones, or gonadotropins, are called *follicle-stimulating hormones* (FSH) and *luteinizing hormones* (LH). The hypothalamus closes the feedback circle by measuring the level of hormones produced by the gonads while at the same time monitoring the release of LH and FSH by the pituitary gland.

This "push-pull" interplay of messages and responses produces the cyclical hormonal environment in the woman that is designed solely to promote pregnancy. A "push-pull" mechanism also occurs in the man with regard to the release of *testosterone*, the male sex hormone. Similar feedback mechanisms regulate other hormonal responses in mammals, such as the functioning of the thyroid and adrenal glands.

There are two primary sex hormones in the female, *estrogen* and *progesterone*; in the male there is only one, testosterone. The pituitary gland releases identical hormones—FSH and LH—to the gonads of both the woman and the man, but the female and male gonads respond differently to these hormones. The level of female hormones fluctuates approximately monthly throughout the menstrual cycle, while male hormone production remains relatively constant.

In men, LH controls the production of testosterone, and FSH, the production and maturation of sperm.

In women, extraneous factors as well as the level of circulating hormones and gonadotropins may influence the body's feedback mechanism. For example, the hypothalamus may be influenced by stress, pain, environmental changes, diseases in the woman's body, birth-control pills, and many forms of medication, including tranquilizers and blood-pressure medication.

The best way to understand this cyclical hormonal process is to trace the woman's hormonal pattern throughout a menstrual cycle. For practical purposes, the menstrual cycle will be considered to begin on the first day of menstruation. The following illustration is based on a 28-day menstrual cycle. However, it is important to remember that many women have somewhat shorter or longer menstrual cycles. In such cases, although the cyclic phases and ovulation occur in the manner described below, their length and timing vary according to the number of days in that particular cycle. For example, a woman with a cycle of 35 days is not likely to ovulate on day 14.

The First Half of the Cycle (the Follicular/ Proliferative Phase)

The body prepares for ovulation during the first two weeks of the menstrual cycle. During this two-week period, the lining of the uterus (endometrium) thickens or proliferates significantly and becomes very glandular under the influence of rising blood estrogen levels. This phase is accordingly often referred to as the *proliferative phase* of the cycle. Because this proliferation of the endometrium occurs at the same time as the development of the ovarian follicle(s), it is often also known as the *follicular phase*. From just prior to the beginning of the menstrual period until the middle of that cycle, the pituitary gland releases the gonadotropin FSH in ever-increasing amounts.

The release of FSH causes the formation of follicles in the ovaries as well as both the production of estrogen and the selection of eggs (usually one per follicle) that are to mature during that cycle. Often as many as 30 or even more follicles begin to develop under the stimulation of FSH,

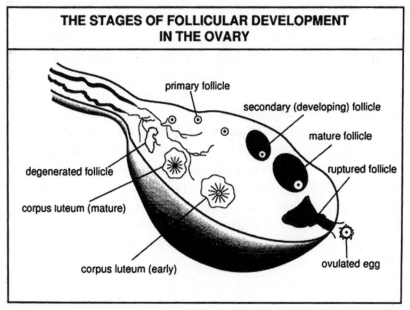

THE STAGES OF FOLLICULAR DEVELOPMENT IN THE OVARY

primary follicle

secondary (developing) follicle

mature follicle

ruptured follicle

degenerated follicle

corpus luteum (mature)

corpus luteum (early)

ovulated egg

Figure 2-11

but in the natural cycle only one and sometimes two follicles progress to ovulation (see figure 2-11). The eggs that do not mature ultimately disintegrate and are absorbed into the ovary. This explains why so many eggs are lost during the reproductive life span, although a woman usually ovulates only one, sometimes two, and, very rarely, three eggs in any particular menstrual cycle.

Responding (usually at the middle of the menstrual cycle) to the rising estrogen levels in the bloodstream, the hypothalamus releases a surge of gonadotropin-releasing hormone (GnRH) when the estrogen reaches a critical level. This rush in GnRH production prompts the pituitary gland to produce a surge of LH, which had been released only in very low, erratic concentrations until this point. It is the sudden surge in LH that actually triggers ovulation.

Ovulation

At ovulation, a muscle connecting the ovary with the end of the fallopian tubes contracts, bringing the fimbriae closer to the follicle containing the egg. The fimbriae then gently massage and vacuum the follicle until the egg, which by this time is protruding from the follicle, is extruded. The fimbriae receive the egg and direct it into the fallopian tube, where contractions transport it toward the uterus.

The follicle collapses once the egg has been extruded and is transformed biochemically and hormonally. It takes on a yellowish color and is then referred to as the *corpus luteum* ("yellow body" in Latin).

All the while that the ovaries are nurturing eggs and producing hormones, the endometrium is developing in preparation for receiving an embryo. By the time ovulation occurs, it is about three times as thick as it was immediately after menstruation. (In Chapter 8 we will discuss in detail the critical role the endometrium plays in successful implantation of the embryo.)

The Second Half of the Cycle (the Secretory/Luteal Phase)

Once the corpus luteum forms, the ovary begins to secrete the hormone progesterone as well as estrogen, and the levels of progesterone begin to rise very rapidly. The progesterone converts the proliferated, glandular endometrium to a moist, receptive structure capable of secreting nutrients that will sustain an embryo, hence the term *secretory phase*. The term *luteal phase* describes the stage of the menstrual cycle during which the corpus luteum produces the progesterone that enhances the secretory environment in the uterus.

The corpus luteum, through the production of both estrogen and progesterone, supports the survival of the secretory endometrium through the second half of the menstrual cycle. The life span of the corpus luteum is about 12 to 14 days if fertilization and implantation of the embryo into the endometrium do not occur. During that period the endometrium is sustained by the estrogen and progesterone produced

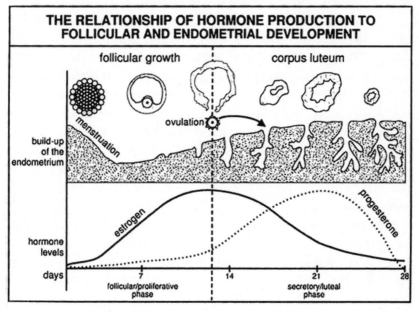

Figure 2-12

by the corpus luteum. Once the corpus luteum begins to die, the hormonal support for the endometrium is lost, and two-thirds of it comes away (often with the unfertilized egg or unimplanted embryo) in the form of *menstruation*. (Figure 2-12 illustrates the relationship of hormone production to follicular and endometrial development throughout the menstrual cycle.)

Should the woman become pregnant, the hormone produced by the implanting embryo and the developing placenta, which is called *human chorionic gonadotropin*, or *hCG*, and has an effect similar to LH on the corpus luteum, prolongs the survival of the corpus luteum beyond its normal 12- to 14-day life span. The corpus luteum, in turn, continues to produce estrogen and progesterone to maintain the secretory environment of the endometrium, which nurtures the growth of the embryo before it makes contact with the blood system of the mother. Because the corpus luteum continues to exist and produces hormones that nurture the endometrium, the woman will miss her next menstrual period and should then suspect that she is pregnant.

The placenta begins to form as the developing embryo establishes a connection with the mother's system. The placenta is both the lifeline between the mother and baby's blood systems and the factory that nourishes the baby as pregnancy advances. Because the placenta is capable of producing estrogen and progesterone, it soon supplants the need for hormone production by the corpus luteum. The placenta itself supports the endometrium's survival after the 60th or 70th day following the last menstrual period. It has been proved that a pregnancy would continue after the 70th or 80th day even if both ovaries were removed because the placental hormones themselves are by then fully capable of sustaining the pregnancy.

After ovulation, the production of both LH and FSH declines significantly. If pregnancy does not occur, the hypothalamus begins to secrete more GnRH when the corpus luteum begins to die, thus initiating the next menstrual cycle. The same procedure is repeated over and over, with each hormonal cycle setting up the following one, much as each wave in the ocean sets up and determines the character and magnitude of the following wave. It is an indication of nature's ability to maintain biorhythms in a bewildering but organized fashion.

MISCARRIAGE IN EARLY PREGNANCY

On average, only about one out of every three embryos implants in the uterus long enough to delay the menstrual period. In other words, in two out of every three pregnancies the woman is not even aware that she has conceived.

Even when a pregnancy has been confirmed by a doctor, there is still a 16 to 20 percent chance of miscarriage (expelling of the products of conception after the death of the embryo/fetus) during the first three months of pregnancy. In most cases, the reason for this is not apparent; but in those situations where a reason is known, the vast majority of miscarriages are attributed to either a chromosomal abnormality in the developing offspring, immunologic factors affecting proper implantation, or hormonal insufficiency.

The use of sophisticated ultrasound techniques to confirm and monitor pregnancies has led to awareness of the phenomenon that not all embryos that implant in the uterus necessarily develop further. (Ultrasound is a painless diagnostic procedure that transforms high-frequency sound waves as they travel through body tissue and fluid into images on a TV-like screen. It enables the physician to clearly identify structures within the body and to guide instruments during certain procedures. There is no evidence that the ultrasound waves cause any damage.)

In some cases of confirmed multiple pregnancies, one (or more) of the implanted embryos are absorbed by the body or miscarried and passed through the vagina, thus reducing the number of surviving embryos. This spontaneous reduction in the number of pregnancies appears to be far more common than previously believed, even in those multiple pregnancies occurring without the use of fertility drugs. See Chapter 14 for additional information on Recurrent Pregnancy Loss (RPL).

An Abnormal Embryo

Early miscarriages usually occur because the embryo is abnormal. Miscarriage is nature's way of protecting the species from an inordinate number of abnormal offspring. These early miscarriages, which mostly occur even before the woman misses her period, are often referred to as biochemical pregnancies or spontaneous menstrual abortions.

The vast majority of such cases are the consequence of embryo aneuploidy. It has been shown that more than 70 percent of early pregnancy losses are attributable to a breakdown in the process of early meiosis.

As previously stated above, as a woman ages, meiosis is far less likely to occur without problems, because an older woman's eggs are not able to divide or be fertilized as perfectly as those of a younger woman. Again, this is why the babies of older women are more prone to Down syndrome and other chromosome abnormalities.

Immunologic Factors (see Chapter 8)

In some cases, the woman develops antibodies against chemicals in the cells that cover the embryo's "root system" or trophoblast (autoimmunity). In other cases, there is a rejection of the conceptus due to the sperm provider's immunologic makeup being too similar to that of the recipient.

Hormonal Insufficiency

In about 5–10 percent of all pregnancies, the embryo fails to implant because the amounts of hormones produced and the timing of their release were not perfectly synchronized. Such miscarriages, which may occur even if the embryo is perfect in every way, are attributed to hormonal insufficiency. This condition is caused by inadequate production of estrogen and/or progesterone during the menstrual cycle.

If hormonal insufficiency occurs because of abnormal hormonal production of estrogen during the follicular phase of the menstrual cycle, it is known as a follicular phase insufficiency. If attributable to inadequate production of hormones by the corpus luteum during the second phase of the cycle, it is referred to as a luteal phase insufficiency. Miscarriages due to follicular or luteal phase insufficiency may be associated with ovulation that occurs at the wrong time (either too late or too early), the production of inadequate amounts of hormones, an endometrium that responds inappropriately, or a combination of these factors.

Hormonal insufficiency may be perpetuated into early pregnancy, when the embryo is dependent on the survival of the corpus luteum before the placenta develops. Obviously, if implantation is imperfect because of improper hormonal stimulation, then placentation (the attachment of the placenta to the uterine wall) might also be defective. Poor placentation might prevent the baby from getting the proper nutrition. As a result, it might grow improperly and could be born too small or too early.

A pregnancy compromised by hormonal insufficiency may delay the onset of the anticipated menstrual period but then result in early miscarriage because of the inadequate hormonal environment. It is sometimes possible; however, to administer certain hormones in early pregnancy to sustain an embryo that otherwise would be lost.

Additional causes of miscarriage include thyroid and other hormonal irregularities, and kidney problems. It is believed that in addition to causing miscarriage, the misuse and abuse of narcotics, psychotropic drugs, alcohol, and nicotine during the first three months of pregnancy, when cell and organ differentiation are taking place, might significantly increase the incidence of birth defects as well as inhibit fetal growth and development.

It is likely that the thickness and quality of the endometrial lining as judged by ultrasound may also be an independent factor that affects the risk of miscarriage. We have come across a number of cases in which there was no apparent cause for recurrent spontaneous abortions (more than three), and the only determinant was that the endometrial lining appeared to be thinner than 9 mm.

It is the start in life that counts most, and in the majority of cases nature will catch its mistakes. The high rate of embryo wastage and early miscarriage when conception occurs naturally may come as a surprise to many couples. However, it should provide a helpful perspective for couples who are considering comparable pregnancy rates offered by IVF and other options.

Until relatively recently, pregnancy was not possible for couples who could not fulfill both requirements of conception: safe transport of the egg and sperm through the reproductive tract and fertilization within a supportive hormonal environment. IVF often solves this problem by bridging anatomical or physiologic disorders that until now have made pregnancy only an elusive dream for many couples.

CHAPTER

3

NATURAL CONCEPTION AND IVF: TWO PATHWAYS TO PREGNANCY

There are five criteria a couple must meet in order for pregnancy to occur naturally:

Ovulation of a mature, healthy egg or eggs at the appropriate time, in association with the proper hormonal environment

Production of strong, healthy, mature sperm that are deposited in or adjacent to the woman's cervical canal around the time of ovulation

A physical-chemical environment that facilitates capacitation (activation) of the sperm as they pass through the woman's reproductive tract

A healthy fallopian tube that will promote the passage of sperm and eggs

A healthy uterine cavity with no abnormalities that might hinder implantation of the embryo, such as fibroid tumors (polyps that protrude into the cavity of the uterus) or scarring, and an endometrium that is thick enough and healthy enough to sustain an appropriate implantation in the uterus. This can be assessed by ultrasound evaluation of the endometrium prior to normal ovulation, by hormonal blood testing, and by a biopsy of the endometrium just prior to the menstrual period.

Couples who cannot fulfill all five criteria are unlikely to conceive or produce a healthy baby. The following section examines some of the ways in which common disease processes may prevent a couple from becoming pregnant. The remainder of this chapter explains how IVF can compensate for many of these deficiencies and thus enable a heretofore infertile couple to have a child.

ORGANIC AND PHYSIOLOGIC PROBLEMS THAT MAY PREVENT COUPLES FROM CONCEIVING NATURALLY

Neither sex contributes more heavily than the other to infertility problems. Roughly one-third of all infertile couples can trace their infertility to the woman, one-third to the man, and one-third to both partners.

Common Causes of Female Infertility

Organic pelvic inflammatory disease (PID) refers to the presence of structural damage in the woman's pelvis due to trauma, inflammation, tumors, congenital defects, or degenerative disease. The most common cause of infertility in a woman is damaged or blocked fallopian tubes that prevent the egg and sperm from uniting. Sexually transmitted diseases are a major cause of tubal scarring and blockage. In addition, scar tissue that forms after pelvic surgery may also lead to fertility problems.

Conditions such as endometriosis, in which the endometrium grows outside the uterus (causing scarring, pain, and heavy bleeding), can also damage the fallopian tubes and ovaries. The presence of even a minimal amount of endometriosis in the pelvis is believed to adversely affect fertility by releasing toxic substances that might reduce the ability of sperm and the potential of the egg to be fertilized. While the presence of minimal endometriosis might not necessarily adversely affect the passage of the egg from the ovary through the toxic environment to the fallopian tube, the toxins might diminish its ability to become fertilized. It has been shown that even the mildest form of endometriosis elicits a local immune response by releasing cells called macrophages, which wander through the pelvis and even into the fallopian tubes, destroying the eggs, sperm, and even the embryo. Accordingly, even the most minimal form of endometriosis may reduce fertility by as much as 70 percent through these mechanisms.

Damaged ovaries might also contribute to infertility. Sometimes an ovary cannot release an egg even though hormonal production is normal and the egg is adequately developed. It is also possible for an egg to be trapped within the follicle by scarring or thickening of the ovary's surface; this relatively rare condition may either be hereditary or induced by the malfunctioning of structures such as the adrenal gland.

More commonly, diseases such as PID or endometriosis, as well as surgically induced scarring, may anchor the ovaries in an awkward position or form a barrier that prevents the fimbriae from applying themselves properly to the ovaries' surface. Although one or both fallopian tubes may be perfectly free and mobile, the corresponding ovary could be inaccessible and unmovable. In such cases, the egg or eggs would be ovulated into the abdominal cavity instead of being retrieved by the fimbriae.

Abnormal ovulation is another cause for female infertility. Some women do not ovulate at all, while others ovulate too early or too late in their cycle for a pregnancy to occur. One of the reasons why normal fertility usually wanes after 35 is because ovulation is more likely to become abnormal later in the childbearing years.

In addition, it is believed that the quality of eggs decreases as women get older because the eggs' meiotic capacities are diminished by the aging process. The quality of the woman's eggs is one of the major determinants of whether a couple can get pregnant. (See Chapter 8 for a detailed discussion of the effect of age on a woman's eggs.)

A woman may also be infertile because disease, surgery, or infections have damaged the lining of her uterus. Damage caused by scarring or the presence of tumors, such as fibroids, may prevent the embryo from attaching to the endometrium and developing properly.

Abnormalities in the size and shape of the uterus can also cause infertility problems. Sometimes women develop an abnormally shaped uterus as a result of exposure to certain drugs their mothers took during pregnancy. A classic example of this disorder is the "T-shaped" uterus and significantly smaller uterine cavity often found in women whose mothers took diethylstilbestrol (DES) during pregnancy.

Some women are unable to produce the cervical mucus that ensures the passage and vitality of the sperm. The production of hostile cervical mucus might be due to infection or abnormal physical and chemical properties in the secretions. Occasionally, surgery or injury to the cervix may have destroyed the glands that produce cervical secretions.

In some cases, women develop antibodies or an allergic response to their partner's sperm. These antibodies may be passed into the cervical secretions and thereby prevent fertilization by destroying or immobilizing the sperm.

(See Chapter 9 for a more detailed discussion of the negative impacts of PID, endometriosis, DES exposure, and other conditions on a woman's fertility.)

Common Causes of Male Infertility

The causes of male infertility are often more difficult to define. Blockage of the sperm ducts is one obvious cause. Generalized blockage may be caused by sexually transmitted diseases. More easily identifiable blockage is caused by a vasectomy (voluntary surgery to occlude the sperm ducts for birth-control purposes). While it is usually possible to surgically reconnect the tubes after vasectomy, some men, especially those who underwent the procedure more than 10 years earlier, remain infertile because in the interim their systems have developed an immune reaction that results in the production of antibodies that destroy or immobilize their own sperm.

Another common cause of male infertility is a varicocele, a collection of dilated veins around the testicles that hinders sperm function by increasing body temperature in the scrotum. In order for the testicles to produce healthy sperm, the temperature in the scrotum must be lower than it is in the rest of the body.

Ideally, the testicles should have descended into the scrotum shortly after birth, but in some cases they do not reach the scrotum for years. In such circumstances it may be necessary to accomplish this surgically when the boy is very young to prevent the testicles from becoming severely damaged, thereby resulting in infertility. In rare cases, abnormal development of the testicles and/or sperm ducts may result from injury, disease, or hereditary abnormalities.

Certain drugs or chemicals in the environment may also inhibit sperm production and function. And as in women, drugs such as DES can produce abnormalities in the male offspring's reproductive system.

Finally, for reasons that are often not readily apparent, some men lack the adequate hormonal stimulation that is required for proper sperm production, or there is an abnormality in sperm parameters.

Unexplained Infertility

For about 10% of all infertile couples, the cause of the infertility cannot be readily determined using conventional diagnostic methods. Such cases are often referred to as "unexplained infertility." The truth however is that in most such cases, the diagnosis of "unexplained infertility" is in fact presumptive because a more in-depth evaluation would have revealed a cause. This having been said, people diagnosed with so called "unexplained infertility" fall into two broad groups: a) those couples who don't have any biological problems interfering with pregnancy and, b) those who do but the reason cannot be found due to insufficient medical information or technology. It is in this latter group that improved testing techniques have made infertility easier to diagnose and treat.

In order to make even a presumptive diagnosis of "unexplained infertility," the answers to the following questions must be in the affirmative.

Is the woman ovulating normally?

Is the couple having intercourse regularly in the periovulatory phase of the cycle?

Are the fallopian tubes normal and open?

Can endometriosis be excluded?

Does the male partner have normal semen parameters (most specifically with regard to sperm count and motility)?

Is the postcoital (Huhner) test (periovulatory examination of cervical mucus, done 6-18 hours after intercourse) normal?

The definitive diagnosis of "unexplained infertility" has a lot to do with the thoroughness of the health care provider in excluding all possible causes. The fewer tests performed, the more likely a presumptive diagnosis. . . . For example:

Abnormalities of the fallopian tubes (adhesions or developmental defects) of the finger-like "petals" at the outer ends of the tubes that help sweep eggs inside (i.e., fimbriae) can prevent eggs from being collected and transported to the awaiting sperm.

Chromosomal Abnormalities of Eggs or Embryos: Eggs must be euploid (contain the right number of chromosomes) to be successfully fertilized, and embryos must also be euploid in order to implant successfully in the uterine lining. Until recently there was no reliable method for determining whether eggs and embryos were euploid. The recent introduction of genetic tests such as comparative genomic hybridization (CGH) now allows for identification of all chromosomes in the egg and embryo. As such CGH represents an important addition to the "infertility" diagnostic armamentarium.

Luteinized Unruptured Follicle (LUF) Syndrome: Here, the eggs can become trapped in the follicle and not be released (trapped ovulation). In such cases routine tests done to detect ovulation (temperature charting, urine LH testing, blood progesterone levels) may be normal, resulting in false interpretation that ovulation is actually occurring.

Ovulation (hormonal) dysfunction: Abnormalities in ovarian hormone production in the preovulatory phase of the cycle (follicular phase defect) and/or in the postovulatory phase (luteal phase defect) can negatively affect preparation of the uterine lining (endometrium), thus thwarting normal implantation.

Immunologic Implantation dysfunction (IID): Sometimes, the woman's or the man's own immune system can attack sperm cells, killing them or causing them to become immobilized. Also, immunologic dysfunction involving the uterine lining can cause the implanting embryo to be rejected so early that the woman does not even recognize that she in fact had conceived.

Cervical infection: Ureaplasma urealyticum infection of the cervical glands can prevent sperm from migrating through the cervix and uterus to reach the egg(s) in the fallopian tube(s). Such infection will usually not be detectable through routine examination and/or cervical culturing methods.

Mild or Moderate Endometriosis: Endometriosis is in 100% of cases associated with the production of "pelvic toxins" that reduce the fertilization potential of otherwise normal eggs by a factor of 3-5. In addition, about one-third of women with endometriosis (regardless of its severity) have immunologic implantation dysfunction (IID). Furthermore mild and often even moderately severe endometriosis can only be accurately diagnosed by direct visualization of the lesions through laparoscopy or laparotomy, and the detection of IID requires highly sophisticated tests that can only be adequately performed by a handful of Reproductive Immunology Reference Laboratories in the United States. Finally, a condition called nonpigmented endometriosis, in which the endometrium may be growing inside the pelvic cavity with many of the same deleterious effects as overt endometriosis, cannot be detected even by direct vision (at laparoscopy/laparotomy). The fertility of these patients may be every bit as compromised as if they had detectable endometriosis.

Psychological Factors: The entire reproductive process is governed by the brain. Thus it should come as no surprise that stress and negativity can interfere with hormonal balance and decrease the ability to conceive.

Successful management of "Unexplained Infertility" requires that a very individualized approach be taken. Wherever possible the underlying cause should first be identified. Problems that involve ovulation dysfunction (hormonal imbalance) require ovulation induction with oral or injectible fertility drugs. Cervical mucous hostility due to infection with ureaplasma (which is transferred back and forth sexually to both partners) requires specific and concurrent antibiotic therapy. In other cases involving younger women (under 39 years) where there is a problem with sperm migration via the cervix and uterus to the fallopian tube(s) intrauterine insemination (IUI) with or without ovulation induction, is indicated. When these treatments fail, in cases with women over the age of 39 years, in women with IID, in men or women who harbor antisperm antibodies in significant concentrations and in cases associated with tubal abnormalities, in vitro fertilization (IVF) is needed. All cases of intractable, moderate or severe male infertility call for injecting sperm directly into the egg to achieve forced fertilization (Intracytoplasmic sperm injection-ICSI).

It is an indisputable fact that most causes of infertility can be diagnosed, and it is a great pity that the diagnosis of "unexplained infertility" is often used as an excuse for not having performed a full and detailed evaluation of the problem. Couples should not simply accept a diagnosis of "unexplained infertility" at face value, since treatment is most likely to be successful when the specific cause of the problem can be fully identified.

HOW IVF DIFFERS FROM NATURAL CONCEPTION

This section provides an overview of how IVF adapts the principles of human reproduction to achieve pregnancy. The procedures are described here in general terms and will be discussed in detail in subsequent chapters.

Fertility Drugs Are Used to Produce More Eggs

The administration of fertility drugs promotes the growth of more ovarian follicles than would develop naturally. These drugs also enable more follicles and eggs to develop and (following administration of hCG or LH) mature instead of regressing prior to ovulation. Increasing the number of mature follicles facilitates the retrieval of more eggs and enhances the chance of creating more healthy embryos. As will be explained in Chapter 5, the hormonal environment created by the regime (protocol) of COS used can profoundly influence egg development, especially in women who have "polycystic ovarian syndrome (PCOS), in older women (over 39 years of age), and in women who, as they get closer to menopause start to run out of eggs [diminishing ovarian reserve (DOR)].

A "competent" embryo is one that upon reaching a receptive uterine environment is most likely to develop into a normal baby. While epigenetic and metabolic factors do play a role, it is by far the "embryo's karyotype" (chromosomal integrity) that is the most important determinant of its "competence." To be "competent" the human embryo must be euploid. An aneuploid embryo is "incompetent." It will either not develop into a blastocyst (the most advanced preimplantation stage of development), will not attach to the uterine wall, will attach temporarily resulting in a transient rise in blood hCG levels and then be lost prior to becoming detectable clinically or through ultrasound examination (i.e., a chemical pregnancy), will be lost after becoming clinically manifest by ultrasound or clinical examination (a clinical miscarriage), or will develop into a chromosomally abnormal baby (e.g., Down syndrome). It is important to bear in mind that in the absence of severe sperm dysfunction, in the vast majority of cases, it is the egg's chromosomal integrity (rather than that of the sperm) that will determine the embryo "competence." The sperm's contribution to embryo aneuploidy increases in cases of significant sperm dysfunction (male factor infertility). It is almost as if, when surrounded by mostly "normal" sperm, the egg has the ability to select an euploid sperm to fertilize it. But when surrounded by mostly aneuploid sperm it is more likely to select those that are 2nd best.

After reaching the uterus naturally, an embryo has approximately a 15 percent chance of surviving. With IVF, the implantation rate of a "microscopically high grade" embryo or blastocyst is profoundly affected by the age of the woman whose fertilized eggs generated the embryo(s). A good grade embryo or blastocyst derived from the egg of a younger woman (under 35 years) might have about a 20-30% and 40-50% (respectively) of propagating a pregnancy while an embryo and blastocyst derived from the egg of a woman in her midforties might be less than 10%. Though the recent introduction of genetic tests such as comparative genomic hybridization (CGH-Chapter 6), which can accurately differentiate between euploid and aneuploid ("competent" and "incompetent") embryos, is a game changer. Now, the transfer of a CGH-normal (euploid/ "competent") blastocyst can generate a viable pregnancy almost 70% of the time, regardless of the age of the egg provider. But CGH embryo testing is quite costly, adding to the already high cost of IVF. As such it is not widely used. Accordingly, many IVF programs, in an attempt to improve the chances of a successful IVF treatment, still transfer several embryos at one time into the uterus. This is the main reason for an explosion in the incidence of IVF multiple births and the unacceptably high rate of maternal complications as well as premature deliveries that has resulted in related neonatal complications.

It may well be that when some women, especially those approaching menopause, are stimulated with fertility drugs, their ovaries, besides producing the eggs and the estrogen hormone that builds the endometrial lining, also might be producing disadvantageous chemicals and hormones that have an adverse effect on the lining. The problem is sidestepped in third-party parenting (ovum donation and gestational surrogacy) when the egg provider and the embryo recipient are not the same person.

As indicated in Chapter 16, it might soon become possible to limit the use of fertility drugs altogether in IVF. The advent of in vitro maturation (IVM), where eggs are harvested without using these expensive and potentially harmful drugs, could change the entire field of IVF. We at SIRM are intimately involved in research aimed at speeding up the process of reaching this point.

The Chance of a Multiple Pregnancy Is Greater with IVF

While the success rate of an IVF procedure is directly related to the quality and number of embryos transferred to the woman's uterus, the more embryos transferred, the greater the risk of twins and high-order multiple pregnancies (triplets or greater). (See Chapter 4 for a discussion of the risks of multiple pregnancies and the options available to couples.)

The risk of multiple babies is not simply a function of the number of embryos transferred but also embryo quality, which in turn is affected by egg quality. Older women who receive several embryos are far less likely to have multiple pregnancies than younger women receiving the same number of embryos. It is simply a question of embryo viability, which may not be detectable microscopically but might be an issue from a chromosomal point of view.

The impact of age on egg and embryo quality is an unalterable parameter that must be figured into the multiple-pregnancy equation. We have seen very few triplet pregnancies in women undergoing IVF over the age of 40, while the multiple pregnancy rate is at least twice as high in women under 35.

Eggs Are Retrieved from the Ovaries by Suction (Needle Aspiration)

Instead of waiting for the eggs to be ovulated naturally from the follicles, the IVF surgeon sucks them out of the ovaries through a long needle in a process known as egg retrieval. The needle can be inserted into the follicles through the vagina while the physician monitors its progress on an ultrasound screen (see Chapter 6).

Prior to the advent of vaginal ultrasound egg retrievals, it was necessary to remove the eggs using a laparoscope inserted through an incision in the navel into the pelvic cavity, enabling the surgeon to see the pelvic organs and also to aspirate the eggs via a needle inserted through separate puncture sites in the lower abdomen. Laparoscopy is rarely performed for egg retrieval today.

Following retrieval, eggs are sent to the laboratory for fertilization. Egg retrieval is particularly appropriate when the fallopian tubes cannot retrieve or transport the eggs, when the woman is not able to ovulate properly, or in cases of unexplained infertility.

IVF Bypasses the Fallopian Tubes

The fallopian tubes are entirely bypassed in IVF because the eggs are retrieved directly from the ovaries and the fertilized embryos are transferred directly into the uterus via the vagina.

Sperm Are Partially Capacitated in the Laboratory Instead of in the Woman's Reproductive Tract

IVF eliminates many of the hurdles that sperm have to overcome, including escaping from the man's semen and passing through the cervical mucus. This is particularly important in cases where the man has an inadequate sperm count or poor sperm function. IVF is also helpful in situations when the woman forms cervical mucus that inadequately promotes capacitation or is hostile to the sperm. During IVF, laboratory procedures are substituted for the role of cervical mucus in capacitation, and the embryos are transferred directly into the uterus through a catheter to avoid exposure to hostile cervical mucus.

An IVF Embryo Is Not Likely to React to Either Partner's Antibodies

The body sometimes develops antibodies to sperm after it has become familiar with the spermatic blueprint. Accordingly, as sperm come into contact with bodily immune systems over time, women may build up sperm antibodies, and men may even develop antibodies to their own sperm.

IVF often evades fertility problems caused by antibodies produced by the woman and/or the man by enabling sperm to safely fertilize the eggs in the laboratory without interference from antibodies that would be present in the woman's reproductive tract. The resulting embryos are not affected by those antibodies because mammalian embryos do not have an immunological blueprint. In other words, embryos and fetuses are immunologically inert prior to birth. Thus, the woman's body, which might produce antibodies against sperm, tolerates the embryo because it is an unfamiliar, immunologically inert structure against which her body has not yet developed antibodies.

IVF Is Both a Treatment and a Diagnostic Procedure

IVF has a built-in diagnostic capability unmatched in nature or by any other method of evaluating or treating infertility. In ideal circumstances there is a 70 percent or greater chance that any one egg will fertilize in the laboratory. This affords the couple a chance to see whether they are capable of achieving fertilization together. IVF technology has brought to light many instances in which a woman's egg cannot be fertilized by her partner's sperm and sometimes not by any sperm. The reason for this is not always readily identifiable; the problem could lie with the egg, the sperm, or both. If several mature eggs fail to fertilize, this information can help couples make important decisions regarding their future plans. Although the test is not 100 percent foolproof, failed fertilization should encourage couples to consider micromanipulation, the use of donor eggs, donor sperm, donor embryos, or adoption (see Chapters 11 and 14). No other method of treating infertility enables a physician to reach this diagnostic conclusion. IVF might be called the ultimate fertility test.

Another diagnostic application of IVF would be when, for no readily apparent reason, the fallopian tubes might be unable to properly receive and/or transport the egg, sperm, and embryos. Because IVF by its very nature bypasses the fallopian tubes, it might, through a process of exclusion, offer an answer and/or a solution to this problem.

The advent of methods such as CGH which can reliably identify embryo aneuploidy now allows identification of "incompetent" embryos. This could afford better discrimination between embryo defects versus implantation dysfunction (uterine lining deficiencies) as a cause of prior, "unexplained" IVF failure.

IVF Requires a Heavy Emotional, Physical, and Financial Investment

The most significant difference between IVF and natural pregnancy is that a couple must sacrifice a great deal of their personal privacy before and during the IVF procedure, whereas natural conception is a private matter. An IVF couple must bare some of their deepest secrets and fears to the clinic staff and allow themselves to be manipulated physically and emotionally as they progress through the procedure. In addition, IVF is inordinately expensive—and there is no second prize if a woman does not conceive following the procedure. The couple will not have another chance at IVF pregnancy without making the same emotional, physical, and financial commitment again. In natural conception there's always next month, and the following month, and hope for the future, without the major costs that IVF exacts.

DOES IVF INCREASE THE RISK OF BIRTH DEFECTS?

In spite of several reports suggesting that IVF babies are more likely to be born with birth defects, there is little evidence to support the implication that the technique of IVF itself increases this risk. Certainly, with more and more women postponing childbearing to a later age and more and more men with sperm dysfunction resorting to IVF, the effect of the woman's age and the increased incidence of sperm chromosomal abnormalities associated with male infertility could increase the risk of both miscarriages and birth defects. However, short of remaining childless, what other recourse would couples with such forms of infertility have other than to resort to IVF? For additional information see Chapter 17.

4

IVF STEP 1: PREPARATION FOR IVF TREATMENT

Most IVF procedures are based on some variation of the following steps: (1) preparation for treatment, (2) induction of ovulation, (3) egg retrieval, and (4) embryo transfer. All successful IVF programs must be highly organized and exquisitely timed, just as in nature the fertilization process is organized and timed.

Each of these four basic steps in an IVF treatment cycle should be regarded as a hurdle that a couple must overcome before proceeding further. (The term *treatment cycle* refers to the menstrual cycle during which a particular IVF procedure is performed.) Occasionally, a couple may successfully negotiate one hurdle but then be unable to surmount the next step, in which case they would usually begin the treatment cycle anew after allowing the woman's body to rest for a month or two. In general, a couple's chances for successful IVF increase as they put each hurdle behind them.

The descriptions of IVF procedures in Chapters 4 through 7 have been designed to provide an overview of what an infertile couple might expect to experience physically and emotionally during the treatment cycle. Because a truly comprehensive IVF program responds to—and often anticipates—the couple's emotional needs throughout the treatment cycle, some of the techniques that an IVF program might use to address emotional needs are included in the description of clinical procedures.

We do not mean to imply that any of these scenarios is the best or the only way that IVF should be performed.

ACCEPTANCE INTO AN IVF PROGRAM

Before being admitted into any IVF program, the couple would probably be required to have a complete medical evaluation. They would most likely undergo all the routine steps of an infertility assessment, usually performed by their own primary physician, in order to rule out the possibility that procedures other than IVF might better address their needs.

The couple would probably be required to forward their medical records to the IVF program and are likely to be asked to provide additional background. They should expect to be encouraged to speak frankly about themselves and their personal habits (including their sexual practices, use and abuse of recreational drugs, general lifestyle, and other parameters that are known to impact fertility). In many programs, the couple also would undergo psychological counseling. Following a thorough evaluation of the materials submitted by the couple and their primary physician, the medical staff would then decide whether the couple is eligible for IVF.

Once accepted into the program, the couple would probably undergo orientation, including an explanation of the emotional, physical, and financial commitments that IVF would require. The orientation process could take place through letters, other written material, e-mail, and/or by telephone. It may also take place on site if the couple are able to visit the clinic prior to commencement of the treatment cycle.

In some IVF programs the couple is required to be at the clinic during the entire process, including induction of ovulation (usually a series of daily injections of fertility drugs). In other programs, couples are encouraged to initiate the induction of ovulation with their own gynecologist and are required to be on site only for the last few days of the cycle prior to egg retrieval and embryo transfer.

ORGANIZATION OF A TYPICAL IVF PROGRAM

In many programs, one or more clinical coordinators play an important role in assisting the physician to ensure that the couple receive proper emotional preparation throughout the process. The clinical coordinator plays a central role and administers many treatment procedures that have previously been agreed upon by the entire medical staff.

In such a coordinator-oriented program, the couple could anticipate spending as much if not more time with a clinical coordinator as with the physician. This is because a clinical coordinator usually functions as the couple's advocate—the liaison between the couple and all the other members of the IVF team, including the physician. However, this is not meant to imply that both the clinical and administrative roles could not be fulfilled by a physician who has a personality and attitude that engenders a feeling of well-being, relaxation, and optimism. In general, though, clinical coordinators contribute significantly to the smooth operation of many IVF programs.

It is the responsibility of the person who guides the couple throughout the treatment cycle, whether that is physician or clinical coordinator, to explain every step along the way so the couple knows exactly what to expect. In addition, the same staff member who is responsible for establishing the initial rapport with the couple should be their contact person throughout their tenure with the program.

In most programs the couple will be introduced to the staff, taken on a tour of the facility, and encouraged to ask a lot of questions. The staff in an IVF program, including the clerical personnel, should be upbeat and encouraging when they deal with infertile couples. The empathic IVF program will provide a relaxing, low-key environment that offers subtle support to both partners during their time of emotional need. Although the couple should be well aware that no program can guarantee a pregnancy, even after several attempts, a congenial atmosphere fostered by the staff should help both partners maintain a mood of guarded optimism.

Some IVF programs provide access to a nurse-counselor with special expertise in the psychological aspects of infertility. Although the participation of a nurse-counselor is not essential in order for a couple to conceive, an IVF team member who can predict the way a couple might react, and therefore help improve their tolerance to the emotional roller-coaster ride of IVF, adds another dimension of caring to the program.

TESTS THAT MAY BE CONDUCTED PRIOR TO IVF

Before the couple has a pretreatment consultation with the physician, it is likely that the partners will be asked to complete some or all of the following tests. (See Chapter 10 for a detailed explanation of most of the tests listed in this chapter as well as others the couple might undergo prior to IVF.)

Tests for Certain Viral Infections

The HIV/AIDS test. A couple should defer pregnancy until they are sure that neither partner carries a disease that can seriously prejudice the health, well-being, and even the survival of the offspring. Although this is a personal decision to be resolved between the man and the woman, the physician enters the picture when IVF is being considered. As the catalyst responsible for creating the circumstances under which a new life might be conceived, the physician has a medical, legal, and moral obligation to make every attempt to ensure that IVF does not lead to the birth of a child who suffers from a life-endangering disease such as acquired immunodeficiency syndrome (AIDS).

Accordingly, many programs require that an HIV (human immuno-deficiency virus; the virus that causes AIDS) test be done on both partners prior to any IVF procedure. Unfortunately, this test still does not completely rule out the presence of HIV infection because a person may not register positive for up to six months after infection by HIV. However, the test does provide a good screen to help protect an IVF program from being instrumental in the birth of damaged offspring. (Another reason for administering the HIV test to all new patients is to protect medical and laboratory personnel who work with the couple.)

Some physicians also test both partners for HIV before the woman undergoes any treatment to enhance fertility, such as reconstructive tubal surgery. This is because if one of the partners is HIV-positive and a baby with HIV is born after successful tubal surgery, the couple might argue that they would not have consented to treatment had they known they could transmit HIV to a baby.

We recognize that the decision to undergo HIV testing is a very personal one and that a physician certainly cannot force anyone to have this test. Nevertheless, we strongly advise that the issue be discussed prior to initiating treatment for infertility.

Some IVF couples have expressed concern that HIV might be transmitted through fertility drugs because some of these drugs (e.g., Repronex, Bravelle) are derived from the urine of menopausal women. Most experts agree, however, that HIV does not survive the purification and extraction process to which these drugs are subjected. Moreover, most of the gonadotropins administered today are genetically engineered products that are free of viral contamination.

Hepatitis B and C infection. Hepatitis B and C, which may be transmitted sexually or through blood, may also be transmitted from an infected mother to her conceptus (the collective term for the embryo, as well as the developing fetus and its placenta). Women who test positive for either of these viruses should be counseled that the risk of transmission could be as high as 10 percent and that many fetuses so infected may succumb, be born with liver damage, or acquire serious congenital abnormalities. Additionally, there is a slight possibility that fertilization of eggs with sperm derived from a man who tests positive will infect the embryo and similarly place the fetus at risk. Since active infection with hepatitis B and C (or a carrier state) is difficult and often impossible to eradicate, couples/individuals so infected often choose to take a calculated risk and proceed with fertility treatment. However, it is incumbent upon the treating physician to relay all relevant information that spells out such risk, so that patients can make a well-informed decision before proceeding.

Syphilis. The incidence of venereal infection with syphilis is on the rise throughout the world. While active infection with this organism will usually not prevent fertilization, it can cause serious congenital abnormalities in the offspring. Thus all men and women undergoing IVF should have their blood tested for syphilis and, if detected, be treated before proceeding with IVF.

Chlamydia and gonorrhea. Infection of the male and/or female partner with chlamydia or gonorrhea is not transmitted to the offspring. However, since these diseases are sexually transmitted and result in major health problems, all parties undergoing fertility treatment should be tested. (See Chapter 9 for a discussion of the impacts of chlamydia on infertility.)

Ureaplasma urealyticum. Ureaplasma is a microorganism that occurs in the reproductive tracts of both sexes and may interfere with sperm transport and/or embryo implantation. It commonly produces no symptoms in either partner. When present in the cervical secretions, it can be transmitted to the uterine cavity during embryo transfer, where it might interfere with implantation. Ideally, the male partner should also be cultured for ureaplasma. If the organism is found in either partner, both should be treated concurrently with the appropriate antibiotic.

Selective testing for genetically transmitted diseases. In some cases it is necessary to test IVF candidates for certain genetic conditions that tend to have a high prevalence in certain population groups. For example, Tay-Sachs disease and other lipoidoses are more common in Ashkenazi Jews, Thalassemia is more common in individuals of Mediterranean extraction, Sickle Cell Disease is more common in non-Caucasians of African extraction, men with congenital absence of sperm ducts (vas deferens) are often carriers of the cystic fibrosis gene, etc. Accordingly in cases where egg and sperm providers have a family history of such conditions or fall into such demographic/ethnic and racial categories, appropriate screening should be conducted.

Sperm Quality

In any IVF program the male partner will almost certainly be asked to submit to a basic semen analysis. The purpose is twofold: (1) to ensure that the sperm's viability and mobility are not abnormal and/or have not changed significantly since the last sperm assessment, which would dramatically affect the couple's rational expectations for successful IVF; and (2) to protect the program from medical-legal liability in case the man has developed an undetected fertility problem since his sperm were last evaluated. The quality of the sperm, along with the age of the woman undergoing egg retrieval, are the two most important factors that enable the physician to predict the likelihood of the couple getting pregnant through IVF.

Sperm Chromatin Structure Assay (SCSA)

Over the last few years it has become known that certain abnormalities in sperm DNA can thwart attempts to achieve a viable pregnancy even in cases where the man has normal sperm parameters. The development of tests such as the SCSA hold great promise for couples who otherwise might have unexplained infertility, IVF failure, or pregnancy loss. Many women do conceive in spite of their partners' abnormal SCSA and give birth to healthy babies. However, an abnormal SCSA markedly reduces the pregnancy rate, increases the risk of first-trimester miscarriages, and reduces the natural as well as the A.R.T. birthrate. It is important to point out that an abnormal SCSA neither results in structural or numerical chromosome abnormalities of the embryo nor impairs fertilization potential or appearance of the embryo.

Sperm Antibody Tests

More and more programs require that the male partner take a sperm test to determine whether he is harboring sperm antibodies, which could affect the ability of his sperm to fertilize an egg and thereby adversely affect the chances of a successful outcome with IVF. Moreover, the presence of sperm antibodies in the man will significantly influence the manner in which sperm is prepared for the IVF process. In some cases, the presence of high concentrations of sperm antibodies could mandate the performance of intracytoplasmic sperm injection (ICSI), where a single sperm is captured in a thin glass needle and injected directly into the egg to promote fertilization, thus avoiding the antibodies.

Pelvic Assessment

A careful pelvic examination is important in order to evaluate for the presence of irregularities in the contour of the uterus or the adjacent pelvic organs. Their presence might suggest the existence of fibroid tumors, ovarian cysts, swollen fallopian tubes, and other conditions that might affect treatment.

Ultrasound Assessment of Endometrial Thickness

The importance of the quality of the endometrium and its potential to promote implantation cannot be overstated. When the zona pellucida breaks open and the cells burst out, the cells then try to sink their way into the lining of the uterine wall; whether this embryo is unable to implant, implants but has stunted growth, or grows into a healthy baby, depends on the quality of the endometrium.

In 1989, we were first to show that in both normal and stimulated cycles, preovulatory endometrial thickness/ultrasound appearance is predictive of embryo implantation potential following IVF. With conventional IVF there needs to be a >8mm (preferably >9mm) sagital thickness and a triple line appearance (Grade A) of the endometrium. Anything less is associated with a significant reduction in live birthrates per ET.

A poor endometrial lining most commonly occurs in women with a history of unexplained recurrent IVF failures or early recurrent miscarriages and is usually attributable to (1) inflammation of the endometrium (i.e., endometritis occurring following a septic delivery, abortion, or miscarriage), (2) adenomyosis (gross invasion of the uterine muscle by endometrial glandular tissue), (3) multiple fibroid tumors of the endometrium, (4) prenatal exposure to the synthetic hormone diethylstilbestrol (DES), and (5) administration of clomiphene citrate for at least three consecutive months without a resting cycle (this effect is self-reversible within four to six weeks of discontinuing clomiphene).

Attempts to augment poor endometrial linings by bolstering circulating blood estrogen levels through increased doses of fertility drugs, aspirin, and by supplementary estrogen therapy have yielded disappointing results. We reported on the ability of vaginally administered Viagra and the addition of oral beta adrenergic agents (e.g., Terbutaline or Ritodrine) to significantly enhance uterine blood flow and estrogen delivery to the endometrium, thereby improving its development and facilitating healthy pregnancies.

If an assessment reveals the endometrium to be poor, the woman should probably opt out of that particular cycle of IVF. She then has three choices: Her eggs can be removed, fertilized, and frozen for the purpose of transferring them to the uterus in a subsequent cycle when she has been treated with Viagra hormonal replacement; she can return for a fresh cycle while Viagra vaginal therapy is used; or her embryos can be transferred into the uterus of a surrogate.

Fluid Ultrasonography/Hysterosonogram (FUS) versus Hysteroscopy

We routinely perform fluid ultrasonography (FUS) or hysteroscopy on women scheduled for IVF if the woman has not undergone the examination for a year or two. FUS involves the injection of a liquid into the uterus via the cervix, allowing ultrasound examination of the uterus and fallopian tubes. Hysteroscopy is the examination of the cervix and inside of the uterus for defects by means of a lighted, telescope-like instrument that is passed through the cervix into the uterus.

FUS or hysteroscopy is not required in cases where the woman has had a hysteroscopy within 18 months in which the uterine cavity was shown to be normal. We would perform FUS or hysteroscopy in cases where a hysterosalpingogram or the advent of disease/symptoms suggest the presence of surface lesions in the uterine cavity might have occurred after a prior FUS or hysteroscopy was performed. In one out of eight cases, surface lesions that might interfere with implantation are detected by the routine performance of FUS or hysteroscopy; these should be treated before the woman undergoes IVF. This often occurs despite the fact that a recent hysterosalpingogram was reported as being normal and/or that the woman shows no evidence of disease.

FUS and hysteroscopy can easily be performed in the doctor's office and do not require any significant postoperative care. We have found this approach to be well received by our patients and are convinced that the routine implementation of FUS or hysteroscopy followed by appropriate treatment, when indicated, has prevented numerous women from undergoing otherwise futile attempts at IVF.

Measurement of Blood FSH, Estradiol, Antimullerian Hormone (AMH) and Inhibin-B Blood Levels

The measurement of the hormones FSH, *blood estradiol* (the concentration of estrogen in the woman's blood, also known as E2), AMH and Inhibin B on the third day of a menstrual cycle preceding IVF helps evaluate the potential ability of the woman's ovaries to respond to fertility drugs. It also provides information that the physician can use to select the ideal dosage and regimen of fertility drugs to achieve an optimal response. For this reason, these hormones should be measured in all regularly menstruating women scheduled to undergo IVF. An FSH level of 9.0 miu/ml or greater in association with a blood estradiol level of less than 70 pg/ml, as well as an Inhibin B blood level of less than 45 ng/ml is predictive of incipient ovarian failure (resistance to stimulation with fertility drugs). AMH levels of <5.0 ng/ml also point to diminished ovarian reserve.

Immunologic Testing (see Chapter 8)

In certain types of female infertility, the embryo fails to attach properly to the endometrial lining because of immunologic problems. In such cases the woman most often loses the pregnancy so early that she does not even know she was pregnant. In reality, this in fact represents a "mini-miscarriage" rather than infertility. Others will conceive but then will go on to have a positive urine or blood test but lose the pregnancy before it can be confirmed clinically or by ultrasound. Alternatively the pregnancy may survive and be diagnosed clinically or by ultrasound examination, but thereupon be lost as a "miscarriage." In almost all such cases the immunologic implantation dysfunction will manifest as increased activation of so-called uterine natural killer (NK)cells. NK cells are large lymphocytes in the uterine lining. In about 20% of women with infertility these NK cells will be found to be "activated," (i.e., producing excessive amount of factors known as TH-1 cytokines that can so damage the early root system (trophoblast) of the embryo as to result in failed implantation or early pregnancy loss. It has been theorized that when in some cases the pregnancy survives such an onslaught the partial damage done to the trophoblast can compromise placental development thus leading to poor growth and development of the baby and even late pregnancy loss.

This problem could thus explain some cases of "unexplained infertility," RPL, intrauterine growth retardation, premature separation of the placenta, and even stillbirth. It follows that since the immunologic problem antedates conception, the advance recognition of such immunologic problems and its treatment could not only lead to pregnancy but could affect the very quality of life after birth. In my opinion, to ignore the role of immunologic factors in pregnancy outcome could not only disenfranchise many women from having a baby but could be harmful and be contrary to the Hippocratic Oath, which basically says to "Do no harm."

In my practice I often call for the NK blood assay (the K-562 Target Cell Test) as a screen and withhold further detailed immunologic testing pending the result. If there is evidence of NK cell activation, then I proceed to order more detailed testing. One word of caution is necessary. There are less than a half a dozen Reproductive Immunology Reference laboratories in North America that can perform many of these sophisticated immunology tests adequately. (See Chapter 8 for more details.)

Measurement of Prolactin

Prolactin is a protein hormone (closely related to human growth hormone) that is secreted by specialized cells in the anterior part of the pituitary gland. In addition, the hormone is also produced and secreted by a broad range of other cells in the body, most prominently various immune cells, the brain, and the lining of the uterus. Most cells respond to prolactin. In fact it is hard to identify any tissue that does not have prolactin receptors.

Although prolactin's major target organ is the breast, where it stimulates development and milk production, the hormone has many other functions. Several hundred different actions have been reported for prolactin.

Immune cells are rich in prolactin receptors and certain types of lymphocytes in fact synthesize and secrete prolactin. These observations suggest that prolactin may to some extent act as a regulator of the body's immune activity.

In an area in the brain known as the hypothalamus, a chemical called dopamine is released. Dopamine suppresses prolactin synthesis and release by the pituitary gland. As such it acts as a "hypothalamic brake set" causing prolactin only to be secreted when the "brake" is released. Several other hypothalamic hormones, including thyroid releasing hormone (TRH) and gonadotropin releasing hormone (GnRH) cause an increase in prolactin secretion. Stimulation of the nipples (including but not limited to nursing) leads to hypothalamic activation and prolactin release. Estrogen also exerts a positive control over prolactin synthesis and secretion.

Common manifestations of increased prolactin secretion (hyperprolactinemia) in women include amenorrhea (lack of menstrual cycles) and galactorrhea (excessive spontaneous breast secretion). Men with hyperprolactinemia may present with hypogonadism, decreased sex drive, sperm dysfunction resulting in infertility, and with impotence. Such men also can show breast enlargement (gynecomastia), but very rarely have galactorrhea.

Causes: Significantly raised blood prolactin levels (>60ng/ml) might point to a prolactin producing pituitary tumor (adenoma) which may be large (macroadenoma), small, or even microscopic (microadenoma). Markedly elevated blood prolactin is also associated with other types of intracranial lesions such as craniopharyngiomas, meningiomas, etc. Prolonged treatment with bromocryptine (Parlodel) or related products will usually effectively lower blood prolactin concentration and lead to shrinkage of pituitary adenomas. Such treatment is also safe during pregnancy. Other intracranial lesions causing hyperprolactinemia are usually treated by surgical removal.

Certain drugs (e.g., tranquilizers, ganglion blocker antihypertensives, antidepressants, thiazides, and narcotics) can also lead to a significant elevation in blood prolactin. Drug-induced hyperprolactinemia can be reversed by modifying or withdrawing the causative medication. In cases where this cannot safely be done, bromocryptine (Parlodel) derivatives can be used.

Elevated Prolactin and Female Reproductive Performance: It is important to recognize that even modestly raised prolactin levels (20ng/ml-40ng/ml) can interfere with response of the uterine lining to estrogen (i.e., endometrial proliferation) as well as ovarian follicle growth and development, thereby reducing reproductive potential, and may require treatment with prolactin suppressants such as bromocryptine.

Unexplained *hyperprolactinemia is sometimes an early indicator of impending or existing thyroid hormone deficiency or hypothyroidism (Hashimoto's disease)* which in most cases results from antithyroglobulin and/or antimicrosomal antibodies that attack thyroid hormone producing glands, replacing them with connective tissue. In about 50% of cases where the woman has such thyroid antibodies in her blood (regardless of whether or not they have concomitant hormonal or clinical evidence of thyroid deficiency) she will also have increased natural killer cell and cytotoxic lymphocyte activity. When this is this case embryo implantation will likely be impaired and the woman will often present with inability to conceive ("infertility"), unexplained IVF failure, or with recurrent pregnancy loss (RPL).

It is my opinion that all women who manifest with such reproductive problems, women who have a personal or family history of hypothyroidism and those in whom hyperprolactinemia or elevated blood levels of thyroid stimulating hormone (TSH) are detected, be tested for antithyroid antibodies cytotoxic lymphocyte (CTL) and NK cell activity (using the K-562 target cell assay) and that women found to have such antibodies as well as NKa, undergo selective immunotherapy with Intralipid (IL) infusions plus steroid (prednisone, prednisilone, dexamethasone) therapy to down-regulate NK/CTL activity. IL is administered intravenously 7-14 days prior to embryo transfer (or about 4-7 days prior to ovulation or egg retrieval) and then repeated once more, immediately upon biochemical confirmation (beta hCG blood test) of embryo implantation. The steroids are continued to the 10th week of pregnancy and then slowly tailed off.

What often goes unrecognized is that treatment of hypothyroidism with thyroid hormone replacement alone, while resolving the hormonal imbalance associated with hypothyroidism will usually not resolve associated reproductive dysfunction due to associated immunologic implantation dysfunction.

Antral Follicle Count (AFC)

The performance of an antral follicle count (AFC) or ultrasound examination of the ovaries, during the first few days of the menstrual cycle will reveal the presence of small antral (fluid-filled) follicles. It is these follicles that can ultimately develop into large egg-bearing follicles with ovarian stimulation. The number of antral follicles suggests the potential number of eggs that could become available for egg retrieval under optimal circumstances.

NUTRITIONAL SUPPLEMENTS IN PREPARING FOR IVF

Good nutrition is indeed an important prerequisite for optimal reproductive function. However, a well-balanced diet that meets food preferences, coupled with modest vitamin, mineral, and antioxidant supplementation (as can be found in many prenatal vitamin preparations) should suffice.

This having been said, conceiving is a delicate process, and eating the right foods is essential to optimize reproductive potential. Indeed, a balanced diet (i.e., a lot of organic and brightly colored foods) will provide most of the nutrients you need. But the truth is that most people do not have a balanced diet and are unwittingly often deficient in important nutrients.

A balanced diet is one that is rich in good quality protein, low in sugar, salt, caffeine, and industrially created trans-fats (trans-fatty acids or partially hydrogenated oils) and soy, uncontaminated by heavy metals, free of nicotine, alcohol, and recreational drugs. This is why routine supplementation with the following nutrients could enhance preconception readiness:

- Folic acid (400 micrograms daily)
- Vitamins A (2565 IU daily); B6 (6mg -10 mg daily); B12 (12-20 mcg per day); C (2,000 mg a day for both men and women); E (both sexes should get 150-200 U daily)
- Co-enzyme Q10 (100mg daily)
- Amino acids such as L-Carnitine (3 grams daily) and L-arginine (1 gram per day)
- Omega 3 fatty acids (1,000-2,400 mg per day)
- Minerals, mainly zinc (15mg per day); selenium (70-100mcg per day); iron (up to 20mg per day); magnesium (400mg per day)

There are likely to be significant reproductive health benefits (including enhanced fertility and intrauterine development) associated with the use of nutritional supplements. However there are also certain potential pitfalls associated with their use. Some supplements are not as safe as they would seem. For example, excessive intake of fat-soluble vitamins (A, D, E, and K) can even be dangerous to your health and may be associated with fetal malformations.

Additionally, numerous supplements have been found to contain contaminants such as toxic plant materials, heavy metals, and even prescription medications that can compromise fetal development. Prior to the passage of the Dietary Supplement Health and Education Act of 1994, supplements (vitamins, minerals, amino acids, and botanicals) were required to demonstrate safety. However, since passage of "the Act," they are now presumed to be safe until shown otherwise, thus establishing a rather hazardous situation where a typical prenatal vitamin that will provide sufficient vitamins and minerals for a healthy early pregnancy and potentially dangerous supplements can and are being sold in the same store without product liability.

What about taking DHEA? I am fully aware of the fact that the use of DHEA is currently being advocated by many as a method by which to "improve" egg development and quality. DHEA is readily metabolized by the ovary to the male hormone, testosterone. While a small amount of testosterone is needed to promote optimal follicle and egg development as well as estrogen production, too much can have a detrimental effect. However, because the ovaries of older women, women who have diminished ovarian reserve (DOR), and women with polycystic ovarian syndrome (PCOS) already tend to over-produce testosterone, the ingestion of DHEA by such individuals would in my opinion, have the effect of "adding fuel to the fire" and should be discouraged.

In summary, maximizing reproductive performance and optimizing outcome following fertility treatment requires a combined strategy involving a balanced diet (rich in protein, low in sugars, soy, and trans-fats), modest nutritional supplementation, limiting/avoiding foods and contaminants that can compromise reproductive potential, and adopting disciplined lifestyle modification such as not smoking, reducing stress, minimizing alcohol intake, avoiding nicotine and recreational drug consumption, and getting down to a healthy weight through diet and exercise.

THE PRETREATMENT CONSULTATION

Once the appropriate tests have been completed, the physician and perhaps the clinical coordinator will discuss with the couple what to expect throughout the treatment cycle. Although the couple may have a general idea, the physician will reinforce what they have already been told and will encourage them to ask questions.

The physician probably will also outline some of the decisions the couple will have to make in the next few days. These include (1) how many eggs they wish to have fertilized, (2) what they want to do with any excess eggs, (3) how many embryos they want to have transferred into the uterus, (4) how they wish to dispose of any excess embryos (i.e., through embryo cryopreservation, also known as freezing, or donation), and (5) how they would deal with a high-order multiple pregnancy. Although these questions do not all have to be answered at the same time, the physician will probably touch on all of the relevant issues during this consultation in order to give the couple ample time to make their decision.

Preparing for the Inevitable Trade-off: The Probability of Pregnancy vs. the Risk of High-Order Multiple Births

Because an embryo's average chance of implanting is about 20–30 percent with conventional IVF in women under 35 years of age, enough embryos must be transferred into the uterus to ensure the highest probable birthrate. It has been our experience at SIRM that in women under 40 with a well-prepared endometrium and with good-quality embryos, placement of two cleaved embryos or one or two blastocysts (embryos that are 5–6 days post fertilization) into the uterus yields about a 40 percent chance of having a baby. (See Chapter 8 for a discussion about the technique and advisability of transferring blastocysts into the woman's uterus.)

However, the couple wishing to maximize their chances of pregnancy by increasing the number of embryos transferred must be prepared to confront the unavoidable tradeoff: The more embryos, the greater the risk of multiple births. Currently in the United States the multiple-pregnancy rate from IVF in women under 40 is twins in about one out of every three and triplets or greater (high-order multiple pregnancy) in about one out of every 20 pregnancies. While twin pregnancies and the resulting babies are at greater risk than are singletons, the risk increases dramatically with high order multiple gestations.

The physician should explain that it is the number of viable embryos transferred to the uterus rather than the absolute number (whether or not they are known to be viable) that determines the risk of multiple gestation. Accordingly, the older patient (over 40) undergoing IVF will likely be advised to have more embryos transferred than would be the case with her younger counterpart. This is because the risk of multiple pregnancies has more to do with the number of viable, chromosomally normal embryos than with the absolute number transferred. The number of embryos transferred, therefore, should be influenced by the woman's age.

The risks associated with high-order multiple pregnancies. The couple must be thoroughly educated on the implications of a high-order multiple pregnancy (triplets or greater) before they decide how many embryos to have transferred. While most women can tolerate a twin pregnancy, a higher-order multiple pregnancy threatens the well-being of both mother and babies. Moreover, the risks become greater to both mother and babies as the number of fetuses increases.

Risks to the mother that are especially acute during a high-order multiple pregnancy include high blood pressure, uterine bleeding, and problems associated with a cesarean section. (The incidence of cesarean sections increases dramatically in multiple pregnancies.)

The primary threat to the physical and intellectual well-being of the babies stems from complications resulting from premature birth. Multiple births often occur prematurely, and the more babies, the more premature their birth. Prematurity can cause one or possibly all of the babies to be born brain-damaged and/or with a dangerously low birth weight that can endanger their survival.

Selective reduction of pregnancy. Because of the serious complications that so often occur in high-order multiple pregnancies, most IVF programs tend to transfer fewer embryos or blastocysts to the uterus than was the case a few years ago and counsel couples on the concept of selectively reducing the size of a multiple pregnancy as a possible life-saving measure for the remaining fetuses.

Selective reduction of pregnancy, which is usually performed prior to completion of the third month of gestation, involves the injection of a chemical under guidance by ultrasound directly into one or more developing fetuses. This causes the involved fetus(es) to succumb almost immediately and be absorbed by the body. Selective reduction of pregnancy can cause a miscarriage in the remaining fetus(es), but this occurs infrequently when the procedure is done by an expert. Experience has demonstrated that the risk of complete miscarriage or damage to the remaining fetuses is very small in cases where the fetuses are not identical (from the same embryo), as is virtually always the case with a multiple pregnancy following IVF. This is because IVF multiple pregnancies are almost always fraternal (from different embryos), having separate placentas and hence separate blood supplies.

We at SIRM advocate against women carrying more than two babies and advise receptive patients to reduce triplets to twins. We would definitely not suggest selective reduction in cases where there are fewer than three babies in the uterus unless indicated by unusual medical circumstances, such as one of twins being affected by a serious genetic/chromosomal defect.

IVF might be considered a pro-life procedure because by its very nature it is the opposite of abortion. Yet many physicians who perform IVF strongly believe that selective termination of pregnancy in the interest of saving life is acceptable or at least presents a possible option. We believe that couples should always be made aware, in an unbiased manner, of the option of selective termination of pregnancy in a pro-choice environment.

Constructing a framework for decision making. Before the couple can decide how many eggs should be fertilized, they first have to decide whether they are willing to risk a high-order multiple pregnancy. At this point, the physician might say to them:

> *"There is a difference of opinion as to how many embryos should be transferred into the uterus. What you need to remember is that there is a trade-off. If you put in more embryos you have a higher chance of pregnancy, but also a greater chance of a high-order multiple pregnancy (triplets or greater), and this can be dangerous for the mother and the babies. We have found that where the egg provider is 35 to 40 years old, two embryos is a safe number to transfer to the uterus. In women over 40, three embryos can reasonably be transferred to the uterus with a relatively low expectation of high-order multiple pregnancies."*

At SIRM we tend to cryopreserve (freeze and store) all remaining (non-transferred) blastocysts deemed to be viable. In most cases, the embryos are first kept in culture for an additional two to three days, and only those that develop into good-quality blastocysts are frozen and stored. In this way, upon transferring thawed blastocysts in a subsequent cycle, we are able to achieve good pregnancy rates.

5

IVF STEP 2: CONTROLLED OVARIAN STIMULATION (COS)

IVF success rates are dependent upon the number of mature eggs and "competent" embryos available for transfer. A woman undergoing IVF is given fertility drugs for two reasons: (1) to enhance the growth and development of her ovarian follicles in order to produce as many healthy eggs as possible and (2) to control the timing of ovulation so that the eggs can be surgically retrieved before they are ovulated. In cases where the woman has previously received fertility drugs, the subsequent treatment protocol is largely based upon her response to the most recent such treatment regime. If a woman is receiving gonadotropins for the first time, the dosage and regimen are determined by her cycle day (CD) 3 blood FSH Antimullerian Hormone (AMH), Inhibin-B concentrations, medical history, and body type.

FERTILITY DRUG THERAPIES

Launching Controlled Ovarian Stimulation (COS) with the Birth Control Pill (BCP)

There are significant advantages to putting the woman on a BCP for 10 days or longer before launching COS for IVF. First, by shortening or lengthening the time on the BCP, it is possible to influence, with relative precision, when menstruation will begin and thus by adjusting the duration of administration, afford convenient control over when precisely COS should begin. Second, it suppresses LH-induced ovarian male hormone (testosterone, androstenedione, etc.) production, which (especially) in older women, DOR, or PCOS can compromise egg development and thus embryo quality. And if prescribed correctly, the BCP does so without any real down side to its use and, third, it reduces the likelihood of Lupron-induced ovarian cyst formation, thereby largely avoiding the need to delay or cancel the IVF cycle of treatment.

Contrary to what most patients believe, use of the BCP to launch a cycle of COS will not suppress subsequent follicle development or compromise egg/embryo quality, provided it is used correctly. Proper use involves administering a GnRHa such as Lupron or Buserelin during the last few days while on the BCP and then stopping the oral contraceptive and awaiting menstruation to commence a few days later when COS with gonadotropins is initiated. If a woman goes directly from using a BCP to COS, without first overlapping the last few days on the BCP with a GnRHa, subsequent follicular response and egg quality is often severely compromised.

Towards the end of a natural ovulatory cycle, starting a few days prior to menstruation, the corpus luteum (the structure that produces estrogen and progesterone after ovulation) starts to fail. This is associated with a rise in blood levels of FSH, which in turn triggers the final stage of egg recruitment and the development of antral follicles. Antral follicle development is an essential step in preparation for COS without which orderly follicle and egg development are unlikely to take place once gonadotropin therapy is instituted. Since the BCP suppresses FSH release by the pituitary gland, and blocks ovulation, antral follicle development will not occur. Administration of GnRHa during the last few days on the BCP triggers FSH release and thus overcomes this suppressive effect. The bottom line is that the use of a BCP to set up a cycle of IVF is advantageous, provided it is always accompanied by overlapping with a GnRHa for a few days before COS begins. If this is done the BCP will NOT suppress or compromise response to COS.

As soon as menstruation begins, blood is drawn, and if the plasma E2 concentration is less than 70 pg/ml, the patient is ready to initiate COS with gonadotropins. If the E2 level is greater than 70 pg/ml, GnRHa therapy is continued at the same (or an increased) dosage for a few more days, whereupon the E2 concentration is re-measured. Subsequent failure of the E2 to fall below 70 pg/ml is an indication for a pelvic ultrasound for the detection of an ovarian cyst, the presence of which usually mandates the performance of an ovarian cyst needle aspiration.

Coming off the BCP and on to Managing the Cycle of COS

As soon as menstruation begins, GnRHa injections are either continued (at a reduced dosage) until regular ultrasound evaluations confirm that the leading follicles are fully developed or, the GnRHa is discontinued and supplanted by low-dose GnRH antagonist (Ganirelix, Orgalutron or Cetrotide). This latter approach is referred to as the agonist/antagonist conversion protocol (A/ACP). At this point (and preferably no later than 10 days after the onset of menstruation, an individualized regime of gonadotropins therapy is initiated. Patients requiring heparinoid (Heparin, Lovenox /Clexane) therapy begin this treatment on the first day of receiving gonadotropins. Patients who have severely diminished ovarian reserve DOR might first receive intramuscular estradiol valerate (Delestrogen) by daily injections for 7-10 days prior to and then during COS, in an attempt to first "prime" the follicles in the hope of achieving an optimal follicular growth response. Patients who have a past history of a poor endometrial lining might be prescribed sildenafil (Viagra) vaginal suppositories in an attempt to improve the development of their uterine lining. Patients who have activated CTL and natural killer cell activity (NKa) as measured by immunophenotype and the K-562 target cell test and/or endometrial cytokine analysis, will receive Intralipid (IL) or IVIg therapy by intravenous infusion 7–14 days prior to embryo transfer. Commencing with the start of COS, all IVF patients receive oral daily corticosteroids (dexamethasone, prednisilone or prednisone). Two days after the initiation of COS with gonadotropin injections, the dosage of gonadotropins is substantially reduced, and is then maintained at this lower level until the administration of the hCG trigger. Gonadotropin dosage adjustments are sometimes made during the course of COS, based upon the patient's response to medication. Commencing seven days after the initiation of gonadotropin therapy, the patient starts undergoing serial ultrasound and plasma estradiol (E2) evaluations to monitor her ovarian response. These assessments are aimed at determining the ideal day for administering 10,000 IU of hCG to trigger the final maturation of the egg(s) and the production of progesterone by the ovaries. Lupron or Ganirelix/Cetrotide/Orgalutron and gonadotropin injections are discontinued on this day and the patient is scheduled for egg retrieval approximately 36 hours after receiving the intramuscular injection of hCG. Subcutaneous heparin injections are discontinued approximately 12 hours prior to the egg retrieval and restarted after the embryo transfer procedure.

Virtually all patients will receive a broad spectrum oral antibiotic beginning about seven days after the initiation of gonadotropin therapy and continuing for a few days after the embryo transfer procedure.

Commonly Used Fertility Medications

Today gonadotropins are used, by and large, across the board in IVF, while clomiphene citrate, once commonly prescribed in the '80s and '90s, has largely fallen out of favor. In general, the woman's response to these drugs will depend on her pattern of ovulation, the degree of ovarian resistance, and her age.

Clomiphene Citrate (Serophene, Clomid)

Clomiphene was the most popular drug used for IVF COS in the 1980s, but because of poor IVF results it is hardly used in the IVF setting any longer. In fact, I rarely, if ever prescribe it to my IVF patients. Clomiphene is a synthetic hormone that deceives the hypothalamus into thinking that the body's estrogen level is too low. In response, the hypothalamus releases GnRH (gonadotropin-releasing hormone), which in turn prompts the pituitary gland to release an increased amount of FSH (follicle-stimulating hormone). As happens in nature, the increased secretion of FSH stimulates development of the follicles, ultimately resulting in ovulation. The growing follicles secrete estrogen into the bloodstream, thus closing the feedback circle that the hypothalamus initiated in response to the anti-estrogen properties of clomiphene citrate. (In the United States, clomiphene is marketed as Clomid and Serophene.)

The administration of clomiphene citrate enhances the normal cyclical pattern of follicular development and ovulation. If initiated as early as day 2 or day 3 of the menstrual cycle, it usually induces ovulation on day 13 or 14 of a regular 28-day cycle. If administered later, such as on day 5, ovulation could occur as late as day 16 or 17, and the length of the cycle may be extended. If the woman does not stimulate appropriately on the original dosage of clomiphene, the dosage may be increased to achieve optimal stimulation.

We sometimes administer hCG (human chorionic gonadotropin) to the woman once ultrasound examinations and hormonal evaluations confirm optimal follicular development. In such cases, ovulation will usually occur about 38-42 hours later. The prolonged usage of clomiphene for more than three consecutive cycles may lead to the accumulation of one of its components (zuclomiphene), which will reduce the amount and alter the quality of the cervical mucus, with negative implications for the passage and capacitation of the sperm. It is also likely to thin the uterine lining and thereby reduce the chances of a healthy implantation. This is the reason why the prolonged usage of clomiphene without at least one month's break every three months is associated with reduced pregnancy rates and a much higher rate of spontaneous abortion, should pregnancy occur. It also explains why 80 percent of births that occur following the use of clomiphene are conceived during the first three months of stimulation and why hardly any pregnancies occur at all in women who have taken clomiphene more than five or six months without a break. One month's hiatus is sufficient to allow for the elimination of zuclomiphene from the body and will restore the potential to respond optimally to clomiphene.

It has been observed that few women as they get older show a declining response to clomiphene. However, in spite of the fact that they appear to ovulate on clomiphene treatment, they frequently develop poor mucus and a poor endometrial lining from the inception of clomiphene administration. We accordingly believe that clomiphene should rarely be prescribed to women over the age of 35 and is relatively contraindicated for women over 40.

Two major advantages of clomiphene are its relatively low cost and the fact that it can be taken orally instead of by injection. A distinct disadvantage is that when administered alone it does not stimulate the growth and maturation of as many follicles as do alternative therapies such as gonadotropins (Follistim, Gonal F, Repronex, Bravelle) or clomiphene plus gonadotropins; accordingly, fewer eggs can be retrieved.

Side effects of clomiphene citrate.   The side effects associated with clomiphene citrate are related to the follicular development this drug stimulates. When administered alone, a luteal-phase defect (inadequate production of progesterone by the corpus luteum to sustain the endometrium) may result if the follicles do not develop properly. This would hinder implantation by preventing the endometrium from responding optimally to the progesterone produced by the corpus luteum. In about 15 percent of clomiphene-treated cycles the hormonal changes associated with ovulation take place along with the commensurate rise in blood progesterone level, but the egg is not released. This form of "trapped ovulation" is referred to as luteinized unruptured follicle syndrome (LUFS). Clomiphene may also interfere with the nurturing effect estrogen must have on the developing endometrium. In addition, traces of clomiphene that might linger in the woman's circulatory system for many weeks may inhibit the normal function of enzymes produced by the developing follicular cells.

Too high a dose of clomiphene may cause follicles to grow too rapidly, producing large fluid-filled collections known as cysts. This may lead to tenderness and swelling of the ovaries, visual disturbances, and hot flashes similar to those at menopause.

Finally, too high a dose of clomiphene may decrease the amount of cervical mucus produced and may also reduce its quality, with negative implications for the passage and capacitation of the sperm. Too high a dosage may also decrease the thickness of the uterine lining.

Safety of clomiphene citrate. Some studies have suggested that clomiphene citrate has caused birth defects or a higher miscarriage rate in laboratory animals and could, therefore, potentially threaten human offspring. Other studies have suggested that clomiphene administered for more than 12 sequential months increases the subsequent risk of ovarian cancer. However, if clomiphene is administered appropriately and is taken under proper supervision, it is a safe and effective method for induction of ovulation.

The fear that clomiphene might cause birth defects arises from the fact that its inner structure, or nucleus, is very similar to that of the hormone DES (diethylstilbestrol), which is known to have caused so many birth defects when administered to pregnant women. Although it is theoretically possible that clomiphene might cause such defects, birth statistics do not indicate an increased birth-defect rate after stimulation with the drug. The laboratory studies mentioned above should not be ignored, however, but should be heeded as a guide to safe, prudent administration of fertility drugs.

Since it is not known with certainty whether clomiphene citrate might adversely affect the developing fetus, we caution that this agent should be taken only when it is absolutely certain that the woman is not pregnant. The appearance of a menstrual period does not provide adequate certainty, because more than 10 percent of women might bleed during early pregnancy. Assessment by a physician, or even a home pregnancy test, provides greater assurance that a pregnancy does not exist.

The administration of clomiphene as a fertility agent over a series of months might promote ovulatory problems. It has been observed that in one out of five cases where clomiphene is administered, the egg remains trapped in the follicle after ovulation. Therefore, the practice of physicians saying to patients, "Here's some clomiphene—take some each month and call me if you miss your period," should be questioned.

But if clomiphene citrate is taken under proper supervision and the woman has previously determined that she is not pregnant, its safety is beyond question. This has prompted many IVF programs to continue using it. Those that do so, however, invariably report a lower pregnancy rate than that which can be achieved by other methods of COS.

Letrozole (Femara)

Letrozole, like clomiphene, is an oral agent that induces ovulation that causes the pituitary gland to release large amounts of FSH as well as LH. The advantage that Letrozole has over clomiphene is that unlike the latter, it is not anti-estrogenic and thus does not compromise development of the uterine lining or adversely affect the production of cervical mucus. However, as is the case with clomiphene, Letrozole causes increased LH release that can lead to overproduction of male hormones (e.g., testosterone) by the ovaries with potentially adverse effect on egg/embryo quality. Thus while Letrozole does have potential advantages over clomiphene, the exaggerated LH-induced testosterone effect, especially in women over 40 years of age and/or those with evidence of diminished ovarian reserve limits its value in the IVF setting.

Gonadotropins

Gonadotropins are hormones produced by the pituitary gland and which stimulate sex hormone production as well as gamete (sperm and egg) production in both men and women. They are also responsible for the expression of secondary sexual characteristics such as hair growth, muscular development, and voice changes and breast development. There are two gonadotropins, Follicle stimulating Hormone (FSH) and Luteinizing hormone (LH). Gonadotropins are excreted in the urine.

Because gonadotropins cannot be absorbed through the stomach into the bloodstream, they must be administered by injection rather than in pill form. While hMg must be injected intramuscularly, FSHr and LHr can be administered subcutaneously, thereby rendering the injections easier to administer and far less painful. The usual injection schedule is from day 2 or 3 through day 8-12 of the menstrual cycle.

One of the most significant attributes of gonadotropins is the safety-valve effect on ovulation. No matter how well stimulated a woman becomes when she takes gonadotropins, she will be unlikely to ovulate until she receives an injection of the hormone Human Chorionic Gonadotropin (hCG). Thus, if for any reason it is determined that the woman should not progress to ovulation, the hCG is simply not administered.

Risks and Side Effects of Gonadotropin Therapy

a) General side effects: Some women taking gonadotropins report breast tenderness, backaches, headaches, insomnia, bloating, and increased vaginal discharge, which is directly due to increased mucus production by the cervix.

b) Ovarian hyperstimulation syndrome (OHS): Potentially serious side effects of gonadotropin administration include over-stimulation that can threaten the woman's well-being including enlargement and "weeping" of the ovaries, a condition in which fluid exudes into the abdominal cavity. OHS is discussed in greater detail later in this chapter.

c) Variations in response to gonadotropins: Some women stimulate well after relatively small doses of gonadotropins. Others require two, three, or even four times that dosage to achieve the same effect. In the past, selecting the proper dosage was a trial-and-error process. There was simply no way to predict how a particular woman might respond. Each woman is unique, and each can be expected to react differently to gonadotropins. However, about 80% of women respond appropriately to an average injection.

Note: We measure FSH (follicle-stimulating hormone) and estradiol (E2) in the woman's blood on the second or third day of a natural menstrual cycle preceding the IVF cycle. We also can measure AMH and Inhibin B to predict the probable way she will respond to a variety of stimulation methods. We believe all these tests to be valuable in selecting the most appropriate dosage and regimen of fertility drugs to be administered.

Despite these refinements, however, stimulation for IVF is still somewhat of a hit-or-miss procedure. For example, when a woman has used up most of her lifetime egg budget and is left with less than a critical number of eggs, she begins to enter a phase of hormonal change known as the climacteric. The climacteric is associated with a loss of fertility, the onset of hot flashes, and mood changes. It ultimately culminates with the total cessation of menstruation between the ages of 40 to 55, a process called the menopause. The ovaries still produce hormones after menopause, but they are released in a constant rather than cyclical manner.

When a woman fails to be adequately stimulated with gonadotropin on the first try, the dosage and even the regime of treatment must be adjusted for her next attempt.

Follicle growth and development, egg maturation, the number of eggs that can be retrieved, and the risk of side effects are directly related to the patient's response as evaluated by blood-estrogen levels and/or ultrasound, and the dosage of gonadotropins. Therefore, it is illogical and ill-founded to fear administering an escalating dose of gonadotropins after a poor response to a standard dosage. What is important is to monitor the individual's response to the drug and then to adjust the dosage and length of administration accordingly.

There are two varieties of commercially available gonadotropins. The first is menotropins or urinary derived Human Menopausal Gonadotropins (hMG) and the second is genetically engineered Recombinant DNA-gonadotropins (FSHr and LHr).

1. <u>Urinary-Derived Gonadotropin (Menotropin) or Human Meno-pausal Gonadotropin (hMG)—(e.g., Menopur, Merional, Niken-hMG, Bravelle)</u>: These are derived from the urine of post-menopausal women. In such cases the pituitary glands, in response to a feedback message that her ovaries are no longer producing enough estrogen, increases the output of both FSH and LH in an effort to re-stimulate her failing ovaries. The excess FSH and LH is excreted in the urine, which is collected, distilled, filtered, and purified whereupon the FSH and LH is extracted.

a. *Menotropins comprising a combination of FSH + LH/hCG Menotropins (e.g., Menopur, Merional, Niken hMG):* These hMGs contain a good source of both FSH and LH and in the case of Menopur, a small amount of LH and hCG is added. Presently one vial of hMG (75 units) costs about $80 in the United States. The average IVF patient might require 25 or more vials per treatment cycle. It has been postulated that the LH/hCG component of hMG directly stimulates the tissue surrounding the ovarian follicles (ovarian stroma/theca), which in response produces male hormones or androgens (predominantly testosterone). The testosterone is then carried to the surrounding follicles where FSH converts it to estrogen (estradiol). A little LH is thus essential for normal follicle growth and development. However, a problem arises when there is too much LH because this can result in excessive ovarian testosterone production, which can be counterproductive, in that this can adversely affect follicle growth and egg development. Excess ovarian testosterone can also access the pelvic/uterine blood and suppress endometrial response to estrogen thereby compromising development and "thickening" of the endometrial lining. Simply stated, modest production of LH-induced ovarian male hormone promotes optimal follicle, egg, and (ultimately thus) embryo development and enhances development of the uterine lining, thereby favoring IVF outcome, On the other hand, excessive LH-induced ovarian male hormones can compromise egg development, thereby compromising egg quality, and might compromise estrogen-induced endometrial growth and development. Since older women and those who have polycystic ovarian syndrome (PCOS), and women who have diminished ovarian reserve often have elevated LH activity and, as a result, their ovaries produce an overabundance of the male hormone testosterone, they should probably not be given large amounts of LH-containing drugs such as Menopur or Merional because this could compromise egg quality and endometrial development.

b. *Predominantly FSH-Menotropin (e.g., Bravelle):* Here, the urinary derived hMG has been processed further to extract most of the LH. Bravelle is less expensive than FSHr (see below) but is not as effective, and there tends to be quite significant batch-to-batch variation in its biopotency. Accordingly I tend to restrict the use of Bravelle in my IVF patients.

2. Recombinant DNA-Derived Gonadotropins

a. *Recombinant FSH [FSHr] (Follistim, Puregon, and Gonal-F):* Human menopausal gonadotropin (hMG) has in recent times largely been supplanted by purified FSHr: derived by way of genetic engineering that makes it possible to induce bacteria to produce the FSH product. Known as recombinant FSH (FSHr), it appears to be more bioactive than urinary derived FSH products such as hMG. FSHr also has advantages in treating selected infertility problems such as PCOS. Instead of influencing the hypothalamus and pituitary gland to produce more of the body's own FSH/LH to stimulate follicular development (as is the case with clomiphene), gonadotropins act directly on the ovaries. If administered in sufficient amounts starting early enough in the cycle, gonadotropins will prompt the maturation of multiple follicles. Although the average number of eggs usually retrieved from a woman younger than 40 after gonadotropin stimulation, provided she has two ovaries, is usually between six and fifteen, retrievals of more than fifty eggs have been reported.

b. *Recombinant LH (LHr) (e.g., Luveris):* Some LH is absolutely essential to provide ovarian testosterone to the granulosa cells that line the follicles for subsequent conversion to estrogen. Thus, since the GnRH agonists and antagonists which are administered during most IVF-COS cycles will suppress the body's own (endogenous) LH, LH must be supplemented if optimal follicle and egg development is to take place. This can be achieved through the daily administration of a small amount of LH/hCG-containing menotropins (e.g., Meonopur) or through supplementation with LHr (Luveris).

3. Combination of Clomiphene + Gonadotropins

This approach was quite common in the mid-'80s and early '90s and resulted in a significant number of IVF babies being born. The main motivation for using this combination was that clomiphene increases ovarian sensitivity to gonadotropins, thereby reducing the dosage and cost of gonadotropins. Another reason was that clomiphene can be taken orally in pill form. But when it comes to IVF, the clomiphene + gonadotropin combination has several drawbacks. Firstly, because clomiphene has the ability to induce ovulation, a combination of clomiphene and gonadotropins may cause spontaneous ovulation even without the administration of hCG. In such a case, egg retrieval might inadvertently take place after ovulation has occurred, resulting in fewer eggs being retrieved. Secondly, the combination of the two drugs makes it difficult to pinpoint the amounts of each that should be changed when the overall dosage must be adjusted in subsequent cycles. While hMg must be injected intramuscularly, FSHr and LHr can be administered subcutaneously, thereby rendering the injections easier to administer and far less painful. The usual injection schedule is from day 2 or 3 through day 8–12 of the menstrual cycle.

One of the most significant attributes of gonadotropins is the safety-valve effect on ovulation. No matter how well stimulated a woman becomes when she takes gonadotropins, she will be unlikely to ovulate until she receives an injection of the hormone Human Chorionic Gonadotropin (hCG). Thus, if for any reason it is determined that the woman should not progress to ovulation, the hCG is simply not administered.

The considerable interpersonal and intrapersonal variations in response to gonadotropins might be attributable to one or both of the following factors. It could be that hormonal and biochemical factors governing the response to gonadotropins vary in the different women or even at different stages of the same woman's life. For example, as we noted earlier in this chapter, age influences the woman's ovarian receptivity to gonadotropins, especially as she nears the climacteric. In addition, some women simply will not respond consistently to administration of the same dosage of gonadotropins from month to month.

It is significant that gonadotropins are highly unlikely to produce any serious persistent side effects until the woman receives the injection of hCG to stimulate ovulation. Thus, the physician has ample time to assess her status and withhold the hCG if it appears that she might develop major side effects. (Such an assessment is made on the basis of blood estradiol values or ultrasound examinations immediately prior to administration of hCG.) This built-in protective advantage shields almost all women being treated with gonadotropins (administered either alone or in combination with clomiphene) from the serious hazards of over stimulation.

> *Note:* Side effects associated with the use of gonadotropins are by and large related to the degree of stimulation as measured by follicle growth and blood estrogen levels. Proper management of the treatment cycle should limit the risks of side effects and optimize the chance of a successful outcome.

OVARIAN HYPERSTIMULATION SYNDROME (OHS)

OHS is a condition where a woman receiving fertility drugs (usually gonadotropins) over-responds by developing a large number of ovarian follicles which upon administration of hCG triggers a series of systemic events that can place the woman at risk.

Moderately severe ovarian hyperstimulation is quite common. Here, the hyperstimulated ovaries are enlarged and there will usually be a moderate amount of free fluid in the abdominal cavity (ascites) without vomiting, diarrhea, compromised kidney function, severe abdominal pain, or shortness of breath.

Severe ovarian hyperstimulation syndrome (OHSS) represents a significant progression and can be a life-endangering condition. It presents with the gross abdominal distention due to fluid collection (ascites) and possible fluid collection in the chest (pleural effusion) with shortness of breath, severe pain, renal failure, blood coagulation failure, and even circulatory collapse. The severity of the ascites can cause such a degree of increased intra-abdominal pressure as to result in part of the stomach sliding through the diaphragmatic opening through which the esophagus passes. This creates a "functional hiatal hernia" causing gastric reflux, pain and vomiting. In addition, marked ovarian enlargement can stimulate the vagus nerve, leading to marked slowing of the heart rate (bradycardia), sweating, and diarrhea.

Women with OHSS require a full hematologic, biochemical, and physical evaluation and depending on the severity of the condition, may need to be admitted to hospital for close observation and management. Pronounced ascites that causes undue pain and difficulty in breathing, may require transvaginal or transabdominal drainage (paracentesis) of the fluid. This usually affords immediate symptomatic relief because it alleviates growing intra-abdominal pressure. It also reduces compression of major blood vessels allowing for improved liver, kidney, and intestinal function.

OHSS is a condition that rarely occurs in normally ovulating women. It is most commonly seen in young women and in those who do not ovulate spontaneously on their own (as with PCOS). An experienced IVF physician will be on the lookout for OHSS in cases where early on in the course of undergoing controlled ovarian hyperstimulation (COH) with gonadotropins, the woman develops >25 ovarian follicles of 14mm-16mm (in mean diameter) in association with a blood estradiol (E2) level of above 2,500 pg/ml prior to the "hCG trigger." He/she will also know that when the blood estradiol (estrogen) level rises to above 4,000 pg/ml, the risk of OHSS escalates, and if it rises above 6,000 pg/ml, the likelihood of OHSS developing will be greater than 80%.

OHSS is a self-limiting condition: The development of OHSS is linked to the effect of hCG on the cells that line the inside of ovarian follicles. Thus it does not occur until the "hCG trigger" is administered. In fact, there is no risk of OHSS until hCG is administered. Accordingly, if the hCG trigger is withheld, then regardless of the peak blood estradiol level the condition will not develop. And even if the "hCG trigger" and OHSS develops but pregnancy does not ensue, the condition will be self-limiting and will most likely resolve within 12–14 days. Conversely, if pregnancy results from the ET, the condition will get progressively worse commensurate with increasing production of hCG by the developing root system (placenta) of the conceptus. The good news is that even if this should happen, the condition will spontaneously resolve beginning 7-8 weeks into the pregnancy.

The challenge in treating OHSS is to try and avoid over-administration of gonadotropins to women known to be susceptible to developing this condition, and in the event of inadvertent overstimulation, to institute measures that will minimize the risk. To achieve this requires that all women with 25 or more ovarian follicles be critically reassessed for OHSS riskfactors prior to receiving the "hCG trigger."

Once pregnancy occurs there is no turning back, as OHSS will then run its own course. Thus, if the warning signs of potential OHSS developing are missed, either the hCG trigger should be withheld or if a judgment is made to administer it, fresh embryos should not be transferred to the woman's uterus. Rather her embryos should be cryostored (frozen) and the ET be deferred to a subsequent hormone-prepared cycle.

Prolonged Coasting (PC). PC is a procedure introduced by SIRM physicians in the '90s. It involves abruptly stopping gonadotropin therapy while continuing to administer the GnRH agonist (e.g., Lupron, Buserelin) and then allowing the blood estradiol level below 2,500 pg/ml) before administering the hCG trigger. A word of caution . . . unless PC is initiated at precisely the right time, it will result in poor quality eggs and embryos. So timing and experience are both cardinal attributes in implementing PC. In most cases, after initiating PC, the blood E2 level will at first continue to rise for 1–4 days. Thereupon, follicle growth will cease and the blood E2 levels will start to decline. Only once the E2 concentration drops below 2,500 pg/ml should the "hCG trigger" be administered. Proper implementation of PC will avert the risks associated with OHSS without seriously compromising egg/embryo quality.

Since I first reported on the benefits of PC in the early '90s, this approach has gained widespread international acceptance as the method of choice by which OHSS can be addressed.

Many IVF physicians are unfamiliar in dealing with full-blown condition OHSS and are so fearful of its consequences that when confronted with even moderately severe OHS and the possibility that the condition might evolve, they either cancel the IVF cycle altogether or administer the "hCG trigger" prematurely in the hope of stopping the process in its tracks. In such cases, the eggs retrieved will almost always be "immature" and be of such poor quality as to yield "incompetent" embryos that are incapable of propagating a pregnancy.

> *Note:* When correctly implemented, "prolonged coasting (PC)" prevents OHSS, protects egg/embryo quality, removes the need to cancel the IVF cycle, and thus avoids canceled dreams.

Gonadotropin-Releasing Hormone Agonists (GnRHa)—Lupron, Buserelin

All gonadotropin-releasing hormone (GnRH) agonists act by rapidly expunging reservoirs of FSH and luteinizing hormone (LH) from the pituitary gland. GnRH agonists (both Lupron and Buserelin) can be administered by intramuscular injection.

I prescribe gonadotropin-releasing hormone agonists (GnRHa) such as leuprolide acetate (Lupron) to launch most IVF-COS cycles.

The reason that agonists are administered to women receiving gonadotropin therapy for IVF is because of their ability to suppress LH and so prevent a premature rise in LH which is most likely to occur in older women or those with diminished ovarian reserve. When this happens the cells lining the follicles undergo premature change (premature luteinization), compromising further follicle development and egg/embryo quality. Such premature luteinization (often referred to as a "premature LH surge") severely compromises further follicle development as well as egg/embryo quality. Women with reduced ovarian reserve (who are resistant to ovarian stimulation) are most susceptible to this happening.

There is often talk of agonists "over-suppressing" ovarian response to gonadotropins. The reason for this concern is that agonists probably compete with FSH for receptor binding sites on the granulosa cells that line the ovarian follicles and produce estrogen…and so can blunt ovarian follicle response to FSH. On the other hand, GnRh-antagonists apparently do not exert the same effect, and thus can be used to supplant agonists prior to starting gonadotropin therapy (see the agonist/antagonist conversion protocol below). While both antagonists and GnRHa block LH activity, antagonists do so much more rapidly (within hours) than agonists (within a few days).

As previously stated, I selectively favor launching COS for IVF by prescribing on a birth control pill (BCP) and then overlapping with the BCP just prior to menstruation. Menstruation will usually occur 4-7 days after stopping the BCP. Thereupon, one of two variations in approach is taken: either the long Lupron approach or the agonist/antagonist conversion protocol (A/ACP).

In patients undergoing egg donation and gestational surrogacy, embryo donation with frozen/thawed embryo transfers (FET) undergo a similar regime of BCP/agonist preparation as do those who undergo ovarian stimulation, except that instead of receiving gonadotropin injections, these women receive daily estradiol valerate injections. Thereupon, progesterone therapy (administered by intramuscular injection and/or by vaginal administration) is added for several days. The combination of estrogen and progesterone therapy prepares the uterine lining for embryo implantation. Lupron therapy is discontinued 5-7 days prior to ET in such cases.

Extensive studies on non-human primates, as well as limited human evaluations, indicate that agonists such as Lupron are relatively harmless to both mother and baby. The drug is eliminated from the system within hours of discontinuing its administration. I favor discontinuing GnRHa therapy 5-7 days prior to transferring embryos/blastocysts to the woman's uterus. The administration of GnRHa is rarely associated with significant side effects. Some women experience temporary fluctuations in mood, hot flashes, nausea, and symptoms not vastly dissimilar from PMS. No serious long-lasting sideeffects have been reported.

The subcutaneous injection of GnRHa is relatively painless. Unfortunately, the drug will incur a modest additional financial burden. GnRHa administration as described above spares women the inconvenience and frustration of unnecessary cancelled treatment cycles with gonadotropins. As such, the use of such therapy in reality reduces the overall cost of ovulation induction.

GnRHa can also be used selective to supplant hCG to trigger ovulation: Because the administration of GnRHa results in a rapid release of LH by the pituitary gland, and an LH surge is the "natural trigger" for spontaneous ovulation, some have advocated supplanting the hCG trigger with administration of a booster intramuscular shot of GnRHa (Lupron or Buserelin) in women at risk of developing OHSS (high responders). Protagonists of this approach argue that an induced LH surge is less likely than hCG to precipitate OHSS. Personally, I am not really convinced of the merit of such an approach. I much prefer to administer a predetermined dosage of hCG to my patients.

Gonadotropin-Releasing Hormone Antagonists: (Ganirelix, Cetrotide, Orgalutron)

Unlike GnRH agonists which expunge most LH and FSH from the pituitary gland, leading to their virtual disappearance from the blood as they are progressively eliminated from the body over a number of days, GnRH agonists work within hours to block the release of FSH and LH. As such they have the following potential advantages over GnRH agonists: (1) GnRH agonists evoke a rapid suppression of pituitary gonadotropins release; in fact, women who receive GnRH antagonists will have minimal blood levels of endogenous gonadotropins (FSH and LH) produced by the pituitary gland within 48 hours of the treatment being initiated; (2) GnRH antagonists do not competitively bind with ovarian FSH receptors and accordingly they allow for a better response to stimulation by a given dosage of gonadotropins; and (3) the use of GnRH antagonist allows for the initiation of COS to begin on short notice in the natural or oral contraceptive-treated cycle, thereby minimizing the need to postpone initiation of COS. (Oral contraceptives are often used to set up the cycle of stimulation.)

EVALUATION OF FOLLICULAR DEVELOPMENT

In order to properly schedule surgical retrieval of eggs, the IVF physician must be sure that proper follicular development has occurred. Because IVF programs rely heavily on the woman's daily blood-estrogen levels and daily ultrasound measurements of follicular developments in order to fine-tune this scheduling, usually by day 9 to 14 of the cycle a go/no-go decision can be made about whether to proceed to egg retrieval.

The Role of Vaginal Ultrasound Evaluation

When undergoing a vaginal ultrasound examination, the woman can feel the pressure of the transducer in her vagina, but she cannot feel or hear the sound waves as they travel through body tissue and fluid, and form images on a TV-like screen. Ultrasound enables the physician to see the woman's ovaries clearly and to identify, count, and measure the fluid-filled follicles as they develop, providing an important indicator of the expected time of ovulation.

The Importance of Serially Measuring Blood Estradiol (E2) and Performing Serial Ultrasound Follicular Assessments for COS

Measurement of the level of the hormone estradiol in the blood gives an approximate indication of how many eggs the physician might expect to retrieve. In general, the higher the estradiol level, the more eggs. This test will usually be done daily during the latter part of the treatment cycle preceding egg retrieval. In some programs, the estradiol level is measured throughout the treatment cycle.

If a woman taking gonadotropins does not stimulate enough after a week or so, she can continue gonadotropin medication for a few more days while her response is monitored by blood tests and/or ultrasound examinations. Such a delay should not significantly decrease her chance of getting pregnant. In certain cases, a woman who has not received GnRH agonist will at first show a steady rise in blood estradiol followed by a drop of >20% over the ensuing 24 hours. When this happens it is suggestive of premature luteinization. Either way, it indicates that the hormone LH has been released prematurely, thus causing an increase in ovarian male hormone (androgen) production which will inevitably compromise the health of the follicles and eggs. Such eggs will either not be fertilizable or, should they fertilize, will propagate poor quality embryos that will result in failed IVF. Thus when such an unanticipated drop in blood estradiol levels is noted prior to the hCG trigger, the cycle is best cancelled and the treating physician should reassess both the method and dosage of stimulation in a subsequent cycle.

THE INJECTION OF HCG (PROFASI, NOVAREL, PREGNYL, OVIDREL)—A SAFETY VALVE

When blood estradiol levels and/or ultrasound assessment indicate that the follicular development of a woman taking gonadotropins is enough to produce an adequate number of eggs but unlikely to cause dangerous side effects, she will be given an injection of 10,000 U of (urinary derived) hCG to ripen the follicles and eggs for ovulation. The hCG "triggers" ovulation, which occurs within 38 to 42 hours, in the same manner as does the surge of LH in nature.

Similar in structure to LH, hCG is favored for the induction of ovulation. (It is also the hormone measured to assess whether a woman is pregnant.) Because hCG is broken down and made inactive when it passes through the stomach if taken in pill form, it must be injected in order to be transported directly to the ovaries.

After the administration of hCG, egg retrieval is scheduled to be performed within about 36 hours (i.e., prior to the anticipated time of ovulation). The follicles will then continue to grow until the eggs are retrieved or ovulation occurs.

Recently a recombinant DNA form of hCG (hCGr) has been marketed as Ovidrel. While potentially Ovidrel works just as effectively as regular, urinary derived hCG (hCGu), I believe that the recommended dosage of administration (i.e., 250 mcg of Ovidrel) is inadequate. However, administration of double the recommended dosage of Ovidrel is as potent as is 10,000 U of hCGu. However, this is much more expensive and probably no more effective than hCGu . . . so why use it at all?

The Need for an "Individualized" Approach to COS?

Most young, ovulating women who have normal ovarian reserve will respond well to a standard, "recipe" protocol of COS. However, older women, women who have diminished ovarian reserve, and those who are high responders (e.g., very young women and women with PCOS) will often not and will produce poorer quality eggs/embryos. Thus in such cases it is imperative that the protocol of COS be individualized or customized in order to protect egg development and thus optimize embryo quality. Unfortunately, too many IVF physicians fail to recognize this important consideration and instead tend to take a recipe or "one size fits all" approach to ovarian stimulation with gonadotropins. Since >70% of women undergoing IVF tend to be ovulatory and have normal ovarian reserve, it follows that they would not be compromised by being put on recipe-type COS protocols. It is the remaining 20%–30% who fall outside the standard curve that will often suffer the consequences of such a "one size fits all" approach. Oftentimes, following several unsuccessful IVF attempts they will be advised to give up on using their own eggs and to resort to IVF using donated eggs. It is my position that in many such cases, the use of a more individualized approach to COS would have allowed many of these women to still achieve a pregnancy with their own eggs.

In order for any organism to attain an optimal state of maturation it must first undergo full growth and development. A plum plucked from a tree before having developed fully, or a poorly developed plum, might still ripen (mature) on the windowsill, and might even look just as enticing, but the underdeveloped fruit will never achieve optimal quality. The same principle applies to the development and maturation of human eggs. Proper development as well as precise timing in the initiation of egg maturation with LH or hCG is no less crucial to optimal egg maturation, fertilization, and ultimately to embryo quality. In fact, in cases where egg maturation is improperly timed (LH or hCG is released/given too early or too late), there is an increased risk of structural and numerical chromosomal abnormalities leading to compromised reproductive performance.

The potential for a woman's eggs to undergo orderly development, maturation, successful fertilization, and subsequent progression to good-quality embryos capable of producing healthy offspring is, in large part, genetically determined. However, the expression of such potential is profoundly susceptible to numerous extrinsic influences, especially to intra-ovarian hormonal changes during the pre-ovulatory phase of the cycle.

During the normal ovulation cycle, ovarian hormonal changes are regulated to avoid irregularities in production and interaction that could adversely influence follicle development and egg quality. As an example, small amounts of ovarian androgens, such as testosterone, enhance egg and follicle development, while overexposure to excessive concentrations of the same hormones can seriously compromise egg quality. It follows that protocols for COS should be geared toward optimizing follicle and egg development while avoiding overexposure to androgens. The fulfillment of these objectives requires an individualized approach to COS and that the administration of hCG or LH to trigger ovulation be timed precisely.

It is important to recognize that LH and FSH, while both playing a pivotal role in follicle development, have different primary sites of action in the ovary. The action of FSH is mainly directed toward proliferation of the granulosa cells, which line the inside of the follicles and produce estrogen. LH, on the other hand, acts primarily on the ovarian stroma, the connective tissue that surrounds the follicles, to produce androgens. Only a small amount of testosterone is necessary for optimal estrogen production; overproduction can have a deleterious effect on granulosa cell activity, follicle growth/development, egg maturation, fertilization potential, and, ultimately, on embryo quality. Furthermore, excessive ovarian androgens can also compromise estrogen-induced endometrial growth and development.

In conditions such as polycystic ovarian syndrome (PCOS), which is often characterized by increased blood LH levels, there is usually increased ovarian androgen production. It is, therefore, not surprising that poor egg/embryo quality and inadequate endometrial development are often features of this condition. The use of LH-containing preparations such as Menopur further aggravates this effect. Thus, I strongly recommend against the exclusive use of such drugs in PCOS patients, preferring FSH-dominant products such as Follistim, Gonal F, and Puregon.

While it would seem prudent to limit LH exposure in all cases of COS, this appears to be more relevant in women with PCOS, in those with diminished ovarian reserve, and in older women, all of whom tend to be more sensitive to LH.

It is common practice to administer GnRH agonists (e.g., Lupron, Buserelin) and, more recently, GnRH antagonists to prevent the release of LH with COS (see discussion of GnRH agonists and GnRH antagonists earlier in this chapter).

Long GnRHa Protocols

The most commonly prescribed protocol for Lupron/gonadotropin administration is the so-called "long protocol." Lupron is administered starting 5–7 days before menstruation in the cycle prior to the IVF treatment cycle, and precipitates an initial rise in FSH and LH levels, which is rapidly followed by a precipitous fall to near zero. Menstruation then ensues, whereupon gonadotropins treatment is initiated to ensure a relatively LH-free environment while daily Lupron injections continue.

"(Micro) Flare" GnRHa Protocols

Another approach to COS is by way of so-called "(micro-)flare protocols." This involves initiating gonadotropin therapy simultaneously with administration of GnRH agonist. The intent is to deliberately allow Lupron to cause an initial surge ("flare") in FSH levels in order to augment ovarian response to the gonadotropins medication. Unfortunately, this approach is a double-edged sword, as the resulting increased release of FSH is likely to be accompanied by a similar rise in blood LH levels that could evoke excessive ovarian stromal androgen production. This could potentially compromise egg quality, especially in older women and in women with conditions like PCOS in which the ovaries have increased sensitivity to LH. I believe that in this way, "flare" protocols could potentially hinder endometrial development, compromise egg/embryo quality, and reduce IVF success rates. Accordingly, I prefer to avoid them altogether.

GnRH Antagonist Protocols

In my opinion, the use of GnRH antagonists as currently prescribed in ovarian stimulation cycles could be problematic, especially in women with high LH and overgrowth (hyperplasia) of ovarian stroma (e.g., women over 40, women with raised cycle day 3 FSH and/or low AMH, women with DOR, other poor responders to gonadotropins, and in some women with PCOS). In such cases, the initiation of pituitary suppression with GnRH antagonists so late in the cycle of stimulation fails to suppress relatively high tonic pituitary LH levels in the earliest stage of follicular growth and development. One of the roles of LH is to promote androgen production, which as previously stated, is essential. Small amounts of LH are essential for optimal follicular growth to take place. High concentrations of LH are deleterious. In such women, the failure of conventional GnRH antagonist protocols to address this issue results in the inevitable excessive exposure of follicles to androgens, mainly testosterone. As discussed earlier, this can adversely influence egg/embryo quality and endometrial development.

Presumably, the reason for the suggested mid-follicular initiation of high-dose GnRH antagonist is to prevent the occurrence of the so-called premature LH surge, which is known to be associated with "follicular exhaustion" and poor egg/embryo quality. However, the term "premature LH surge" is a misnomer, and the concept of this being a terminal event or an isolated insult is erroneous. In fact, the event is an end point in the progressive escalation in LH ("a staircase effect") with increasing ovarian stromal activation and commensurate growing androgen production. A more appropriate term would be "premature luteinization." Trying to improve ovarian response so as to stave off follicular exhaustion by administering GnRH antagonist (Ganirelix, Cetrotide, Orgalu-tron) during the final few days of ovarian stimulation is like trying to prevent a shipwreck through removing the tip of an iceberg. The use of such late-period follicular phase GnRH antagonists in younger women or in normal responders will probably not produce such adverse effects because the tonic endogenous LH levels are low (normal) in such cases, and such normally ovulating women rarely have ovarian stromal hyper-plasia. A better question would be: Do such women in fact require any form of pituitary suppression at all? We doubt that they do.

So, I favor prescribing 125 mcg Ganirelix, Orgalutron, or Cetrotide (i.e., half the usual dosage) starting on the day that FSHr (Follistim, Gonal F, Puregon) stimulation is initiated, thus intentionally allowing a very small amount of the woman's own LH to enter her blood while preventing a large amount of LH from reaching her circulation. This is because while a small amount of LH is essential to promote and optimize FSH-induced follicular growth and egg maturation, a large concentra-tion of LH can trigger overproduction of ovarian stromal male hor-mones (predominantly testosterone) with an adverse effect on follicle/egg/embryo quality. Moreover, since testosterone also down-regulates estrogen receptors in the endometrium, an excess of testosterone in the pelvic circulation can also have an adverse effect on endometrial growth.

Estrogen "Priming" Protocols

Older women, women who have demonstrated a prior reduced ovar-ian response to COS, and those who by way of significantly raised cycle day 3 FSH and reduced AMH levels are considered likely to be poor responders and are first given GnRH agonist for a number of days to effect pituitary down-regulation. Upon menstruation and confirmation by ultrasound and blood estradiol measurement that adequate ovarian suppression has been achieved, the dosage of GnRH agonist is drasti-cally lowered (or the agonist is replaced with a GnRH antagonist) and the woman is given twice-weekly injections of estradiol for a period of seven to ten days. COS is then initiated using a relatively high dosage of FSH-dominant gonadotropins (such as Follistim, Puregon, or Gonal

F) that is continued along with daily administration of GnRH agonist/ antagonist until the hCG trigger is injected. A recently completed study has demonstrated the efficacy of this protocol and the ability to significantly improve ovarian response to gonadotropins in many hitherto resistant patients.

Agonist/Antagonist Conversion Protocols (A/ACP)

As established above, the use of GnRH antagonists as currently prescribed in ovarian stimulation cycles (i.e., the administration of 250 mcg daily from the sixth or seventh day of stimulation with gonadotropins) may be problematic, especially in women with high LH and overgrowth (hyperplasia) of ovarian stroma.

It is my position that some form of pituitary blockade, either in the form of a GnRH agonist or a GnRH antagonist is an essential component in ovarian stimulation of "poor responders" undergoing IVF. However, GnRH agonists have somewhat of a suppressing effect on ovarian response to gonadotropin stimulation. Thus, switching over from an agonist such as Lupron to an antagonist such as Ganirelix, Orgalutron or Cetrotide at the onset of the Lupron-induced menstrual period (just prior to initiating ovarian stimulation with gonadotropins) could have significant benefits, especially in the treatment of "poor responders."

With the A/ACP, low-dose GnRH antagonist (125 mcg daily) is commenced at the onset of spontaneous menstruation or bleeding that follows initiation of GnRH agonist (e.g., Lupron) therapy using a long-down-regulation protocol arrangement and continuing until the day of the hCG trigger.

There is one potential drawback to the use of the A/ACP: The sustained use of a GnRH antagonist—from the beginning of COS, the stimulation phase of the cycle—appears to compromise the predictive value of serial plasma estradiol measurements as a measure of follicle growth and development. The estradiol levels tend to be much lower in comparison to cases where agonist (Lupron, Buserelin) alone is used or where a "conventional" GnRH antagonist protocol is employed (i.e., antagonist administration is commenced six to eight days following initiation of gonadotropin stimulation). Rather than being due to reduced production of estradiol by the ovary(ies), the lower blood concentration of estradiol seen with prolonged exposure to GnRH antagonist could be the result of a subtle, antagonist-induced altera-tion in the configuration of the estradiol molecule, such that currently available commercial kits used to measure estradiol levels are rendered much less sensitive/specific. Thus when the A/ACP is employed, we rely much more heavily on ultrasound growth of follicles along with observation of the trend in the rise of estradiol levels than on abso-lute estradiol values. Thus I commonly refrain from prescribing the A/ACP in "high responders" who are predisposed to the development of OHSS and accordingly where the accurate measurement of plasma estradiol plays a very important role in the safe management of their stimulation cycles.

It is remarkable that while using the A/ACP + E2V in "poor responders" whose FSH levels were often well above threshold limits, the cycle cancel-lation has consistently been maintained below 10 percent (i.e., much lower than expected). Many of these patients who had previously been told that they should give up on using their own eggs and switch to ovum donation because of "poor ovarian reserve" have subsequently achieved viable preg-nancies at SIRM using the A/ACP with "estrogen priming."

I currently prescribe the A/ACP to most of my IVF patients regard-less of whether they are "normal responders" or "poor responders." Preliminary results suggest a significant improvement in the yield of mature (M2) eggs and egg/embryo quality as well as in implantation and viable IVF pregnancy rates. The A/ACP has, however, proven to be most advantageous in "poor responders" where additional enhancement of ovarian response to gonadotropins may be achieved through incorporation of "estrogen priming." I have reported on the fact that the addition of estradiol for about a week following the ini-tiation of the A/ACP, prior to commencing FSH-dominant gonado-tropin stimulation, appears to further enhance ovarian response, presumably by up-regulating ovarian FSH-receptors. I refer to this as the A/ACP + E2V.

MOVING ON TO EGG RETRIEVAL

The woman who is optimally stimulated through COS will, in my opinion, usually demonstrate a continuing rise or at least maintain a sustained level of blood estradiol while receiving gonadotropins. This would confirm that the follicles and eggs are continuing to develop optimally. It has been demonstrated that a large drop in the blood estradiol level after gonadotropins are discontinued is often associated with poor-quality eggs.

The optimum time for egg retrieval is about 36 hours after the hCG "trigger" injection is administered.

The average number of eggs retrieved varies from program to program, depending on the patient population and the protocol of stimulation. We average between ten and twenty eggs per retrieval attempt (and can usually successfully fertilize about 70 to 80 percent of the mature eggs that we retrieve).

Overcoming the induction-of-ovulation hurdle is particularly significant in IVF. But in IVF, as in other important events in life, things don't always go as planned. Therefore, a reputable IVF program should counsel couples in preparation for the possibility that they may experience a poor stimulation cycle.

However, couples able to negotiate the COS hurdle have a right to be guardedly optimistic about their overall chances of success. This is how one IVF physician encourages his patients and at the same time helps them maintain realistic expectations:

While the level of hormones and the ultrasound findings roughly correlate with the chances of retrieving a large number of eggs, this doesn't always hold true. Sometimes the follicles don't want to give up the eggs, or scar tissue may prevent us from reaching the ovary. And just because we retrieve an egg doesn't mean it will fertilize or that a fertilized egg will produce a "good-quality embryo." If we get a lot of eggs, that's great. I always emphasize that we have had many pregnancies result from the transfer of just one embryo.

6

IVF STEP 3: THE EGG RETRIEVAL

Arrival at Step 3 represents a major accomplishment for IVF candidates because it means that the woman has been optimally prepared, both physically and emotionally, for egg retrieval. Now, for the first time in the treatment cycle, she and her partner have a realistic expectation of conceiving, because the IVF pregnancy rate is usually based on the chance of getting pregnant after undergoing egg retrieval. Their chance of success is now the pregnancy rate quoted by the program they have selected.

The egg retrieval phase exacts the greatest physical, emotional, and financial investment the couple will be expected to make in the entire treatment cycle. From egg retrieval onwards, the financial investment in IVF escalates sharply by the hour, largely because of the costs involved in the egg-retrieval procedure, laboratory fees for fertilization, and the embryo transfer. This outlay is particularly burdensome in the United States, where most couples must assume the entire expense, since few insurance companies will fund these procedures.

THE PRE–EGG RETRIEVAL CONSULTATION

Prior to egg retrieval, the couple should have a refresher consultation with the physician who will actually perform the procedure. They should also meet with the rest of the IVF team that will be involved, including the nurses who will provide postoperative care.

The physician should explain the procedure in detail and describe how the woman might expect to feel afterwards. In addition, the physician should point out that although serious complications are highly unlikely, no one should undergo any kind of surgical procedure with the idea that it is devoid of risk. Although extremely rare, complications may include infection, bleeding, and injury to surrounding structures such as the bowel, bladder, or major blood vessels.

Because women who receive fertility drugs very often have corpus-luteum insufficiency, from the day of egg retrieval onwards many programs administer injections or vaginal suppositories containing progesterone to augment the production of progesterone by the corpus luteum. The physician who does so will probably discuss it with the couple at this point.

A consultation should also take place with the couple's anesthesiologist, who should review the woman's medical history, looking for conditions that could complicate the procedure. In the event that any such factors are detected, the anesthesiologist may call for an electrocardiogram, blood or urine tests, or other appropriate diagnostic measures in order to ensure that the surgery can proceed safely.

Finally, prior to the administration of any medication, the woman and her partner should be asked to decide what to do with the retrieved eggs and the embryos. The physician should reiterate the various scenarios previously discussed during the initial consultation, including a reminder that the more embryos transferred, the higher the pregnancy rate—with the concurrent risk of multiple pregnancy. The couple will usually be expected to issue a directive as to how many eggs they want fertilized, how many embryos (if any) should be frozen, and how many eggs or embryos (if any) may be donated. Finally, both partners will be asked to read and sign an informed-consent form that indicates they understand the egg-retrieval procedure and the risks associated with it.

ULTRASOUND-GUIDED EGG RETRIEVAL

Needle-aspirated egg retrieval under guidance by ultrasound can be performed in a doctor's office or in an outpatient surgery center environment.

Ultrasound-guided egg retrieval should be performed under conscious sedation and/or with the use of paracervical block for pain relief. A paracervical block is a procedure in which local anesthetic is injected on each side of the cervix to numb the nerves surrounding the uterus and cervix. At the same time, local anesthetic is also injected into the upper part of the vagina surrounding the cervix. Some patients prefer to undergo the egg retrieval with the use of paracervical block alone, while the majority will prefer conscious sedation. (It is advisable than an anesthesiologist be present at the time of the egg retrieval.)

During ultrasound-guided egg retrieval, which is done transvaginally, the physician will introduce a long ultrasound probe into the vagina. The probe is the projector that transmits the clearly identifiable image of each ovarian follicle to the ultrasound-viewing monitor. The physician will then pass a sterile needle via a sleeve alongside the probe through the top of the woman's vagina into the ovarian follicles. The physician should be able to accurately direct the needle into each follicle by visualizing its progress on the ultrasound screen.

In the past, after the contents of the follicle were aspirated, the follicle was usually reinflated with a physiological solution in an attempt to flush out any egg that might otherwise have adhered to the wall of the follicle. Since this added a great deal of time to the procedure, it also created the necessity for prolonged conscious sedation. In addition, the injection of fluid through the aspiration needle would often reinject an egg lodged in the bore of the needle back into the follicle, making it far more difficult to aspirate a second time.

We believe that this flushing procedure is redundant in the vast majority of cases. Most important, it seldom improves the chances of harvesting more eggs. The rare exception might be in cases where the woman only has one or two follicles in her ovaries. Under such circumstances, the flushing process might ensure that the few eggs present will all be recovered.

Immediately following the procedure, the woman and her partner are informed as to the number and quality of eggs that have been retrieved. The egg retrieval procedure takes about 20 to 30 minutes, with approximately one hour of postoperative recovery. The woman can usually return to normal activity within a few hours of being discharged. The risk is very low.

OBTAINING A SPERM SPECIMEN TO FERTILIZE THE EGGS

The laboratory will need a semen specimen for insemination or intracytoplasmic sperm injection (ICSO), which occurs a few hours after egg retrieval. Although most men are able to produce a masturbation specimen upon demand, some may be unable to produce a specimen under the stress of the situation. If it is thought that this might happen, a backup specimen could be collected well in advance and frozen in liquid nitrogen or stored temporarily in special media.

The advantage of collecting a specimen a few days prior to egg retrieval is that the woman can assist her partner by creating circumstances in which he is more likely to be successful. In cases where obtaining a specimen by masturbation is difficult or inappropriate for religious or other reasons, the man can use a special condom while having intercourse so the specimen can be retrieved from the condom, or coitus interruptus can be performed.

Although it has been suggested that thawed sperm usually fertilize eggs as well as a fresh specimen would, we have found that a fresh specimen is better, especially in cases of male infertility. We therefore recommend that even if the man has a frozen semen specimen available, he should attempt to produce a fresh specimen around the time when his partner's eggs are to be fertilized.

If the man has very poor sperm quality, it may be necessary for him to produce several daily specimens so they can be concentrated and frozen in case he cannot produce enough on the day of egg retrieval. In such cases it may also be advisable to enhance the quality of the sperm to improve their fertilizing capacity prior to capacitation in the IVF laboratory.

THE LABORATORY'S ROLE IN IVF

The IVF laboratory acts as a temporary womb that supports the delicate gametes and nurtures the newly formed embryos until they are transferred to the woman's uterus.

Examining the egg and its 1st polar body (PB-1)

Even though the egg is the largest cell in the body (about the size of a grain of sand), it is too small to be seen in the follicular flushings without a microscope. However, it is usually embedded in the collection of cells known as cumulus granulos a and collectively termed the cumulus complex. In the mature egg, the appearance of this complex often looks like "rays" radiating outward from its outer envelopment (zona pellucid). Hence the term *corona radiata* (see Chapter 2). The egg and its cumulus complex can often be identified in the follicular fluid with the naked eye. In other cases its detection requires microscope examination.

A mature and fully "competent" mature egg is one that upon fertilization and (the resulting embryo) reaching a receptive uterus is most likely to result in a normal pregnancy. Such an egg will usually have a normal size, be of rounded shape, have a well defined but thinnish zona pellucida and a well defined single PB (PB-1) below its envelopment. Moreover, the cytoplasm should be clear, non-granular light and be free of pools of fluid (vacuoles).

This having been said, it is not possible, using a regular microscope, to reliably and accurately identify a "competent egg." This is because you cannot identify chromosomes this way and it is predominantly the chromosomal integrity of the egg, rather than the sperm, that determines embryo "competence." Most human eggs start off with 46 chromosomes, but within 24–36 hours of the LH surge or an hCG shot the normal egg undergoes chromosomal division (meiosis) with the objective of halving this number to 23. An egg that ends up with more or less than 23 chromosomes is "incompetent." Similarly, a "competent" embryo is one that has 46 chromosomes (the sum of the 23 from the egg and 23 from the mature sperm). An egg or embryo that has more or less than 23 and 46 chromosomes (respectively) is referred to as aneuploid and aneuploid embryos are "incompetent." While egg aneuploidy is the main cause of embryo "incompetence," it is not the only factor. Epigenetic and metabolic factors play a role too (albeit a much lesser one).

Examination of the egg allows for examination of:
1. *Overall appearance:* Its shape, color, size, consistency, the absence of vacuoles, and the thickness of the zona pellucida.
2. *Assessment of the 1st polar body(PB-1):* The presence of a single PB-1 indicates that the egg has gone through initial maturational development (meiosis-1), in an attempt to halve its chromosome number (from 46 to 23) so as to prepare for fertilization. The detection of a single PB-1 thus suggests that such an egg is "mature" (M2). The absence of a PB-1 suggests that the egg is chromosomally "incompetent" (aneuploid) and thus incapable of propagating a competent embryo, while the detection of more than one PB (polyploidy) likewise points to aneuploidy and egg "incompetence."
3. *Full chromosomal analysis (complete karyotyping):* Proudly, because of research largely conducted through SIRM and supported by several publications, we are now able, by performing comparative genomic hybridization (CGH), to fully karyotype both the egg and the embryo. Since the number of chromosomes in PB-1 is a mirror image of the chromosome number within the egg, CGH allows for accurate assessment of egg "competence." We have reported that the transfer of an embryo derived through fertilization of a mature (M2) egg that has a normal chromosome number (i.e., 23) will result in a normal live birth about 70% of the time. While CGH analysis of the eggs potentially has decided advantages when it comes to selective donor-egg banking for female fertility preservation (FP), when it comes to selecting "competent" embryos for transfer, it is by far preferable to fully karyotype the embryo. The reason is that such an evaluation takes the contribution of both the egg and the sperm into consideration.

Nurturing the Eggs and Embryos

When the egg has reached optimal maturity it is placed in a petri dish in a nourishing liquid called an insemination medium. The insemination medium, which contains serum supplements, is a liquid environment that bathes and nourishes the eggs and embryos, just as in nature where the woman's body fluids nurture them in her reproductive tract. Each dish is carefully labeled with the couple's name, number, and perhaps even a colored label to guard against any mix-up.

The insemination medium contains a common household product—baking soda, or sodium bicarbonate—which maintains the acid-alkaline balance (pH) of the medium at the same level as that found in the body. Without sodium bicarbonate the pH level would fluctuate because eggs and embryos, like any other living cells, convert oxygen, water, and food into waste products and excrete them into the surrounding environment. Sodium bicarbonate neutralizes these acidic and alkaline wastes so they do not threaten the well-being of the eggs and embryos.

Because sodium bicarbonate cannot perform this vital function without an adequate supply of carbon dioxide, the eggs and embryos are kept inside an incubator whose air supply contains a constant carbon-dioxide level of 5 percent. Under these conditions the sodium bicarbonate combines with the carbon dioxide to produce the chemical reaction that maintains the proper pH level in the insemination medium.

The embryos remain inside the incubator for the entire time they are in the laboratory, except for brief periods when they are temporarily removed in order to be microscopically examined and graded, changed to a new medium, or prepared for transfer to the uterus.

Sperm Washing and Capacitation

Freshly ejaculated sperm cannot fertilize an egg without undergoing capacitation. In the laboratory, sperm are washed in a special medium to induce capacitation before the insemination of the egg. As explained in Chapter 2, capacitation involves altering the plasma membrane covering the acrosome on the sperm's head, thus releasing enzymes that will be needed for penetration and fertilization of the egg. Natural capacitation is performed by the fluids in the woman's reproductive tract, especially by the cervical mucus. In the laboratory, capacitation is accomplished by washing and then incubating the sperm at 37°C (body temperature) for about an hour.

The male partner's semen specimen can be prepared for insemination in a variety of ways. One way is to wash the semen in medium and process it in a centrifuge to separate the sperm from the seminal fluid. The sperm gravitate to the bottom of the container, and the seminal plasma is poured off and discarded. Additional medium is then added to the sperm, which are re-centrifuged until they again collect at the bottom of the container. At this point the used medium is discarded. New medium is added, and the washed sperm are placed in the incubator to complete the capacitation process.

Sometimes, the sperm are allowed to swim through special columns of fluid that contain a substance called Percoll. The healthiest sperm can in this way be harvested from the bottom of such columns and used for insemination.

Caffeine-like substances are sometimes added to enhance sperm motility—to "wake them up," in effect. And incubation in follicular fluid obtained from one or more of the woman's follicles at the time of egg retrieval or in a special protein medium called test yolk buffer may improve the ability of the sperm to penetrate the egg.

Insemination

During insemination, the embryologist adds a drop or two of the medium containing capacitated sperm to the petri dish containing the egg(s). The egg, now surrounded by about 50,000 swimming sperm (the number contained in just two drops of fluid), is returned to the incubator and left undisturbed until the following morning. Fertilization, the actual entry of the sperm into the egg, normally occurs within the first few hours after insemination. In reputable laboratories, each harvested mature egg has a better than 70 percent chance of fertilization. However, if most or all of them fail to fertilize, one might suspect the existence of a previously undiagnosed fertility problem. This is an example of the dual role—both therapeutic and diagnostic—that IVF fulfills.

INTRACYTOPLASMIC SPERM INJECTION (ICSI)

ICSI involves the direct injection of a single sperm into each egg under direct microscopic vision. The successful performance of ICSI requires a high level of technical expertise. In centers of excellence, when ICSI is employed, the IVF birthrate is unaffected by the presence and severity of male infertility. In fact, even when there is an absence of sperm in the ejaculate such as occurs in cases of congenital absence of the Vas deferens, when a man is born without these major sperm collecting ducts, in cases where the vasa differentia are obstructed (such as following vasectomy or trauma), and in some cases of testicular failure or where the man has impotency, ICSI can be performed with sperm obtained through Testicular Sperm Extraction (TESE), or aspiration (TESA). In such cases, the birthrate is usually no different than when IVF is performed for indications other than male infertility.

The introduction of ICSI has made it possible to fertilize eggs with sperm derived from men with the severest degrees of male infertility and in the process to achieve pregnancy rates as high as, if not higher than that which can be achieved through conventional IVF performed in cases of non-male factor related infertility.

Is ICSI Recommended in All Cases?

The performance of ICSI in cases of "male factor infertility" has been shown to slightly increase the risk of certain embryo chromosome deletions (leading to a slight increase in early miscarriages) as well as the potential for a resulting male offspring to have male infertility in later life; there is no evidence of any significant increase in the incidence of serious birth defects attributable to the ICSI procedure itself. More relevant is the fact that when ICSI is performed for indications other than male infertility there is NO reported increase in the risk of subsequent embryo chromosome deletions, miscarriages, or in the incidence of subsequent male factor infertility in the offspring.

A study was performed some years ago in Sweden, in which 542 children conceived naturally were compared with 941 children conceived through IVF/ ICSI (440 by conventional IVF and 541 by ICSI). The following parameters were assessed at birth and during the first 5 years of life:

1. Birth health and obstetrical complications
2. Birth defects or malformations
3. Family relationships
4. Physical development
5. Mental, psychological, and social development

No major differences in birth weight, growth, total IQ, motor development, and behavior problems or parental stress were found between the children conceived with infertility treatments and those conceived naturally.

About 12–15% of conventional IVF is associated with unanticipated absent or poor fertilization. This has led many to conclude that male infertility may be an "occult phenomenon" in some men. In fact a relatively new test, the sperm chromatin structure assay (SCSA), has demonstrated that DNA damage may be present in sperm from men with both normal and abnormal semen analyses and that male infertility is equally prevalent in such cases. Thus disappointments associated with unanticipated failed fertilization might in some cases be avoided through routine performance of ICSI. There simply does not seem to be any practical downside to this approach, which is now routine throughout the SIRM system.

There is no convincing data suggesting that ICSI should not be performed in all cases of in-vitro conception. In all cases, the routine use of ICSI could potentially bypass most sperm dysfunctions and so eliminate many barriers to fertilization. If in spite of ICSI, using motile sperm, fertilization does not occur, then there is a greater chance of it being due to a severe and intractable genetic egg or sperm factor. The performance of ICSI, since it requires initial removal of the cumulus complex allows evaluation for and examination of PB-1. This allows for evaluation of egg maturity and opens the door to the performance of CGH karyotyping of PB-1 (see above).

MICROSCOPIC EMBRYO GRADING AND GENETIC EMBRYO ASSESSMENT

No other factor in the IVF process influences success as directly as choosing the "right" embryo for transfer to the uterus. This is due mainly to the fact that aneuploidy, an irregular numerical chromosomal configuration of the embryo, is responsible for the majority of IVF failures. Aneuploidy generally results in either: 1) the failure of the embryo to develop to a stage capable of attaching to the uterine wall, 2) miscarriage after implantation, or 3) a chromosomal birth defect such as Down syndrome. The selection of one or more "competent" embryos for transfer is thus central to IVF success.

Unfortunately, most methods currently used to select the best embryos for transfer are relatively inconsistent – yielding on average less than a 20% pregnancy rate per embryo transferred. This fact has in large part been responsible for the tendency to transfer multiple embryos in hope of increasing the prospect of attaining a pregnancy. Unfortunately, such practice has led to IVF being the largest contributor to the explosion that has taken place in the incidence of high-order multiple pregnancies (triplets or greater), which is associated with substantial risks to both the mother and the babies. The methods currently being used to assess and select embryos (for transfer) include:

1. **Microscopic Embryo Grading:** This is by far the commonest method in use. There are numerous systems being applied. Almost all involve a single microscopic evaluation done on day 2, 3, or 5–6 post fertilization and they all lack reliability. In the year 2000, SIRM introduced an improved method for microscopically grading embryos. The method, Graduated Embryo Scoring (GES) employs sequential evaluation (rather than a single day 2 or 3 assessment) of several milestones in embryo development. The method involves scoring out of a total of 100 points. A cumulative GES score of a day 3 (post-fertilization) embryo of 70 or higher in a woman under 35 years of age, suggests that there is at least a high (but age dependent) chance that the embryo will develop into a blastocyst (>30% when the eggs were derived from women under 39 years, and about 5–15% in

women over 43). The chance that such a blastocyst will develop into a clinical pregnancy is about 30% for women under 39, and 10% for women of 42 years and around 5% in women over 43. This having been said, all methods of microscopic embryo grading have one significant limitation in common, and that is that while they can identify those embryos that are most likely to be able to propagate a pregnancy, they are NOT able to identify competent embryos, since chromosomally abnormal embryos are often identical in appearance to those that are normal.

2. **Assisted Hatching:** In selected cases where it is felt that the zona pellucida (the envelopment of the embryo/blastocyst) is unusually tough or thickened, a process known as assisted hatching (AH) may be employed. The process involves deliberately making a small aperture in the wall of the embryo (usually with a laser) so as to promote hatching (rupturing) and thereby facilitate implantation. It remains controversial as to whether AH actually improves pregnancy rates.

3. **Blastocyst Embryo Transfer:** Following fertilization, the cells in an embryo divide progressively over several days until reaching what is known as the blastocyst stage on day 5–6 (only about 40% of embryos make it this far). With very few exceptions, embryos that fail to progress to the blastocyst stage are in fact chromosomally abnormal and therefore "incompetent." By waiting until the blastocyst stage to select and transfer the embryo(s) to the uterus, they are in effect "self-selecting" by culling out many of the abnormal embryos prior to transfer. SIRM data suggests that embryos that fail to develop into good quality (expanded) blastocysts are aneuploid in more than 95% of cases and should probably not be transferred. Moreover, we have demonstrated that embryos that fail to develop into blastocysts in the incubator would rarely (if ever) have propagated a normal pregnancy anyway. Thus the old adage that it is better to transfer an embryo to the "natural environment" of the uterus earlier, than to take the risk that it would not survive

to the blastocyst stage is blatantly erroneous. Accordingly, in my personal IVF practice I strongly advocate preferentially in favor of blastocyst transfers.

4. **PGD Using Fluorescence In-Situ Hybridization (FISH):** This method involves the extraction of a cell from the embryo, followed by a test to evaluate up to 12 of the 23 chromosome pairs in the embryo for abnormalities. Recent attempts at testing all 23 chromosome pairs using this technique have been disappointing. The results seem to lack reliability. FISH, while it is very accurate when it comes to evaluating for gender and has an excellent ability to identify structural abnormalities (e.g., deletions or translocations) in the chromosomes identified, it presently cannot reliably access and account for all 46 (23 pairs) of the embryo's chromosomes (i.e., full embryo karyotyping). Thus presently, even when FISH results are reported as normal, there remains at least a 45% chance that an aneuploidy involving one or more of the remaining (untested) chromosomes might still be present and what is more, this lack of reliability increases with the age of the egg provider.

5. **Comparative Genomic Hybridization (CGH):** This very promising method of egg and embryo selection, introduced into the clinical arena a few years ago by SIRM, has steadily gained traction and popularity. Today numerous IVF programs are using this method to select the most "competent" embryos for transfer. CGH allows identification of all chromosomes, providing a much more complete analysis than does FISH. CGH performed on day 3 or on day 5-6 post-ICSI embryos overcomes the inadequacies of previous methods of embryo selection. A recently published SIRM study demonstrated a pregnancy rate of 60–70% in women who received just one or two blastocysts (day 5–6 post-ICSI) that were derived from embryos biopsied on day 3 post-ICSI and found to be chromosomally normal by CGH testing. Subsequently, others have shown similar results when CGH is performed on several cells removed from a day

5–6 blastocyst. However, whether embryo biopsy is performed on day 3 or day 5-6 embryos, the time needed to perform the CGH requires that the blastocysts be frozen (vitrified, see below) and cryobanked while awaiting the results of such testing. As such, embryo transfer must be delayed for a subsequent cycle when the blastocysts are thawed and transferred into a hormonally prepared uterus. The vitrification process appears not to harm such embryos whose viability and pregnancy generating ability is at least as good as when "fresh" blastocysts are transferred. With CGH, the ultimate goal of "one embryo/one baby" is closer than ever to becoming a reality. CGH-based embryo selection also eliminates the current incentive to transfer multiple embryos at a time in order to improve the chance of success. Embryo selection by CGH holds the potential to decrease the cost per IVF baby and lead to a reduction in overall reproductive health care costs.

6. **PGD Using Polymerase Chain Reaction (PCR):** Using PCR and applying certain gene-specific markers, it is becoming possible to identify an ever increasing number of genetic disorders such as Tay Sachs disease, cystic fibrosis, familial breast cancer, multiple polyposis (which leads to colon cancer), early onset Alzheimer's, etc., in the embryo. By avoiding the transfer of such affected embryos, the disease is prevented from occurring in the offspring.

Note: Since embryo karyotyping (whether by FISH or CGH) has an error rate of about 5–7%, I strongly recommend that Prenatal Genetic Diagnosis, including (but not necessarily limed to) 1st trimester chorionic villus sampling (CVS) and/or 2nd trimester amniocentesis be carried out in all cases where pregnancy occurs following the transfer of such karyotyped embryos.

EMBRYO/BLASTOCYST CRYOPRESERVATION AND
THE INTRODUCTION OF VITRIFICATION

When deciding what to do with the embryos in excess of those that will be transferred to the uterus, the couple undergoing IVF may have chosen cryopreservation.

Cryopreservation of human embryos has been a routine procedure since the early 1980s. Conventional techniques (which are still being widely used by most IVF centers) involve slow freezing, which unfortunately results in ice crystal formation inside the cell(s), damaging them and reducing embryo viability. The relatively recent introduction of ultra-rapid freezing or vitrification changed all this. This innovative technology rapidly freezes the cells (literally within the blink of an eyelid), thereby avoiding intracellular ice from forming and preventing cell damage.

Vitrification involves rapid freezing of embryos and eggs in a tiny amount (less than 0.1 microliters) of a special vitrification solution, before storing them in liquid nitrogen. When compared to the older conventional slow embryo freezing method survival rate for human embryos of about 50–75%, vitrification improves post-thaw (warming) embryo survival to >90%.

It is my personal preference to only cryopreserve blastocysts. This is based upon our reported research, which clearly demonstrates that embryos failing to develop to the blastocyst stage are virtually always chromosomally abnormal (aneuploid) and thus not worthy of keeping, let alone transferring.

While the treating RE recommends when the embryos should be frozen, it is in the final analyses, always up to the patient/couple to make a final decision. I recommend freezing only good quality (Grade 1 or 2) blastocysts (120-144 hours post egg retrieval). Regardless of when the freezing process is done however, I personally advocate that all embryos frozen prior to the blastocyst stage be thawed and then be allowed to develop to the blastocyst stage before being transferred to the uterus. Frozen blastocysts are warmed/thawed and then transferred soon thereafter (a few hours later).

All available evidence suggests that the replacement of warmed/thawed blastocysts does not increase the risk of birth defects.

Vitrification represents a major "paradigm shift" in the field of human ART. Now for the first time, cryopreservation of embryos can be performed with relative impunity. Furthermore, vitrification also provides a much needed "shot in the arm" for the field of human egg banking offering promise of better egg survival rates and subsequent post-warming pregnancy-generating potential. This will undoubtedly hurry on the widespread of egg banking for fertility preservation (FP).

CHAPTER

7

IVF STEP 4: EMBRYO TRANSFER

U ndoubtedly, embryo transfer (ET) is a rate-limiting step in IVF. It takes confidence, dexterity, skill, and a soft touch to do a good transfer. Of all the procedures in ART, this is arguably the most difficult to teach. It is a true art and we have seen many women fail to conceive simply because this procedure was not performed optimally.

Although embryo transfer is the shortest step in an IVF procedure and appears at first glance to be the simplest, it is really the most critical phase of the entire process. Successful clearance of (preceding) hurdles means nothing if there is a bad transfer with bleeding, pain, and/or damage to the embryos. These problems can occur if too much time elapses between removal of the embryos from the incubator and their transfer into the uterus. A problem-free embryo transfer is so important that we even grade transfers in our setting on the basis of comfort, technical difficulty, and elapsed time so the staff can gauge their success. (In this chapter the term *embryo transfer* also refers to the transfer of blastocysts.)

Most embryo transfers are performed 72 to 144 hours after insemination or ICSI, but while the timing depends largely on the progression of the leading embryo(s), it is ultimately the patient's decision to make.

THE PRE-TRANSFER CONSULTATION

The patient's first step on the day of embryo transfer is a conference with the embryologist and the physician, with or without the clinical coordinator. The discussion will include the number and quality of the embryos and their cleavage state. The patient will already have discussed with the physician the number of embryos that should be transferred to the uterus, given the woman's age. Some vacillation over what to do with all the embryos is to be expected up to this point, but now it is time for the couple to come to terms with the aforementioned trade-off—success rate vs. high-order multiple pregnancy—as well as with the disposition of any remaining embryos.

The physician should describe what the couple can expect during the procedure (details vary widely from clinic to clinic). Some programs, particularly those located in hospitals, perform the embryo transfer in an operating room or a special procedure room, after which the woman is wheeled out on a gurney to a holding area until she has been discharged. Other programs prefer to perform the embryo transfer in the room where the woman will remain for an hour or two.

At SIRM we invite the woman's partner to observe the transfer. We believe this facilitates the bonding process.

The physician should explain that the embryos are transferred with a thin catheter threaded through the cervix into the uterus. In programs such as ours, where the depth of the woman's uterus has been determined some days prior to the embryo transfer, the woman should be told that the embryos will be transferred to a specific depth just short of the top of the uterus to avoid injuring the endometrium. The intent here is to avoid any injury that might cause bleeding, which has a detrimental effect on the uterus.

THE EMBRYO TRANSFER

Shortly before the transfer, the embryos are put in a single petri dish containing growth medium. The laboratory staff then informs the clinical coordinator that the embryos are ready for transfer, and the coordinator prepares the patient and informs the physician that a transfer is imminent.

Day 3 (Cleaved Embryo) versus Day 5–6, Blastocyst Transfer (also see Chapter 6)

The presumption has always been that it is better to transfer healthy embryos into the uterus sooner rather than later once the best ones for transfer have been identified. It is against this background that attention has been focused on the transfer of more-developed embryos (blastocyst stage). Since the late 1990s, this process, known as blastocyst transfer, has become increasingly prevalent among IVF programs. The transfer of good-quality blastocysts is associated with a high rate of pregnancy, but it carries with it the risk of multiple pregnancies if more than one is transferred.

Prior to the first cell division, the freshly fertilized pre-embryo displays two pronuclei, one derived from each parent, and which contain the genetic material. From 24 to 30 hours after fertilization (day one), the embryo should have divided into two cells, by day two it should have four cells, and by day three, there should be five to nine cells. Until day three, all the cells are identical. Embryonic development is controlled by maternal genes in the egg until around the eight-cell stage, when the potential for further development comes under the control of the embryo itself. By day five the cells have started to differentiate into specific types, each with a specialized function. The outer cells comprising the trophectoderm (TE) will eventually form the placenta and fetal membranes. Secretions from inner cells collect in a central cavity, called the blastocele, and become the amniotic fluid. Specialized cells on the inner surface of the morula form the inner cell mass (ICM) that eventually develops into the fetus. This complex creation is now called a blastocyst. As the cavity fills with fluid, the blastocyst expands and eventually "hatches" from the zona pellucida. The hatched blastocyst then implants into the endometrium six to seven days after ovulation.

The issue of whether it is better to transfer early cleaved embryos rather than blastocysts continues to rage. Here I wish to focus on the reasons why I strongly favor transferring day 5-6 blastocysts rather than earlier (day 2-3), cleaved embryos.

What we do know for sure (and reported on in 2008) is that cleaved embryos (day 2-4, post-fertilization) that fail to develop into blastocysts are with few exceptions aneuploid and "incompetent." So had such cleaved embryos been transferred they almost certainly would not have developed into blastocysts and would not have propagated a pregnancy anyway. Clearly, there is no validity to the often quoted assertion an embryo would develop better and have a greater chance of propagating a baby by being inside the uterus earlier than it would by being allowed to first develop into a blastocyst in an incubator.

Don't get me wrong! I am not saying that there is no place for doing earlier pre-blastocyst transfers. Indeed, were it possible to determine with confidence, through microscopic grading, which embryos would develop into blastocysts and which would not, then it would not now matter whether such embryos were transferred sooner or later. What we do know is that cleaved day 3 embryos that through karyotyping (CGH) are found through CGH to have a full quota of 46 chromosomes (i.e., are euploid) will in about 90% of cases, develop into expanded blastocysts (regardless of the age of the egg provider). By comparison, even in young women, untested embryos (where it is not known whether the embryo is aneuploid or euploid) have but a fraction of the chance (at best 40%) of developing into blastocysts. While chromosomal integrity of the embryo is not the sole determinant of "competency" (epigenetic and metabolomic factors also play a role), it is certainly the most important variable, by far.

There are strong arguments in favor of blastocysts transfers: By waiting to day 5-6 many unworthy, aneuploid and "incompetent" embryos can be culled out, thereby allowing for the transfer of fewer embryos and minimizing the risk of high-order multiple pregnancies.

Diagnostic advantages include the following:

- Failure of the expected number of cleaved embryos to advance to this stage of development suggests either inherent embryo "incompetence" (which is usually a function of the age of the egg provider, the effect of the "biological clock," and/or may be due to the wrong protocol of ovarian stimulation being applied).

- It facilitates the performance of CGH to identify and then selectively transfer only the most "competent" (euploid) blastocysts. In such cases the transfer of a single blastocyst (SBT) should yield upward of a 60% baby rate provided there is no underlying uterine implantation dysfunction.

Of course, after all that IVF patients go through, it is much easier and far less stressful on the treating IVF physician not to have to confront patients with there being no surviving embryos available to transfer. Undoubtedly, this is one of the main reasons why many IVF practitioners still prefer to transfer cleaved embryos rather than blastocysts. But as far as I am concerned, this is no justification to do what ultimately might not be in the patients' best interest. Rather, it is about doing what serves patients best and what they choose after being fully informed regarding associated risks and benefits.

Ultrasound-Guided Embryo Transfer—A Must!

Today all embryo transfers should be performed under direct ultrasound guidance to ensure proper placement in the uterine cavity. This practice, properly conducted, will significantly enhance embryo implantation and pregnancy rates.

We prefer to perform all embryo transfers when the woman has a full bladder. This facilitates visualization of the uterus by abdominal ultrasound and triggers a reflex nerve response that relaxes the wall of the uterus, reducing the likelihood of contractions occurring that could expel the embryo(s). The patient is allowed to empty her bladder 10–15 minutes following the embryo transfer.

It is important that the woman be as relaxed as possible during the embryo transfer because hormones, such as adrenaline, that are released during times of stress can cause the uterus to contract. Accordingly, we offer the woman undergoing IVF in our program 5 mg of oral diazepam (Valium) about a half hour prior to the embryo transfer to relax her and reduce apprehension. Some IVF programs believe that imagery helps the woman relax and feel positive about the experience, thereby reducing the stress level. In such a program a counselor and/or clinical coordinator may help the woman focus on visual imagery for a few minutes immediately prior to embryo transfer so as to enhance her relaxation. As one clinical coordinator explained, couples may select a variety of creative images to visualize during embryo transfer:

> *I encourage patients to visualize the uterus and the embryo growing within it. Some people imagine little embryos with suction cups on their feet—one woman imagined embryos with Velcro-covered feet. Some like to visualize a white light coating the baby or a peaceful blue halo surrounding the embryo, or a baby blanket giving the baby a hug, or little soldiers marching into the uterus and digging foxholes in the endometrium. No matter what our counselor or I suggest, the best visualization is what the woman thinks up for herself.*
>
> *And I'm continually amazed at some of the lucky charms people bring along to the transfer. I have seen them bring drawings and paintings of babies. Some patients wear fertility charms, such as frogs or African face-mask pendants. Some listen to positive-reinforcement tapes. Women have told me they have worn their lucky dresses. You can't help getting caught up in this process.*

When the woman is sufficiently relaxed, she is helped into the appropriate position and made as comfortable as possible. (In programs that rely on relaxation therapy, a counselor or nurse is usually present at the woman's bedside, coaching her in relaxation exercises during the procedure.)

The physician first inserts a speculum into the vagina to expose the cervix and then may clean the cervix with a solution to remove any mucus or other secretions. An abdominal ultrasound transducer is placed on the lower abdomen, and the uterus is clearly visualized. The physician then informs the embryology laboratory that the transfer is imminent and awaits the arrival of the transfer catheter loaded with the embryos.

The physician gently introduces the catheter through the woman's cervix into the uterine cavity under ultrasound guidance. When the catheter is in place, the embryologist carefully injects the embryos into the uterus, and the physician slowly withdraws the catheter. The catheter is immediately returned to the laboratory, where it is examined under the microscope to make sure that all the embryos have been deposited. Any residual embryos would be re-incubated, and the transfer process would usually be repeated to deliver the remaining embryos.

An embryo-transfer procedure usually takes only a few minutes from start to finish, although it naturally takes longer if the embryos must be re-incubated prior to a second or third transfer attempt.

In rare situations where it is determined that it would be highly traumatic to pass the catheter through the cervix, the physician might then elect to perform a transmyometrial embryo transfer. In this procedure, with the patient under general anesthesia, the physician, using a vaginal ultrasound probe, introduces a relatively wide-bore needle transvaginally through the wall of the uterus into the uterine cavity. The catheter containing the embryos is passed through this needle into the uterus, the embryos are delivered into the uterine cavity, and the needle and catheter are withdrawn.

Post-Embryo Transfer Management

Immediately prior to being discharged following the embryo transfer procedure, an exit interview is conducted, whereby the patient/couple is given directions. Hormonal supplementation usually involves the administration of intramuscular, oral, or transvaginal injections of progesterone and/or vaginal suppositories (comprising estradiol valerate and micronized progesterone) until a blood pregnancy test is performed approximately eight days later (the chemical diagnosis of pregnancy). In selected cases, such progesterone treatment can be replaced with Crinone or Endometrin vaginal applications, once or twice daily. If the pregnancy test is negative or the plasma hCG levels fail to rise appropriately in the ensuing days, all hormonal support is abruptly discontinued.

A positive pregnancy test, followed by an appropriate rise in the plasma hCG concentration, is usually an indication to discontinue daily progesterone injections in favor of three times weekly intramuscular injections of hCG 5000 IU, along with daily vaginal estradiol and progesterone suppositories until the 8th week of pregnancy. In patients who experience an exaggerated response to ovarian stimulation with gonadotropins, hCG administration is withheld (for fear of increasing the risk of severe ovarian hyperstimulation), and intramuscular progesterone injections are continued along with vaginal estradiol and progesterone suppositories until the 8th week of pregnancy. Following an appropriate rise in hCG concentrations, heparinoid (heparin, Lovenox, Clexane) and corticosteroid (dexamethasone, prednisolone, prednisone) are continued until the 10th week of pregnancy. Thereupon, the heparinoid is abruptly stopped and the corticosteroid it is tapered down and stopped within a week or so. An ultrasound examination is performed approximately 2-3 weeks after the chemical diagnosis of pregnancy, at which time, designated patients with viable pregnancies receive a final administration of Intralipid. (In some cases additional monthly doses of Intralipid must be administered.)

Embryo (Freezing) Cryopreservation

There have been dramatic advances in the technology of freezing and storing human embryos for future use. We cryopreserve (freeze) embryos as blastocysts. The recent introduction of "ultra-rapid freezing" (vitrification) which so rapidly freezes the embryo that it avoids ice formation in the blastomeres has revolutionized embryo freezing. Now, very few chromosomally normal embryos are lost in the freeze/thaw process and pregnancy rates with thawed pre-vitrified blastocysts are hardly different from those reported following the transfer of fresh blastocysts. In fact recent research suggests that the transfer of pre-vitrified/warmed blastocysts might even yield higher implantation/pregnancy rates than would be the case following the transfer of "fresh blastocysts."

The Frozen Embryo Transfer (FET)

The following represents my personal approach to conducting FETs: The recipient's cycle is initiated with a BCP, which is later overlapped with Lupron daily for 5-6 days. Thereupon the BCP is withdrawn and daily Lupron injections are continued until the onset of menstruation, when the Lupron dosage is administered in a reduced dosage and intramuscular estradiol valerate (Delestrogen/E2V) is administered every 3 days. The objective is to achieve and sustain an optimal plasma E2 concentration of 500pg/ml-1000pg/ml to generate a 9mm endometrial lining as assessed by ultrasound examination. Daily, vaginal Viagra is used in cases of an inadequate endometrial lining and is discontinued with the initiation of progesterone therapy. Intramuscular and/or intravaginal progesterone is administered daily starting about 6 days prior to the FET and continued along with twice weekly Delestrogen IM until the 10th week of pregnancy or until pregnancy is discounted.

At SIRM, oral daily dexamethasone commences with Lupron start and continues until a negative pregnancy test or until the completion of the 8th week of pregnancy whereupon it is tailed off over a week or two and then discontinued. Oral folic acid is taken daily commencing with the first estradiol valerate injection, and is continued throughout gestation. The recipient also receives prophylactic oral antibiotics starting with the initiation of Progesterone therapy, until the day after ET. Usually we would warm/thaw vitrified blastocysts with the objective of having 2 or3 for transfer.

Commencing on the day following the ET, the patient inserts a vaginal progesterone suppository daily and this is continued until the completion of the 8th week of pregnancy or until pregnancy is discounted. Selective immunotherapy (heparin and/or IVIg) is otherwise administered when indicated as with conventional SIRM-IVF patients.

For blastocyst FETs, the blood pregnancy tests are performed 13 days and 15 days after the first progesterone administration is commenced. Contingent upon positive blood pregnancy tests, and subsequently upon the ultrasound confirmation of a viable pregnancy, administration of IM progesterone and/or Crinone 8% and twice weekly Estradiol Valerate (E2V) are resumed and continued until the completion of the 10th week of pregnancy or until a pregnancy is ruled out.

Note: As an alternative regimen for women who cannot tolerate intramuscular Progesterone PIO, we prescribe one (1) vaginal application of Crinone 8% administered on the 1st day (referred to as luteal phase day 0–LP-0). From the next day, (LP-1) Crinone 8% is used twice daily (AM and PM) until the day of embryo transfer. Crinone 8% is withheld on the morning of the embryo transfer and is thereupon resumed straight after the FET.

After the Transfer

The woman's partner or another companion is expected to remain with her for emotional support and otherwise tend to her needs for the one hour she remains recumbent.

What the woman should expect to experience physically after embryo transfer is another important issue the physician would have discussed with the couple so they do not become unnecessarily concerned that the transfer has failed. For example, it is not unusual for the woman to experience minor lower-abdominal pain or a slight discharge after the transfer. This discharge may merely be due to the emission of fluid retained in the vagina as a consequence of cleaning the cervix in preparation for embryo transfer.

THE EXIT INTERVIEW

The exit procedure varies from program to program, but every couple is entitled to an exit interview prior to leaving the IVF clinic. An exit interview prepares and reassures couples for their return home and also provides valuable feedback to the IVF program. During the exit interview, the couple and the physician and/or clinical coordinator discuss follow-up care, including permissible daily activity, work, travel, and when the couple can resume sexual intercourse. The woman would be advised at this time whether the program recommends hormone supplementation until the pregnancy test confirms or rules out successful IVF. Some programs telephone patients after they have returned home to inquire about their emotional stability and physical well-being. The staff of such programs would likely emphasize that whether or not the procedure has been successful, they would still like to maintain contact with the couple and would be available for consultation at all times.

FOLLOW-UP AFTER THE EMBRYO TRANSFER

The Quantitative Beta hCG Blood Pregnancy Test

About 11 days after the egg retrieval, the woman should have a quantitative beta hCG blood pregnancy test, which can diagnose pregnancy even before she has missed a period. It does so by determining the presence of the hormone hCG, which is produced in minute amounts by the implanting embryo. If hCG is detected, the test is usually repeated two days later in order to see if there has been an appreciable rise in hCG since the first test. (We usually recommend that these blood samples be drawn 11 and 13 days following the egg retrieval.) A doubling of the initial value usually suggests that an embryo is implanting and is a good indication of a possible pregnancy. The laboratory then notifies the IVF clinic of the test results.

Because an IVF program usually cooperates closely with the referring physician, it is customary for the clinic staff to call the referring physician with the results of the pregnancy test and ask the physician to notify the couple. Thereupon, the clinic staff may also contact the couple. Obviously, if the couple had selected the clinic themselves rather than on referral, the staff would call them directly with the test results.

Sometimes the physician or clinical coordinator will work through the referring physician to arrange for the pregnancy tests, and the program may also forward a detailed report about the entire procedure to the referring physician. If the couple wishes to make their own arrangements, the program should give them detailed instructions about the necessary tests.

Hormonal Support of a Possible Pregnancy: Progesterone vs. hCG Supplementation

If the two blood-pregnancy tests indicate that one or more embryos are implanting, some programs advocate daily injections of progesterone or the use of vaginal hormone suppositories for several weeks to support the implanting embryo(s). In cases following COS-IVF cycles or natural IVF, some prefer to give hCG injections three times a week for several weeks until the pregnancy can be identified by ultrasound. A relatively small number of IVF programs do not prescribe any hormones at all after the transfer.

This is by no means a clear-cut issue. Just as ovulation occurs following the spontaneous LH surge and/or the administration of gonadotropins following COS, resulting in a corpus luteum that produces both progesterone and estrogen, a similar but exaggerated response follows IVF, where COS with hCG-induced ovulation results in the formation of numerous corpora lutea. The greater the original number of mature follicles, the greater the progesterone/estrogen production is likely to be. Since ovarian stimulation in women who have abnormal or no ovulation patterns at all (e.g., cases of PCOS) tends to result in the growth of many more follicles than when performed in normally ovulating women, it follows that such women also tend to develop many more corpora lutea and accordingly have exaggerated progesterone/estrogen blood concentrations.

The hCG injection following embryo transfer exerts a protracted influence on ovarian progesterone/estrogen production that is sustained for at least one week. A few days later, provided that embryo implantation takes place, the early trophoblast (root system of the conceptus, which subsequently develops into the placenta) begins to produce its own progesterone/estrogen, as well as hCG, in ever-increasing amounts.

There is compelling evidence to show that hCG promotes the release of corpus luteum progesterone following ovulation as well as trophoblastic growth and development following embryo transfer; therefore, hCG enhances both progesterone and estrogen production while simultaneously promoting further hCG as well as progesterone/estrogen production by the trophoblast. As such, hCG might be considered a self-propagating hormone.

When hCG is administered following embryo transfer, the dosage is 5000 units by injection three times weekly beginning after early biochemical confirmation that implantation is taking place; hCG (whether self-produced or administered by injection) enhances the propagation and release of both ovarian and trophoblastic progesterone, which promotes further development of the uterine endometrial lining, trophoblastic growth, uterine relaxation, and adaptation of the reproductive immune response.

The trophoblast produces progesterone/estrogen in ever-increasing amounts so that by the eighth to ninth week of pregnancy it replaces the ovaries as the dominant source of production. Thus, there is probably little benefit through either hCG or progesterone administration after the completion of the 10th week of pregnancy. It follows that a low progesterone blood level is much more likely to be the consequence rather than cause of a failing pregnancy. This is the reason why many authorities believe that progesterone supplementation in such cases will not rescue a failing pregnancy.

Even the most adamant supporters of hCG supplementation recognize that its administration in some cases could bear risk. One such example is when, following COS with gonadotropins, the woman inadvertently becomes severely hyper-stimulated, placing her at risk of developing life-endangering complications associated with severe ovarian hyperstimulation syndrome (OHSS). In such cases, the administration of additional hCG often exacerbates the condition, thus increasing risk. We would prefer to administer progesterone in such cases although it is questionable whether there is any clinical benefit in doing so. A situation where progesterone rather than hCG clearly should be given is where the woman is an embryo recipient (e.g., ovum donation, embryo adoption, gestational surrogacy, or frozen-embryo transfer). In such cases, ovarian hormonal activity is dormant, and any attempt to promote progesterone/estrogen production would be fruitless.

Once reliance upon the corpus luteum to sustain the pregnancy completely transforms into total self-maintenance of the pregnancy by the placental trophoblast, supplementation with either progesterone or hCG is probably of limited, if any, benefit to the maintenance of the pregnancy. This is why after the completion of the eighth week of pregnancy, supplemental hormonal therapy is slowly tailed off and stopped altogether.

Women undergoing third-party parenting through IVF surrogacy or ovum donation will usually receive estrogen and progesterone injections, often in conjunction with vaginal hormone suppositories, for eight to ten weeks following the diagnosis of implantation by blood-pregnancy testing.

We believe it could, in special circumstances, be beneficial to administer hCG prior to performing the beta hCG test for pregnancy diagnosis in order to provide better support for the possible pregnancy. This has been practiced selectively in our setting as well as in other IVF programs, and the results are encouraging. The problem with this approach is that administration of hCG prior to the test delays the ability to diagnose pregnancy because hCG is the very hormone that is measured to see if the woman is pregnant.

Confirming a Pregnancy by Ultrasound Examination

Although a positive beta hCG blood-pregnancy test indicates the possibility of a conception, pregnancy cannot be confirmed until it can be defined by ultrasound (see Chapter 11 for a discussion of the various definitions of pregnancy). Two to three weeks after embryo transfer, ultrasound can confirm that a pregnancy exists, that it is viable through detection of a heartbeat, and that it is not ectopic.

What to Do If Spotting Occurs

The woman may experience a minimal degree of spotting (vaginal bleeding) after IVF, whether or not she is pregnant. If spotting occurs, she should call her physician immediately and rest in bed. Spotting can be caused by a variety of factors: (1) One of the embryos could be burrowing into the endometrium, (2) one could be attaching while another is detaching, (3) the menstrual period may have begun, or (4) the woman may have an ectopic pregnancy. Although there is no way of knowing in the very early stages exactly what is causing the spotting, certain tests can help isolate the problem.

Some women who spot after a positive pregnancy test are undergoing a spontaneous reduction of a multiple pregnancy. For example, many IVF as well as natural pregnancies start off as twins or even triplets and then spontaneously reduce themselves to a singleton or twin pregnancy. Painless bleeding might occur in the process, which could be falsely construed as an indication that the pregnancy is about to be lost.

All women should take the beta hCG pregnancy test after IVF no matter how much they bleed. As one nurse-practitioner explained:

We had one patient who took her first pregnancy test, but since it was low she didn't take the second one. She kept spotting and spotting, and then went back to her aerobics—three hours every day. After about four weeks I called her up and asked how things were going. She said she had never really had her period and was having these pregnancy symptoms. . . . It turned out that she had conceived in spite of everything!

Women who do not get pregnant and want to make another attempt at IVF should wait until they have had at least one full unstimulated menstrual cycle in order to prepare themselves emotionally and give their ovaries a rest before the next procedure.

When an IVF pregnancy has been confirmed by symptoms and by ultrasound examinations, the woman should seek prenatal care as soon as possible. Thereafter, an IVF pregnancy can be expected to progress no differently from any normally conceived pregnancy given the woman's health, age, and related conditions.

CHAPTER

8

THE FIVE ULTIMATUMS FOR SUCCESSFUL IVF CANDIDATES

Years ago, if a woman was pregnant over the age of 35, she was often considered to be at high risk for childbirth. Not only was it almost unthinkable that a woman over 40 would have a baby, it was strongly discouraged. Now many women in their forties and even in their fifties are having babies, often through the use of donated eggs. The point to be emphasized is that in order to get good success rates with IVF, it is important to eliminate as many as possible of the variables that might impact adversely on outcome before actually undertaking the IVF process itself. This chapter discusses these variables—which we refer to as "The Five Ultimatums":

1. Quality of the Woman's Eggs: The First Ultimatum
2. Quality of the Man's Sperm: The Second Ultimatum
3. Quality of the Embryo: The Third Ultimatum
4. Receptivity of the Uterus: The Fourth Ultimatum
5. Quality of the Embryo Transfer: The Fifth Ultimatum

In this chapter we will describe these ultimatums and explain how they may impact a couple's fertility. In Chapter 9 we will describe the diseases that can impact fertility and in Chapter 10 we will discuss tests that might be administered to both partners to determine the scope of their infertility. Chapter 10 suggests how a couple can use this knowledge to help determine what they can reasonably expect from IVF.

QUALITY OF THE WOMAN'S EGGS: THE FIRST ULTIMATUM

The Influence of Age on Egg Quality

Age is one of the most powerful variables to impact the five ultimatums, as well as other factors leading to a successful pregnancy. In fact, all forms of ART, including IVF, are associated with a reduced pregnancy rate in women over 40. Moreover, the cost of treatment is likely to be greater for older women because they often require more IVF cycles before there is likely to be a successful outcome. Infertile couples in which the woman is 40 or over must often overcome two hurdles when they seek fertility treatment: (1) desperation brought about by the realization that time is running out and (2) IVF programs that turn away women over a certain age. Advancing age associated with a progressive decline in a woman's natural fertility understandably induces an overwhelming sense of urgency to achieve a healthy pregnancy before time runs out. Less reasonable is the practice by some programs of turning away older women because their anticipated lower pregnancy rates could decrease the program's overall statistics so dramatically. Fertility drugs might only help a woman produce a greater number of eggs, not necessarily improve their quality. Thus, egg quality is a limiting parameter that must be met if the woman is to conceive. However, we do not believe in assigning arbitrary limits, such as an age-cutoff point beyond which we will not accept IVF candidates. We believe it is far more effective to enable each woman to estimate the probability of conceiving based on how the factors that impact fertility apply to her.

After the very onset of a woman's menstruation (i.e., the menarche), eggs are used up monthly until the number remaining in the woman's ovaries falls below a certain critical threshold, at which time ovarian function starts to decline and the woman becomes relatively resistant to ovarian stimulation with fertility drugs. This phase of the woman's reproductive life, the climacteric, is heralded by gradually increasing blood concentrations of FSH and a decline in Inhibin B levels. The climacteric continues for six to eight years until virtually all remaining eggs have been used up, at which time ovulation and menstruation cease altogether, and the woman has reached menopause.

The timing of the onset of the climacteric varies from person to person. Genetic factors, exposure to environmental toxins and radiation, disease, drugs, and pelvic disease associated with severe periovarian adhesions that compromise blood flow to the ovaries can all influence timing of the onset of both the climacteric and menopause. Most American women will enter the climacteric in their early to mid-40s and go into menopause around ages 45 to 55.

Reduced egg quality is directly related to the woman's age. In contrast, reduced ovarian response to fertility drugs results from progressively declining ovarian function. As a woman advances beyond 30, each mature egg becomes progressively less likely to be "normal." In other words, with every advancing year fertilization is more likely to produce embryos that have an abnormal chromosome number (aneuploid). By age 35 approximately two in three embryos are likely to be aneuploid, while at 40 aneuploidy affects about 70-80 percent of the embryos. At age 42 approximately 80-90 percent of embryos are so affected, and at 45 the incidence of aneuploidy could be as high as 95 percent. Interestingly, in the absence of sperm dysfunction more than 80% of most embryo aneuploidy stems from chromosomal abnormalities originating in the egg. It is almost as if when surrounded by predominantly normal sperm, an egg has the ability to select the best one to be fertilized by. However in cases of male infertility where the egg is surrounded by a high percentage of aneuploid sperm, it might inadvertently select an aneuploid sperm. That is why in cases of severe sperm dysfunction the sperm can play an ever increasing role in determining the "competence" of an embryo.

Since it is nature's intent to protect the integrity of the species through natural selection, abnormal embryos usually will fail to implant into the uterine lining or will be rejected in the first three months of pregnancy as a miscarriage. (In the case of failed implantation, the woman would probably not even be aware that she was actually pregnant for a very brief time.) Infrequently, nature will make a mistake and allow a chromosomally defective fetus to continue on to delivery, resulting in conditions such as Down syndrome (Trisomy 21).

The negative effect of advancing age on egg quality not only explains why there is a gradual increase in the incidence of infertility, miscarriage, and chromosomal birth defects, it also illustrates why treatment of infertility, regardless of the chosen method, becomes progressively less successful with advancing maternal age.

The only way to optimize IVF birthrates while avoiding high-order multiple pregnancies in both younger and older women is to select two or less "competent" embryos for ET (see full karyotyping by CGH—see Chapter 8).

For women whose advancing age and/or ovarian resistance makes having a baby with their own eggs unappealing or unlikely, ovum donation (using donated eggs from a young donor, usually compatible and anonymous) is a highly successful option.

Approach to Ovarian Stimulation (Chapter 6)

As explained in chapter 5, the induction of ovulation with LH or hCG should be conducted against the backdrop of optimal follicle and egg development, and must occur at precisely the right time in order for the egg to achieve optimal maturation. Otherwise, the egg will be dysmature and unlikely to develop into a viable embryo capable of initiating a healthy implantation and pregnancy.

It is often claimed that women who develop ovarian hyperstimulation syndrome (OHS) inherently have poor egg quality. This is not necessarily the case. The fact is that such women, many of whom have PCOS (see Chapter 5), have an inherent tendency to overproduce ovarian testosterone, placing them at increased risk of having poor-quality eggs. The tendency to prescribe high doses of LH-containing gonadotropins in such cases and to administer hCG prematurely in the hope of arresting further follicle growth and development so as to reduce the risk of OHSS often leads to poor egg development. The remedy is to allow the required time for optimal egg development to take place before giving hCG. The method whereby this is achieved can best be through prolonged coasting (see Chapter 5).

IVF May Be the Only Way to Identify Inhibiting Factors in Eggs

While the chromosomal integrity of the egg is far and away the most important determinant of egg and (subsequently) embryo "competency" it is by no means the only factor. Metabolic and epigenetic factors can also play a role. In fact, unexplained infertility is caused in many cases by some physical-chemical, biochemical, or immunological factors within the eggs that prevent the sperm from undergoing the acrosome reaction (being attracted to and then penetrating the zona pellucida). One way to determine whether such inhibiting factors might exist is by observing the interaction of eggs and sperm in the petri dish during IVF.

Expertise of the Embryology Team

It is sad yet true that when confronted with poor-quality eggs there is a tendency to lay the blame on the most convenient scapegoat, namely the embryologist(s). But in fact, poor embryology (deficient expertise, methodology, and technique) is rarely the cause of poor embryo quality and/or failed IVF. And most embryologists are much more disciplined and experienced in proven methodologies than are physicians.

QUALITY OF THE MAN'S SPERM: THE SECOND ULTIMATUM

Sperm Chromosome Structure Assay (SCSA)

The standard sperm analysis, which measures sperm count, motility and morphology, has been around for more than one hundred years. The only difference is that, rather than counting sperm on a grid ("Coulter counter") or under a microscope and then assessing sperm movement and progression from one point to another (motility) and determining sperm appearance (morphology), today we rely on the computer to much more accurately and reliably define these parameters for us. But what has not changed is that while (regardless of how it is performed) an overtly abnormal sperm analysis indeed allows for the diagnosis of male infertility, intermediate values are often difficult to interpret. And what makes matters even worse is the fact that some men with perfectly normal standard sperm parameters are nevertheless infertile.

The introduction of the Sperm Chromatin Structure Assay (SCSA), which measures sperm nuclear integrity, when interpreted in association with standard sperm parameters (count, motility, and morphology), has vastly improved the ability to accurately evaluate male fertility. And when it comes to A.R.T., SCSA results have been found to correlate well with the potential of sperm from a given male, upon fertilizing an egg, to propagate embryos that would be "competent" to produce a live birth. As such the introduction of these tests into the IVF arena represents an important advance.

This having been said, it is important to know that SCSA data will not always correlate well with standard sperm parameters (count, motility and morphology). In most (but certainly not all) cases of overtly abnormal sperm parameters, the SCSA results will be abnormal, and in some cases, overtly abnormal SCSA results will be encountered in cases where the standard sperm analysis is normal.

What is true is that the SCSA is a measure of sperm DNA damage and does predict male sub/infertility and poor reproductive performance. The SCSA measures the degree of abnormalities in the genetic material of the sperm, expressing it numerically as the DNA Fragmentation Index (DFI). It is true that varying degrees of DNA damage may be present in sperm from both fertile and infertile men. However a quantitative expression of the DFI often will reveal a hidden abnormality of sperm DNA and as such unveil infertility in cases where prior standard sperm parameters failed to reveal underlying male infertility. Optimal sperm chromatin packaging seems necessary for full expression of male fertility potential. SCSA emerges as a predictor of the probability to conceive and carry the pregnancy to viability.

Since an abnormal SCSA assay is more likely to occur in cases of abnormal standard semen parameters, it is ideally suited to assessing the fertility potential and predicting embryo development as well as effects of reproductive toxicants. Since SCSA parameters are independent of conventional semen parameters, results may allow physicians to identify those cases of male infertility where the performance of IVF and intracytoplasmic sperm injection (ICSI) would be less likely to result in "competent" embryos that are likely to propagate normal babies.

Certain cancer treatments involving chemotherapy and radiation therapy are known to adversely affect male fertility. In such cases, a reduction of sperm output may arise from cytotoxic effects upon the sperm-producing cells in the testicles. However, even if these cells survive such cancer therapy there remains a risk to reproduction that could express in a variety of forms of reproductive dysfunction ranging from infertility to miscarriage. Such risk could theoretically even be transgenerational (i.e., expressed in the sperm or eggs of the offspring of patients so treated).

Current information on the clinical role of the SCSA testing in patients undergoing IVF suggests the following:

1. The IVF birthrate could be as much as 2 times lower in women under 33 years of age whose husbands have patently abnormal SDI assays (with a DFI of >30%). Results seem to become progressively worse with advancing maternal age such that at 35 years+, the viable pregnancy rate could be as much as 2-3 times lower.

2. Although it is possible for abnormal SCSA results to sometimes spontaneously revert back to normal, this probably occurs quite infrequently.

3. Although abnormal SCSA results are detected in men with apparently normal semen analyses, abnormal results are more commonly seen in cases of men who have abnormal sperm parameters (abnormal sperm count, motility and/or morphology).

4. Abnormal SCSA augers poorly for the outcome of fertility treatments in general and for IVF/ICSI in specific. In the latter cases, fertilization and pregnancy rates are reduced and the chance of early pregnancy loss appears to be increased. However it

is important to stress that an abnormal SCSA result does not preclude a successful pregnancy. In fact we have seen many IVF pregnancies occur in spite of abnormal SCSA results . . . even when the DFI was elevated above 60%.

5. The likelihood of a successful outcome with IVF/ICSI in cases where the SCSA is abnormal worsens progressively as the age of the egg provider advances beyond 35 years.

6. While abnormal SCSA results rarely revert spontaneously to normal this can and does happen on occasion, especially following surgical or interventional radiological treatment of varicoceles (a collection of distended veins surrounding one or both testicles in the scrotum). In addition, there is some suggestion that the use antioxidant/vitamin blends such as "ProXeed" or "Proceptin" (my preference) if taken for 8-12 weeks (the sperm life cycle) will sometimes improve the SCSA.

Sperm Antibodies

The presence of sperm antibodies reduces male fertility significantly, but does not usually prevent conception altogether. Rather, the effects are graduated; i.e., the larger the immunologic response (concentration of antibodies), the less likely it is that a pregnancy will occur, and when the blood level rises above 40%, natural conception is highly unlikely to occur.

Like any other kind of antibody manufactured by the body, sperm antibodies are formed in response to antigens. These antigens are proteins, which appear on the outer sperm membranes as the young sperm cells develop within the male testes. In the man's own body, his sperm are regarded as foreign invading proteins and as such would normally be targeted for attack. However, under normal conditions, direct contact between the man's blood and sperm is prevented by a cellular structure in the testes called the blood–testis barrier. This barrier is formed by so-called Sertoli cells, which abut very closely against each other, forming tight junctions that separate the developing sperm cells from the blood and prevent immunologic stimulation. However, the blood–testis barrier can be broken by physical or chemical injury or by infection. When this barrier is breached, sperm antigens escape from their immunologically protected environment and come in direct contact with blood elements that launch an immunologic attack.

Once sperm and blood come in contact, whether in the male or female, specific antibodies are produced against them by specialized blood cells call T- and B-lymphocytes. The three main types of sperm antibodies produced are Immunoglobulin G (IgG), Immunoglobulin A (IgA), and Immunoglobulin M (IgM). These antibodies bind to the proteins (antigens) on the sperm head, midpiece, or tail. The antibodies formed may be of the circulatory type (in the blood serum) or secretory type (in the tissue). This is important because high levels of antibodies in the blood serum do not invariably mean that the antibodies will find their way to the semen where they can affect the sperm. For example, the concentration of IgG is much lower in secretions of the reproductive tract than it is in the blood. Conversely, the local level of IgA is higher in the reproductive secretions than in the blood. This is an important point, which we will return to later.

Once sperm antibodies have formed, they can affect sperm in several different ways. Some antibodies will cause sperm to stick together or agglutinate. Agglutinated sperm clump together in dense masses and thus are unable to migrate through the cervix into the uterus. Other antibodies mark the sperm for attack by natural killer (NK) cells of the body's immune system (i.e., opsonizing antibodies). Some antibodies cause reactions between the sperm membrane and the cervical mucus, preventing the sperm from swimming through the cervix (i.e., immobilizing antibodies). Antibodies can also block the sperm's ability to bind to the zona pellucida of the egg, a prerequisite for fertilization (i.e., blocking antibodies). Finally, there is recent evidence that the fertilized egg shares some of the same antigens that are found on the sperm. It is possible that sperm antibodies present in the mother can react with the early embryo, resulting in its destruction by phagocyte (i.e., phagocytic antibodies) cells.

There are a number of diagnostic tests available to detect the presence of sperm antibodies. These are performed by flow cytometry and the ELISA (enzyme-linked immunoabsorbent assay), the Franklin-Dukes sperm agglutination assay or the Immunobead Binding Test (IBT), to name a few. At SIRM, the indirect Immunobead Binding Test (IBT) is used to detect antibodies present in the blood serum, in cervical mucus or on the sperm surface.

In the male, IgA and IgG are found in the semen although there is controversy as to whether they originate locally (secreted by testicular cells) or cross over from the circulation. Antibodies of the IgM class are not found in semen.

Like the source of some antibodies, the question of the critical levels of sperm antibodies is also hotly debated among clinicians. There seems to be general agreement that blood levels above 30% by the IBT are associated with significant fertility problems.

Studies have shown that pregnancy is highly unlikely following natural intercourse or intrauterine insemination when either the woman or the man harbors significant antisperm antibodies.

While there have been isolated reports that administration of corticosteroids (e.g., dexamethasone, prednisone) will temporarily suppress antibody production, pregnancy rates are poor. Besides, corticosteroid therapy carries with it the risk of significant side effects, some of which (although infrequent) can be serious. As an example, in the man spontaneous fractures (especially of the neck of the femur) have been reported in 2% of cases. I do not recommend this treatment.

In vitro fertilization (IVF) with intracytoplasmic sperm injection (ICSI) is the best option. Here each egg is injected with a single sperm, and whether there are antibodies attached to the outer surface of the sperm becomes irrelevant. In fact, pregnancy and birthrate are the same as in cases where IVF is performed for reasons other than male factor infertility. IVF/ICSI success rates are also not unaffected by the concentration of antisperm antibodies.

> *Note:* Intrauterine insemination (IUI) of processed sperm is contraindicated in cases of moderate or severe male immunologic infertility because it does NOT improve pregnancy rates over no treatment at all.

QUALITY OF THE EMBRYO: THE THIRD ULTIMATUM

At this time, standard microscopic techniques for predicting the health and viability of embryos are far from optimal. Such limitations, coupled with pressure to maximize the chance of pregnancy, have typically resulted in a tendency to transfer too many embryos at a time. While such practice has led to improved IVF birthrates, the transfer of multiple embryos at one time has resulted in an unacceptably excessive rate of high-order multiple births (triplets or greater). This in turn has resulted in an alarming escalation in the incidence of prematurity-related neonatal complications that are all too often both life-threatening and life-enduring.

Of the approximately 4 million babies born annually in the U.S., about one in 500 is afflicted with a sex-linked disorder that occurs when a genetically defective Y (male) chromosome is transmitted to the offspring. Another one in 300 newborns has an autosomal genetic disorder, an abnormality of one or more genes involving the 44 remaining autosomes (non-sex chromosomes). This means that approximately one in 20,000 babies born annually in the U.S. will have one or another genetic or chromosomal disorder. In addition, about one in 50 babies is born with an identifiable major genetic abnormality. In other words, more than 80,000 babies are afflicted by severe genetic disease annually in this country. Many couples who parent a child with a severe birth defect will subsequently elect not to have another child and may adopt. These facts and figures offer a glimpse at the magnitude of the challenge confronting the medical profession, government, and society in general.

The Human Genome Project, a 15-year effort to draw the first detailed map in human DNA, will inevitably lead to the widespread implementation of human gene therapy for the treatment and prevention of disease. We are on the verge of nothing less than a biomedical revolution the likes of which has not been encountered before. The human genome project will also lead to profound changes in the ability to manipulate genes. It will change the way we are born, how we exist, how we view ourselves in relation to our destiny, and how we die.

Before us lies a difficult transition. Most people have begun to wonder about the cost; and while many are profoundly divided or even ambivalent about genetic research and its applications, most feel strongly that the introduction of human genetic engineering for the purpose of curing disease is well justified. If the use of genetic engineering to cure and prevent disease in an existing human being is justified, then surely the potential to eradicate certain lethal diseases through preimplantation diagnosis is similarly vindicated.

Gender Selection

You may know someone who desperately wants to have a girl . . . or a boy. Perhaps a couple has several children of one gender already and would like to have another, but only if the odds of having a baby of the other gender could be greatly skewed in their favor. Or maybe the couple wants a baby of one gender to avoid passing on one of the more than 500 sex-linked genetic diseases. Gender selection is discussed here because it can reduce the probability of X-linked diseases being passed on through the embryo.

Given that upon fertilization a sperm with a Y chromosome makes a boy and one bearing an X chromosome makes a girl, and any given sperm sample contains an even amount of X- and Y-bearing chromosomes, aspiring parents have no greater than a 50 percent chance of getting a baby of the desired sex. In ancient Greece, men believed that lying on their right side during intercourse increased the likelihood of a male child. A Chinese birth calendar buried over 700 years ago in a tomb outside Beijing is said to predict gender by when conception occurred. In 18th-century France, men would tie off their right testicle to "guarantee" having a boy. Sometimes, couples wanting a child of a particular gender use methods such as timing of intercourse.

Many methods for selecting sperm that would bias towards one gender or the other have been tried. Presently, in spite of wild claims of success, none has been proven to be fully reliable. Currently the only reliable alternative is for the woman to undergo IVF, have her eggs fertilized and then have the resulting embryos tested using PGD (FISH or CGH). In this way the specific gender of the embryo(s) can be determined and thereupon, the embryo(s) of chosen gender can be transferred to the uterus.

Preimplantation Genetic Diagnosis (PGD) to Identify "Competent" Embryos

PGD is a technique used for the early diagnosis of chromosomal/genetic disorders in embryos or blastomeres (cells of the developing embryo). It involves conducting biopsies on the polar body of egg(s) or upon one or more cells (blastomeres) removed from the embryo. PGD incorporates the latest techniques in assisted reproduction and molecular genetics to identify many chromosomal and genetic disorders prior to the initiation of pregnancy, thereby providing real hope to many desperate couples who might transmit a potential genetic catastrophe to their offspring. Embryos shown to be free of the chromosomal or genetic disease under investigation can thereupon be selectively transferred to the uterus.

Polar body biopsy. Polar body biopsy, which involves the removal of egg-derived chromosome populations known as polar bodies, can be performed relatively non-traumatically on the first body of the egg and on the 2nd polar body, within 36 hours of in vitro fertilization.

Blastomere biopsy. Blastomere biopsy involves the removal of one or more blastomeres (cells) from the embryo. It is usually performed on 5 to 9 cell embryos on the 3rd day following in vitro fertilization. It is conducted for the purpose of: (1) Gender selection for "family balancing" or for identifying gender so as to avoid certain sex-linked genetic disorders, (2) to diagnose single or multiple gene disorders, and (3) to recognize certain structural and numerical chromosomal abnormalities. Blastomere biopsy has a distinct advantage over polar body biopsy because it permits assessment of chromosomes and genes derived from both the egg and the sperm. This is especially important when it comes to the diagnosis of embryo aneuploidies. Needless to say, since the sperm contributes the X or Y chromosome, egg polar body biopsy cannot determine embryo gender.

Unfortunately, PGD, as currently performed, commercially using FISH, is only capable of reliably identifying up to 12 out of a possible 23 chromosome pairs. Thus it is not able to fully evaluate the egg or embryo for aneuploidy. Thus, even if PGD were to reveal that the

12 chromosome pairs evaluated were normal, this would not completely rule out embryo aneuploidy.

Furthermore, blastomere biopsy for FISH requires complete removal of an intact blastomere and this is a potentially time-consuming and traumatic process that might compromise the embryo's subsequent implantation potential. For these reasons, PGD/FISH does not represent an optimal method by which to evaluate embryos for aneuploidy.

The use of PGD for the prediction of genetic disorders requires blastomere biopsy and testing through the use of polymerase chain reaction (PCR) technology. PCR involves identification and amplification of one or more gene loci on chromosomes. It is expensive, requires the prior anticipation of an increased risk of the disorder occurring in the offspring, and is very limited by the lack of availability of genetic markers for all but a handful of genetic disorders.

Comparative Genomic Hybridization (CGH). As previously discussed, we were the first to introduce CGH into the human clinical IVF arena in 2005. Its benefit lies in its ability to identify all the chromosomes present and as such is ideal for assessing egg and embryo aneuploidies. We, and others, have demonstrated that the transfer of up to two CGH-normal embryos into a "receptive uterine environment" results in a 60-70% birthrate. There are different methods of CGH. The one referred to is a metaphase CGH (mCGH) and the other is array CGH (aCGH). Both are highly reliable. However, in my opinion, unlike mCGH, which can be performed reliably on the minute mount of DNA derived from a single blastomere, aCGH requires access to much more DNA to perform. Thus I presently believe mCGH is more suited to performance on the polar body (PB) of an egg or on a single blastomere biopsied from a day 3 embryo. Since we introduced egg/embryo CGH assessment into the clinical IVF arena (in 2005) its popularity has grown rapidly. In fact, presently, when it comes to assessing eggs and embryos for their (chromosomal) "competency," CGH has all but replaced FISH in the diagnosis of aneuploidy.

Again, while there is good reason for optimism, it should be recognized that PGD is by no means 100 percent accurate. Conventional FISH only permits 9-12 of the 23 chromosomal pairs to be reliably assessed. Moreover, neither FISH nor CGH techniques are flawless. Errors occur in 5-7% of cases. Accordingly when following such testing and ET a viable pregnancy occurs, a thorough prenatal genetic testing screen involving level-3 ultrasound examination, biochemical testing, and chorionic villus sampling (CVS)/mid-trimester amniocentesis should always be undertaken to exclude the risk of misdiagnosis through PGD.

UTERINE RECEPTIVITY: THE FOURTH ULTIMATUM

It is an unfortunate reality that many IVF programs attach little importance to factors that affect embryo implantation in general, and immunologic implantation dysfunction (IID) in particular (see below). Perhaps the lack of attention given to evaluating IVF patients for factors that adversely affect the receptivity of the uterine lining (endometrium/decidua) is due to the fact that in humans, IVF failure and miscarriage are both four times more likely to be due to embryo "incompetence" than to dysfunctional implantation, and thus a high measure of IVF success can still be achieved in spite of ignoring less common (complex) factors such as IID. But for the 20% of IVF patients with problems relating to lack of endometrial receptivity it becomes a different matter altogether. For them the emotional, physical, and financial roller-coaster ride goes on and on. Often after spinning their wheels and enduring repeated IVF failures many of them will be advised to move on to egg donation . . . only to fail there as well. Optimal implantation is not only important for embryo survival; it is also a major factor in determining normal intra-uterine growth and development and as such is a major determinant of the very quality of life after birth.

Contour of the Uterine Cavity (see Chapter 4)

It has long been suspected that anatomical defects of the uterus might result in infertility. While fibroids confined to the uterine wall are unlikely to cause infertility, an association between their presence and infertility has been observed in cases where they distort the uterine cavity or protrude as submucous polyps through the endometrial lining. It would appear that even small submucous fibroids (ones that protrude into the uterine cavity) have the potential to prejudice implantation.

It is likely that any surface lesion in the uterine cavity, whether an endometrial, placental, or fibroid polyp (no matter how small) or intrauterine adhesion, has the potential to interfere with implantation by producing a local inflammatory response not too dissimilar in nature from that which is caused by a foreign body such as an intrauterine contraceptive device. Unfortunately, a hysterosalpingogram (HSG) will miss the diagnosis in approximately 30 percent of cases. The only reliable methods for diagnosing even the smallest of such lesions are saline sonography, also known as fluid ultrasonography (FUS), or hysteroscopy.

If performed by an expert, FUS is highly effective in recognizing even the smallest lesion and can replace hysteroscopy under such circumstances. FUS is also less expensive and less traumatic. Its only disadvantage lies in the fact that if a lesion is detected, the subsequent performance of hysteroscopy may be required to treat the problem. Diagnostic hysteroscopy involves the insertion of a thin, lighted, telescope-like hysteroscope into the uterus, which is first distended with a sterile solution or with carbon dioxide gas. As is the case with FUS, diagnostic hysteroscopy facilitates examination of the inside of the uterus under direct vision for defects that might interfere with implantation. We have observed that approximately one in 10 candidates for IVF has lesions that require attention prior to undergoing IVF in order to optimize the chances of a successful outcome. We strongly recommend that all patients undergo therapeutic surgery (usually by hysteroscopy) to correct the pathology.

Thickness of the Endometrium (see Chapter 4)

The Immunologic Factor (see Chapter 14–RPL)

Immunologic acceptance of the implanting embryo by the uterus of the mother is both highly complex and magnificent. Not only is it essential for pregnancy to occur, but it also sets the scene for our body's own cells, tissues, and organs to be shielded from attack by our immune systems. For a moment, consider how, when confronted by foreign proteins (bacteria viruses, foreign tissue grafts/transplantation), the body's immune system goes on the attack but yet an embryo that is partially derived from proteins that come from another individual (the sperm or paternal antigen), usually safely implants in the pre-pregnancy uterine lining and then grows into a healthy baby. This phenomenon has come to be referred to as the "immunologic riddle of pregnancy."

For such a complex arrangement never to fail would be without precedent in human biology. To argue to the contrary is, in my opinion, an absurdity, bordering on arrogance. It can and does go wrong in about 15–20% of women with reproductive failure and when it does, it sometimes presents as failed implantation (presumed by the patient to be infertility), as miscarriage, or (much less frequently) as placental failure and compromised fetal development or intrauterine death. It all depends on the timing, nature, and severity of the immune assault.

It is well known that the reason the implanting normal embryo thrives in the womb is that unique immunologic adjustments convert the pre-pregnancy uterine lining (decidua) into a "privileged site" where the embryo and the fetus come to be regarded as "bodies own" ("self") and as such are protected from immune attack. This initial acceptance of the embryo as "self" or "friend" rather than "non-self" or "foe" (in spite of it being a semi-allograft) is one of the miraculous adaptations of nature and is in large part responsible for our survival as a species.

As soon as implantation begins, the paternal genetic contribution to the embryo (so called DQ alpha genes) initiates a signal to the pre-pregnancy decidual immune system which thereupon determines whether the embryonic allograft should be welcomed (i.e., be accepted as "friend") or be regarded as "foe" and be rejected through immune attack. The process is referred to as "alloimmune recognition." Given that with the exception of monozygotic twins, interpersonal differences in genotype are inevitable, it follows that maternal and paternal DQ alpha gene combinations will usually also differ in the vast majority of cases. Thus, preservation of the human species required that in spite of such immunogenetic dissimilarities, the immune system of the pre-pregnancy endometrium (decidua) adapt and recognize the embryo as "self" or "friend" rather than as "non-self" or "foe."

Upon reaching the uterine environment, the "genetically competent" embryo, hatches and thereupon, within 12–24 hours starts sending its root system (trophoblast) into the decidua. The trophoblast has both villous (root-like) and extravilous (diffuse) components. The extravilous trophoblast, which diffusely permeates the decidua, expresses several so-called major histocompatibility complex (MHC) class 1 genes [e.g., histocompatibility leukocyte antigen (HLA-) C, E, and G]. These HLA genes, (primarily HLA-G) regulate primarily two types of lymphocytes present in the decidua. These are uterine natural killer (NK) cells and cytotoxic lymphocytes (CTL). NK cells comprise approximately 75% of decidual lymphocytes and CTL comprise about 10%. They both likely play a vital role in regulating the normal implantation process by controlling the penetration and functioning of the trophoblast.

The recognition of proteins as "self" ("friend") or "non-self" ("foe") is propagated by highly specialized immune lymphocytes known as regulatory T-cells. These so-called Treg cells can "turn off" immune reactions even once they have been started by conventional immune cells. They play a pivotal role in the immune system's ability to prevent rejection of an embryo whether due to an autoimmune or alloimmune response. Other immune cells known as dendritic cells, introduce antigenic proteins to these Treg cells, whose concentration increases when the antigen is recognized as "self" and decreases when recognized as "foe." MHC (primarily HLA-G) signaling, through the Treg lymphocyte mechanism working in combination with other regulatory proteins, influences the production and release of so-called cytokines by the NK and CTL cells. There are three varieties of cytokines, two of which play defining roles in the maintenance of implantation: The first is TH-2 cytokines, which encourage growth and expansion of the trophoblast and promote proliferation of blood vessels (angiogenesis). The second, TH-1 cytokines, promote destruction (cytolysis) of trophoblastic cells and also cause blood to clot (procoagulant effect). A balance between TH-1 and TH-2 cytokines is essential for normal implantation and development of the placenta (placentation).

Over-activity (dominance) of TH-1, the hallmark of NK cell and CTL activation, leads to damage of the trophoblast, implantation dysfunction, and reproductive failure.

Alloimmune Implantation Dysfunction

Every human being has two DQ alpha genes. One is contributed by the father and the other by the mother. When (albeit in a small percentage of patients undergoing IVF) paternal-maternal DQ-alpha gene similarities occur, it will, following repeated exposures to such genetically matching embryos, provoke activation of the decidual immune system. Usually, this will, through the mechanisms described above, ultimately lead to NK/CTL activation and reproductive failure (i.e., infertility, and pregnancy loss) in most cases. We refer to this phenomenon as *alloimmune implantation dysfunction.*

This is how alloimmune implantation dysfunction happens: Immunogenetically triggered HLA-G signaling on the part of the implanting embryo leads to a reduction in Treg cells and eventually to a destabilization of NK/CTLs with domination of TH-1 over TH-2 activity. The severity with which this occurs is an important determinant of whether total implantation failure will occur or whether there would remain enough residual trophoblastic activity that would allow the pregnancy to limp along until the nutritional supply can no longer meet the demands of the pregnancy, at which point miscarriage or pregnancy loss occurs. With paternal-maternal DQ alpha matching it will often take the passage of several pregnancies for NK cell activation to build to the point that woman with alloimmune implantation dysfunction will present with clinical evidence of implantation dysfunction. Sometimes it starts off with one or two pregnancies surviving to birth of a baby, whereupon NK/CTL cell activity starts to build, leading to one or more early miscarriages. Eventually the NK /CTL activity is so high that subsequent pregnancies can be lost before the woman is even aware that she was pregnant at all. At this point she is often diagnosed with secondary, "unexplained" infertility and/or "unexplained" IVF failure.

Autoimmune Implantation Dysfunction

With *autoimmune implantation dysfunction*, NK cell activation is already well established by the time the embryo reaches the uterus. Accordingly, in such cases the pregnancies is usually lost before its presence can be established by a blood pregnancy test or an early ultrasound examination (i.e., it presents as a negative pregnancy test or a chemical gestation).

So how is autoimmune implantation dysfunction established? The initial recognition of the non-DQ alpha matching embryo as "friend" or "self" sets the stage for the cells/tissues of our tissues not coming under immune attack. However under certain circumstances, genetic, infective, toxic, and degenerative influences can result in our own body's proteins coming to be regarded as "non-self" ("foe"). When this happens the immune system starts to produce antibodies that are directed against our body's own proteins. These so-called autoantibodies then start attacking the body's own cells/tissues/organs creating pathologic states (diseases) such as can be seen with certain (autoimmune) disease states—e.g., lupus erythematosus, autoimmune hypothyroidism (Hashimoto's disease), and rheumatoid arthritis, etc. There are also certain reproductive diseases such as endometriosis, where cell membrane phospholipids are often altered by the disease process and then combine with proteins to evoke the production of so-called antiphospholipid antibodies (APA). Certain types of APAs can both directly damage the trophoblast and can also lead to a reduction of Treg lymphocytes, culminating in activation of NK/CTLs. This type of reaction—albeit due to a predisposition to autoimmune diseases such as lupus erythematosus, Hashimoto's disease, or reproductive conditions such as endometriosis—is referred to as autoimmune implantation dysfunction. Autoimmune implantation dysfunction is much more common than alloimmune implantation dysfunction. In fact it is responsible for more than 85% of reproductive failure due to immunologic implantation dysfunction. The three most common types of autoantibodies involved are antiphospholipid antibodies (APA), antithyroid antibodies (ATA), and possibly, antiovarian antibodies (AOA).

Since autoimmune implantation dysfunction is often genetically transmitted, it is not surprising that this condition is more likely to exist in women who have a family (or personal) history of primary auto-immune diseases such as lupus erythematosus, scleroderma, clinical or subclinical hypothyroidism, rheumatoid arthritis, etc. Reactionary (secondary) autoimmunity can occur in conjunction with any medical condition associated with widespread tissue damage. One such gyne-cologic condition is endometriosis.

As previously stated, autoimmune implantation dysfunction is often immediately lethal to the implanting embryo and accordingly most often presents as "unexplained " infertility and/or "unexplained" IVF failure, rather than as miscarriage. This is because NK/CTL activation is present prior to implantation and as such the embryo's root system is severely damaged from the get-go. Autoimmune implantation dys-function is readily amenable to reversal through timely, appropriately administered, selective immunotherapy (see below).

Diagnosing Immunologic Implantation Dysfunction

Whether alloimmune or autoimmune in origin, it is only when specialized immune cells in the uterine lining known as natural killer (NK) Cells and CTL become activated and TH-1 cytokine dominance is established that IID occurs. Thus a full evaluation of IID requires that DQ alpha, APA, ATA, as well as NK/CTL activation be evaluated. This requires highly specialized blood and possibly also endometrial tests that can only be adequately performed by a handful of specialized reproductive immunology laboratories in the United States.

Alloimmune ID is diagnosed by testing the blood of both the male and female partners for matching DQ alpha genes. A sufficient degree of matching clinches the diagnosis. Since matching DQ alphas will not cause reproductive failure unless there is concomitant NK/CTL cell acti-vation, it is important to also test the embryo recipient for this. NK cell activation is best tested for through a blood K-562 target cell test. CTL activation can be evaluated by a blood immunophenotype and HLA-DR measurement. Some reproductive immunologists might also test blood Treg cell concentration and/or recommend an endometrial biopsy to histolochemically evaluate uterine NK cells or assess the local TH-1/TH-2 balance. The performance of blood TH-1 and TH-2 cytokines to assess for TH-1 dominance is controversial and is of unproven value.

Treating Immunologic Implantation Dysfunction

In the United States, effective treatment of NK/CTL activation associated with either alloimmune or autoimmune implantation dysfunction requires the administration of intralipid (IL) or intravenous immunoglobulin-G (IVIg). Such treatment is much more likely to be successful in the case of autoimmune implantation dysfunction where the NK/CTL activation is present in advance of the uterus being exposed to the embryo. It is not nearly as effective for the treatment of alloimmune implantation dysfunction where a DQ alpha-matching embryo will exert a sustained activation of NK/CTLs over several months of gestation. It is presently not yet possible to recognize paternal DQ alpha in the embryo. Accordingly, in cases where the paternal DQ alpha genes only match with one of the mother's DQ alpha's (i.e., a partial match) there is a one out of two chance that a transferred embryo will inadvertently be a match with at least one of the mother's DQ alpha genes. Thus IL and IVIg therapy will only prove half as likely to propagate a viable pregnancy in cases of partial DQ alpha matching as it can achieve in the treatment of NK/CTL activation associated with autoimmune implantation dysfunction. Thus I prefer to transfer only one embryo (rather than multiples) at a time in such cases, for fear of there being one DQ alpha matching embryo in the mix and so "muddying the waters" for the non-DQ alpha matching that otherwise might have propagated a healthy baby.

A real problem arises in cases of a complete match, where both paternal DQ alpha genes match with at least one of the mother's DQ alpha's. Here, every embryo will express a paternal DQ alpha gene that matches that of the mother's. In such cases, IL and/or IVIg therapy will rarely work. The reason is that such treatment cannot match the sustained provocation of NK/CTL activity brought about by an ever-present DQ alpha "clash." In cases of a complete DQ alpha matching (with associated NK/CTL activation), where all the embryos will inevitably carry one or both paternal DQ alpha that match(es) the mother, there is in my opinion little hope of success, even with intalipid/IVIg/steroid therapy. In such cases, gestational surrogacy or the use of non-DQ alpha matching donor sperm may offer the only reasonable chance of a successful IVF outcome. Some patients ask whether using an egg donor might not offer another solution in such cases. The answer is no! The matchup is between the paternal DQ alpha contribution (in the sperm) and the mother's uterus. It is not between the sperm and the egg.

IVIg or IL therapy should be administered in combination (with corticosteroids) at an adequate dosage, 7–14 days prior to planned embryo transfer, and with alloimmune implantation dysfunction it should (ideally) be maintained, at least through the 1st half of pregnancy. The goal is to down-regulate NK/CTL activation and thereby reinstate a TH-1: TH-2 cytokine balance in advance of a "competent" non-DQ alpha matching embryo reaching the uterus. Treatment of autoimmune implantation dysfunction requires that IL and/or IVIg (with corticosteroids) be administered only twice, once 7–14 days prior to embryo transfer and then one more time when the beta hCG blood level has shown evidence of an appropriate rise, thereby suggesting that healthy implantation could be in progress. Supplementation with heparinoid is indicated when there is evidence of concomitant APAs.

Heparinoid Therapy: There is compelling evidence that the subcutaneous administration of heparin twice daily or low molecular heparin (Clexane, Lovenox) once daily, (starting with the onset of ovarian stimulation) can improve IVF birthrate in women who test positive for APAs.

What About Taking a Baby Aspirin a Day? In my opinion, aspirin has little (if any) value when it comes to IID, and besides, could even reduce the chance of success. The reason for this is that aspirin thins the blood and increases the potential to bleed. This effect can last for up to a week and could complicate an egg retrieval procedure or result in "concealed" intrauterine bleeding at the time of embryo transfer, thereby potentially compromising IVF success.

IVIg and Intralipid Therapy: In the past, the only effective way to accomplish this was through the intravenous administration of a blood product known as immunoglobulin-G (IVIg). However, although never documented in first-world-produced IVIg, the administration of a blood product initially raised concern with regard to the potential of transmitting viral infections such as HIV and hepatitis C.

Several years ago, researchers at SIRM and an affiliate Reproductive Immunology program in Chicago, IL, reported on the use of intalipid (IL), a synthetic product which, upon being administered intravenously a week or longer prior to embryo transfer, elicits a similar down-regulatory effect on NK/CTL activation as does IVIg. We subsequently conducted confirmatory internal trials in 2007. Thereupon, several SIRM programs began prescribing IL preferentially to patients with CTL/NK activation. To date we have treated more than 1,000 cases in this way and results have been very encouraging. Against this background I have now all but abandoned the use of IVIg for IID associated with NK/CTL activation, supplanting it with IL. On very rare occasions, where IL alone does not achieve the desired result, we would recommend combined IVIg and IL therapy.

IVIg is very expensive and it does elicit immediate and delayed side effects and complications in about 20% of cases. IL on the other hand, provided that it is prescribed and administered appropriately, is virtually devoid of risk and/or significant side effects. It is also safe to the developing conceptus and it comes at a fraction of the cost of IVIg.

Corticosteroid Therapy (e.g., Prednisone, Prednisolone, and Dexamethasone): Corticosteroid therapy has become a mainstay in the treatment of most women undergoing IVF. It is believed by most to enhance implantation overall. This is more than likely due to an over-all immunomodulatory effect. Some IVF programs prescribe daily oral methyl Prednisilone (Medrol) while others prefer prednisone or dexamethasone, commencing a week or two prior to egg retrieval and continuing until pregnancy is discounted or until after the ultrasound confirmation of pregnancy.

TH-1 Blockers (Enbrel, Humira): I was one of the first to advocate using TH-1 cytokine blocker, Enbrel (and Humira) for treating NK cell activation, only to find it to be relatively ineffective in the IVF setting. There has to date, to the best of my knowledge, not been a single publication in an accredited medical journal that has shown TH-I blockers to be of real benefit in patients undergoing IVF. These blockers might have a role in the treatment of a threatened miscarriage thought to be due to CTL/NK activation, but in my opinion, not for IVF. The reason is that the very initial phase of implantation requires a cellular response involving TH-1 cytokines. To block them (rather than simply restore a TH1: TH-2 balance as occurs with IL or IVIg therapy) so very early on could in my opinion compromise rather than benefit implantation.

What about Leukocyte Immunization Therapy (LIT)? The subcutane-ous injection of the husband's lymphocytes to the mother is thought to enhance the ability for the mother's decidua (uterus) to recognize the DQ alpha matching embryo as "self" or "friend" and thereby avert its rejection. LIT has been shown to up-regulate Treg cells and thus down-regulate NK cell activation and thereby improve decidual TH1: TH-2 balance. Thus there could be a therapeutic benefit from such therapy. However, in my opinion, such benefit is no greater than can be achieved through the use of IL plus corticosteroids. Besides IL is much less expensive and the use of LIT is prohibited by law, in the United States.

Note: The evaluation for immunologic dysfunction as well as for other factors that can affect implantation should form part of the evaluation of patients preparing to undergo IVF, and especially so in women with endometriosis, recurrent pregnancy loss (RPL), women with a personal or family history of autoimmune conditions, and women with "unexplained" infertility or unexplained IVF failure(s).

EMBRYO TRANSFER: THE FIFTH ULTIMATUM

It cannot be overstated that embryo transfer is the single most determinant factor in IVF outcome. The procedure requires gentle placement of the embryo(s) within 1 cm of the roof of the uterine cavity under direct ultrasound visualization.

The selection of embryos most likely to implant and the timing of embryo transfer, both critical to the transfer process, have been greatly enhanced by use of the following three elements in the embryo transfer protocol: 1. Graduated Embryo Scoring (GES), 2. Blastocysts transfers, and 3. CGH embryo selection.

9

OTHER CONDITIONS THAT COMPROMISE FERTILITY

CONDITIONS THAT NEGATIVELY IMPACT A MAN'S FERTILITY

Inadequate Secretion of FSH by the Pituitary Gland

In a relatively small number of cases of male infertility, the failure to produce an adequate quality of sperm is associated with reduced secretion by the pituitary gland of those hormones necessary to stimulate sperm production. The pituitary gland in the man produces two important hormones with regard to testicular function: follicle-stimulating hormone (FSH) and luteinizing hormone (LH). LH's predominant function is to act on the Leydig cells in the testicles, which produce the male hormone testosterone. A sustained reduction in FSH production, therefore, is capable of resulting in male infertility. Usually, if there is a reduction in either LH or FSH, the other one will also be low. Men produce sperm in cycles of approximately 90 days, from initiation to the production of the most mature forms of sperm. Accordingly, any treatment administered to the man in order to improve sperm production can only be properly assessed after waiting about three months. In order to assess the potential of a male to respond to fertility drugs, it is therefore necessary to first measure both FSH and LH as well as the male hormones testosterone, androstenedione, dehydroepiandrosterone, and prolactin. Measurement of these hormones gives an indication as to whether the man is likely to respond to treatment with FSH or FSH/LH.

There are three approaches to treating male infertility that are potentially responsive to therapy:

1. **Clomiphene citrate.** As mentioned earlier, clomiphene citrate is a hormone that stimulates the pituitary gland to produce large amounts of FSH and LH, which is essential to the production of sperm. The first step in this simple treatment is to perform a baseline semen analysis, FSH, LH, and male hormone measurements immediately prior to initiating therapy. Then 25 mg of clomiphene citrate is administered every day for 90 days, and all of the tests are repeated serially throughout the treatment period. The administration of clomiphene citrate is essentially harmless to the man, who may experience some minor side effects such as spots in front of the eyes, dryness of the mouth, headaches, slight changes in mood, and, rarely, hot flashes. All of these side effects abate upon discontinuation of therapy.

2. **Gonadotropin therapy.** In cases where clomiphene citrate therapy is not successful or in certain situations where it is not possible for clomiphene to stimulate the pituitary gland into action, FSH alone or in combination with LH can be administered in the hope of stimulating the testicles directly. This therapy might also include the administration of hCG in order to further stimulate the production of male hormones in cases where failed masculinization is associated with reduced sperm production. These drugs are usually administered three times per week, again for about 90 days, and the same hormonal and sperm assessments as stipulated for clomiphene therapy would apply. The treatment is, again, relatively harmless, and the minor side effects that might occur cease upon discontinuation of therapy.

3. **Other medical therapies.** There is some evidence that the administration of certain vitamin preparations and antioxidants are of benefit in the treatment of male infertility associated with

an abnormal SCSA and/or reduced sperm motility. In some cases, systemic conditions affecting other areas of the body might indirectly impact upon the pituitary gland's ability to produce the hormones necessary to stimulate testicular function. In cases of thyroid deficiency, severe diabetes mellitus, and collagen diseases, selective therapy with thyroid hormone, insulin, or corticosteroids may be of benefit. Sometimes the pituitary gland produces too much prolactin, which in turn inhibits the ability of FSH and LH to act on the testicles. In such cases, it may be necessary to administer a drug called bromocryptine to suppress prolactin production, thereby removing its restraining effect on the action of FSH upon the testicles. There are, of course, many other such examples in which treatment of unrelated conditions might improve overall male fertility. Such approaches as the use of temperature-lowering devices on the testicles and prevention of exposure to dangerous chemicals have been reported to be preventative and even curative, but in our opinion they are of dubious value.

If the previously infertile man is indeed fortunate enough to respond to one of the above treatment modalities for enhancement of sperm production, then it is possible for a number of masturbation specimens of sperm to be collected and frozen in liquid nitrogen so there will always be relatively good-quality sperm on hand, even if the fertility treatment is discontinued and the man again produces relatively poor sperm. It is, of course, not practical to permanently treat an individual on potent medications such as clomiphene, FSH, LH, or hCG.

CONDITIONS THAT NEGATIVELY IMPACT A WOMAN'S FERTILITY

Pelvic Inflammatory Disease (PID)

Pelvic inflammatory disease (PID) results from infection of pelvic structures, especially the fallopian tubes, via which the uterus, fallopian tubes, ovaries, bowel, and the smooth membrane that lines the surface of the pelvic cavity (the peritoneum) may also be infected. PID's damage to pelvic structures can inhibit the passage of eggs, sperm, and embryos in a timely manner to and from the uterine cavity, thus compromising fertility.

It has been estimated that about 1.5 million women develop PID annually in the United States. Less than one-third of these women present with acute pelvic inflammatory disease, and the remaining cases usually go undetected until the woman presents with symptoms of infertility. In fact, more than 70 percent of patients who undergo surgery or IVF are unaware of any history of acute PID. It is an unfortunate irony that although many of the sexually transmitted organisms are readily eradicated through appropriate antibiotic therapy, because their presence produces no overt symptoms infected women rarely seek treatment.

Grades of severity.   Acute PID usually prompts the woman to seek immediate medical attention because of fever, severe lower abdominal pain, a yellow- or blood-stained nonirritating vaginal discharge, and vomiting. More commonly, the onset of sub-acute PID is gradual, less severe, and often goes unnoticed until superimposed acute PID occurs or chronic incapacitating symptoms prompt the woman to seek medical attention. Chronic PID, a consequence of untreated or unsuccessfully managed acute and/or subacute PID, presents with symptoms of pelvic pain, heavy and painful menstrual periods, pain with intercourse, and infertility.

Causes.   PID results from (1) sexual transmission via the vagina and cervix of infecting organisms, (2) contamination from other inflamed structures in the abdominal cavity (e.g., appendix, gallbladder, kidneys, etc.), (3) a foreign body inside the uterus (e.g., an IUD), (4) contamination of retained products of conception following abortion or childbirth, and, rarely, (5) blood-borne bacterial transmission (e.g., pelvic tuberculosis, which is common in developing countries but rare in the United States).

Factors that facilitate development of PID include (1) exposure to infection immediately prior to menstruation because menstrual blood provides an excellent growth medium for bacteria, (2) relatively ill health and poor nutritional status, which is why PID is rampant in lower socioeconomic groups, and (3) high susceptibility to re-infection of women with a history of PID. While sexually transmitted PID is certainly capable of causing endometritis (infection of the uterine lining), the fallopian tubes rather than the uterus itself are usually the main focus of the inflammatory process in such cases because menstruation tends to remove infected tissue monthly, thereby preventing the inflammation from causing permanent damage to the endometrium.

In contrast, PID (endometritis) that occurs following childbirth or abortion primarily targets the uterine lining because the delayed onset of menstruation after both childbirth and abortion enables the inflammatory process to take hold in the products of conception that are sometimes retained in the uterus. This sometimes leads to the development of scar tissue in the uterine cavity and can cause opposing surfaces of the endometrium to fuse (Asherman's syndrome); produce scarring that obliterates the junction into the fallopian tubes and might also damage a small, adjacent segment of the tubes; and cause the fallopian tube(s) to separate from the uterine wall. Less commonly, post-childbirth and post-abortal endometritis can result in salpingitis, or infection of the entire fallopian tube(s), causing partial or complete blockage and/or spreading into the pelvic cavity.

PID may also result from the use of the intrauterine contraceptive device (IUD) for contraceptive purposes. This most commonly occurs in cases where the device is inserted into the uterus of women concurrently infected with gonorrhea or chlamydia. The IUD causes local irritation that compromises the defense mechanisms normally protecting against infection. At the same time, the IUD string, which protrudes through the cervix into the vagina, may act as a wick via which infecting organisms gain entrance to the uterus. IUD-related uterine infection causes the same damage as post-abortal and post-childbirth endometritis. IUD-related PID is a potentially life-endangering condition capable of causing formation of a pelvic abscess, peritonitis, systemic infection, and shock.

In cases where the ends of the fallopian tubes are blocked, pus can collect and distend the tube(s). The pus is usually absorbed over time and replaced by clear straw-colored fluid, resulting in occluded, fluid-filled, distended, and often functionless fallopian tube(s), referred to as a hydrosalpinx. This fluid, which contains dead cells and other noxious products, is believed to be toxic to embryos and can hinder implantation following IVF. Difficult as it may be to accept, women with hydrosalpinges should strongly consider having their tubes removed or ligated prior to undergoing IVF. This is because the presence of hydrosalpinges renders the tubes non-functional; and even if the tubes could be opened, the likelihood of pregnancy occurring would be remote.

Sexually transmitted PID almost invariably affects both fallopian tubes. Even in cases where hysterosalpingogram or laparoscopy (see explanation of tests in the following chapter) indicates that only one fallopian tube has been infected, the other tube is almost invariably involved.

Pelvic Tuberculosis

Pelvic tuberculosis is an uncommon cause of infertility in the United States although its incidence is on the rise as a result of the influx of immigrants from Asia, particularly India, and other underdeveloped countries where poor nutrition and general ill health contribute to its formation.

Pelvic tuberculosis is often a "silent disease" that may exist for 10 to 20 years without producing any symptoms. Infertility is often one of the reasons—and sometimes the only reason—to investigate for the presence of the condition; and because of its rarity as a cause of infertility in the United States, the diagnosis is often missed.

Pelvic tuberculosis usually presents with one or more of the following symptoms: (1) pelvic pain, pain with menstruation, pain with intercourse, chronic lower abdominal pain or discomfort, chronic back pain; (2) abdominal distention, usually due to the collection of free fluid in the abdominal-pelvic cavity; (3) local tuberculous lesions on the external genitalia, cervix, and/or vagina; (4) tuberculous salpingitis (tubal disease), which occurs in 75 percent of cases; (5) ovulation dysfunction, which often presents with absent, excessive, or noncyclical menstruation, largely attributable to ovarian involvement (40 percent of cases); and (6) uterine (endometrial) tuberculosis (30 percent).

Diagnosis.   The diagnosis is made on the basis of evidence of con-comitant, pulmonary tuberculosis; the detection of calcifications on pelvic X-rays; a typical tubal pattern on hysterosalpingogram (dye X-ray test); findings at laparoscopy or laparotomy and the subsequent pathologic examination of biopsy material obtained during these proce-dures; and blood tests such as a differential blood count and erythrocyte sedimentation rate.

Microscopic and bacteriologic examination is the primary method for diagnosing pelvic tuberculosis. Most commonly, a dilatation and curettage (D&C) of the uterus is performed a few days prior to men-struation. The surgeon uses a physiologic salt solution to cleanse the vagina and cervix while preparing for the D&C lest an antiseptic kill any tuberculous bacilli present in the specimen, thereby rendering a falsely negative culture result. Upon collection, part of the specimen of uter-ine curettings is cultured by the microbiology lab, and some is used for guinea pig inoculation for detection of the acid-fast tuberculosis. Biopsy specimens of lesions on the external genitalia, vagina, cervix, and pelvic cavity can also be studied by culturing, by guinea pig inoculation, and by histopathologic examination. Even in the presence of established tuberculosis, histopathologic examination will only be positive about 50 percent of the time. Cultures, although more reliable, can also yield false-negative results. Accordingly, it is often necessary to repeat such tests several times if the diagnosis is strongly suspected.

Treatment.   Treatment is primarily directed towards eradicating the inflammation by selective administration of antibiotics. Pelvic surgery (other than to remove distended or infected lesions and damaged fallo-pian tubes) has little therapeutic benefit. Provided that the tuberculous process has not destroyed the uterine lining, IVF following successful antibacterial treatment is the only rational method of treating infertility associated with pelvic tuberculosis.

Endometriosis

Endometriosis is a condition where the endometrium grows on pel-vic structures outside the uterine cavity. In early-stage endometriosis there is usually little, if any, visible evidence of anatomical distortion sufficient to compromise ovulation or transportation of the egg from the ovary to the fallopian tube. In contrast, more advanced endometriosis is characterized by the presence of pelvic adhesions sufficient to distort normal pelvic anatomy and interfere with fertilization as well as egg/embryo transportation mechanisms.

Endometriosis often goes unnoticed for many years. Frequently, such women are erroneously said to have so-called unexplained infertility until the diagnosis is finally clinched through direct visualization of the lesions at the time of laparoscopy or laparotomy. Not surprisingly, many patients with unexplained infertility are eventually diagnosed with endometriosis.

Recent medical research has helped shed light on how reproductive problems associated with endometriosis evolve and offers promise with regard to the future treatment of infertility/reproductive failure associated with this condition. One of the most interesting breakthroughs is the finding that endometriosis appears to have a genetic component. In the future, the development of genetic markers might provide an important diagnostic tool.

Grading endometriosis. In the case of advanced endometriosis, inspection at laparoscopy or laparotomy will usually reveal severe pelvic adhesions, scarring, and "chocolate cysts" causally linked to the infertility. The quality of life of women with advanced endometriosis is usually so severely compromised by pain and discomfort that having a baby is often low on the priority list. Accordingly, such patients are usually more interested in relatively radical medical and surgical treatment options that might preclude a subsequent pregnancy, such as removal of ovaries, fallopian tubes, and even the uterus as a means of alleviating suffering. Women with moderately severe endometriosis have a modest amount of scarring/adhesions and endometriotic deposits, which are usually detected on the ovaries, fallopian tubes, bladder surface, and low in the pelvis, behind the uterus. In such cases, the fallopian tubes are usually opened and functional. Women with mild endometriosis are often erroneously labeled as having unexplained infertility because of the insignificant distortion of pelvic anatomy.

How endometriosis impacts fertility.   To hold that infertility can only be attributed to endometriosis if significant anatomical disease can be identified is to ignore the fact that biochemical, hormonal, and immunological factors profoundly impact fertility. Failure to recognize this salient fact continues to play havoc with the hopes and dreams of many infertile endometriosis patients. The questions that should be asked are why, in the absence of any other apparent cause of infertility, women with mild to moderate endometriosis experience up to a six-fold reduction in spontaneous conception rate compared to women who do not have endometriosis; normally ovulating women with mild to moderate endometriosis do not experience a much-improved pregnancy rate following Controlled Ovarian Stimulation (COS) with clomiphene citrate or gonadotropins, regardless of whether intrauterine insemination (IUI) is done. Surgery performed on normally ovulating women to remove small endometriotic deposits is unlikely to improve pregnancy rates very much.

The causes of these problems are "toxins" in the peritoneal fluid ("the peritoneal factor") and the immunologic rejection of the early embryo as it attempts to implant into the uterine lining. Toxins that impair fertilization of the egg are present in the peritoneal secretions of most women who have endometriosis, regardless of its severity. This explains why women with endometriosis are three to four times less likely to conceive per month of trying and why procedures such as intrauterine insemination do not increase the chances of pregnancy. It also explains why IVF, which entails removing eggs through aspiration of the ovarian follicles before they can be affected by peritoneal toxins, improves pregnancy rates dramatically and, accordingly, is the treatment of choice for most endometriosis patients with infertility. (See Chapter 8 for a discussion of the role of therapeutic immunomodulation.)

Treatment.   The following basic concepts apply to management of endometriosis-related infertility:

- Ovulation induction with or without intrauterine insemination: Because toxins in the peritoneal secretions of women with endometriosis exert a negative effect on fertilization potential regardless of how sperm reaches the fallopian tubes, it follows that intrauterine insemination will not improve the chances of pregnancy much (over no treatment at all) in women with mild to moderate endometriosis.

- Surgery: Surgery aimed at restoring the anatomical integrity of the fallopian tubes neither counters the negative influence of toxic peritoneal factors that inherently reduce the chances of conception in women with endometriosis nor addresses the immunologic dysfunction commonly associated with this condition. For this reason, we believe that pelvic surgery is relatively contraindicated for the treatment of infertility associated with endometriosis when the woman is over 35 years old. Impending diminution of ovarian reserve (with premenopause approaching) in such women means that they simply do not have the time to waste on less efficacious alternatives and that IVF is needed. In contrast, younger women with endometriosis, who have time on their side, might consider surgery as a viable option. Approximately 30 to 40 percent of such younger normally ovulating women will conceive within three years following corrective pelvic surgery.

- Sclerotherapy of ovarian endometriomas in preparation for IVF: An endometrioma is a cystic collection of altered menstrual blood in the ovary that interferes with optimal follicle/egg development such that eggs harvested from the affected ovary are often compromised in their development, yielding poor-quality embryos following IVF. It is for this reason that ovarian endometriomas must be removed prior to ovarian stimulation for IVF. Simple aspiration of endometriomas is unsatisfactory because they will recur. Conventional surgical treatment, which involves either an abdominal incision or laparoscopic drainage of the cyst contents with subsequent removal of the cyst wall, can also be unsatisfactory because, unfortunately, in many cases normal ovarian tissue is inadvertently removed along with the cyst wall, which may decrease the number of eggs available for subsequent fertility treatment. Additionally, visualization of anatomic structures may be obscured by pelvic adhesions, leading to inadequate surgical removal with frequent cyst recurrence and the increased risk of surgical complications. Many patients with recurrent ovarian endometriomas are uncomfortable with the prospect of repeat surgery, and its avoidance is often a factor in the decision to proceed with IVF. We have performed sclerotherapy on more than 200 women with endometriomas who were preparing for treatment with IVF. Sclerotherapy for ovarian endometriomas involves needle aspiration of the liquid content of the endometriotic cyst, followed by the injection of 5 percent tetracycline into the cyst cavity. Treatment results in disappearance of the lesion within six to eight weeks in more than 80 percent of cases so treated. In the remainder, a simple cyst may remain, which in the vast majority of cases resolves permanently following a single aspiration. Ovarian sclerotherapy can be performed under local anesthesia or under general anesthesia. It has the advantage of being a low-cost, ambulatory office-based procedure with a low incidence of significant post-procedural pain or complications and avoidance of the need for laparoscopy or laparotomy. Since sclerotherapy for endometriomas is associated with a small but yet realistic possibility of adhesion formation, it should only be used in cases where IVF is the only treatment available to the patient. Women who intend to try and conceive through fertilization in their fallopian tubes (e.g., following natural conception or intrauterine insemination) will be better off undergoing laparotomy or laparoscopy for the treatment of endometriomas.

- In vitro fertilization: IVF is the treatment of choice for women over 35 or where surgery and treatment with fertility agents has proven to be unsuccessful. We anticipate that approximately 70 percent of such women under the age of 40 will achieve the birth of one or more babies within two IVF attempts (including associated frozen embryo transfers).

It is possible and perhaps even likely that women who fit this profile might conceive on their own spontaneously and have a baby in spite of (rather than due to) treatment. Failure to recognize this possibility carries the risk of unjustified complacency brought about by the perception that if a pregnancy occurred with or without treatment, it can be expected to happen just as easily again. Not so. The chances for pregnancy remain three to four times lower than for non-endometriotic, healthy ovulating women of a similar age, whether so treated or not.

While the exact cause of endometriosis remains an enigma, it is now apparent that immunologic dysfunction is a significant feature of this disease. Whether immunopathology is causally linked to this condition or whether it occurs in response to endometriosis is unknown. Regardless, the underlying immunologic disorder adversely impacts on implantation. However, it is possible, by means of thorough and meticulous evaluation, to quantify, typify, and, thereupon, selectively treat the underlying immunopathology. In so doing, IVF pregnancy rates can be significantly improved.

Asherman's Syndrome

Asherman's syndrome is a condition characterized by the presence of intrauterine adhesions that often destroy most of the basal layer of the endometrium from which, under the influence of estrogen and progesterone, the endometrium develops. When most of the basal endometrium is incapacitated so that virtually no regeneration of the endometrium can take place, cessation of menstruation and infertility follow.

Asherman's syndrome most commonly results from postpartum or postabortal endometritis; but it can also occur following uterine surgery, such as removal of fibroid tumors that encroach upon or penetrate the uterine cavity.

Treatment involves a procedure called hysteroscopic resection, whereby a telescope-like instrument is introduced via the vagina and cervix into the uterine cavity to allow direct surgical resection of scar tissue. The objective is to remove as much scar tissue as possible and to free adhesions that fuse the walls of the uterine cavity, so as to uncover and enable viable basal endometrium to resume growth and progressively cover as much of the surface of the uterine cavity as possible. Postoperatively, a small balloon is often placed in the uterine cavity for a day or two to keep the opposing surfaces separated in the hope of preventing recurrence of adhesions. The woman usually receives supplemental estrogen to encourage endometrial growth.

Endometritis severe enough to produce Asherman's syndrome usually scars and blocks the uterine entrance to the fallopian tubes. However, sometimes one or both tubes remain open (although there is usually some degree of damage to the inner lining). While in such cases the uterus is often incapable of allowing proper embryo implantation, implantation could occur in a fallopian tube, leading to an ectopic pregnancy.

Unfortunately, with Asherman's syndrome there is such widespread destruction of the basal endometrium that improving blood flow with (vaginal) Viagra is often unsuccessful in improving estrogen-mediated endometrial development sufficient to achieve adequate endometrial growth. In such cases, the women should consider stopping all treatment and adopting or attempting gestational surrogacy.

Diethylstilbestrol (DES) and Reproductive Failure

It is well recognized that prenatal exposure to diethylstilbestrol (DES) sometimes results in reproductive failure. Tubal (ectopic) pregnancies, miscarriages, premature labor, and both male and female infertility are all relatively prevalent in the offspring of women exposed to DES during the first half of pregnancy. It is important to recognize however, that only 30% of women prenatally exposed to DES experience these problems.

Diethylstilbestrol is a synthetic (man-made) hormone with profound estrogen-like properties. However, its chemical structure bears no similarity whatsoever to that of natural estrogen. Natural estrogen is a lipid (fatty) substance with a "steroid structure" while DES is a non-lipid chemical containing a "stilbene nucleus." DES is very similar in structure to the fertility agent clomiphene.

In order for a natural hormone such as estrogen to exert a biological effect, it must first engage the cell surface at specialized sites called receptors. These receptors are uniquely specific for each hormone. It so happens that DES paradoxically has great affinity for estrogen receptors and is even capable of displacing estrogen from its own receptor sites. It is, accordingly, not surprising that the development of reproductive structures such as the upper vagina, cervix, uterus, and fallopian tubes, and sperm ducts in the male, all of which are dependent upon maternal estrogen for their development, are adversely influenced by exposure to DES. The structures referred to above share a common embryologic origin. They are all derived from the Mullerian system, which undergoes maximal development during the third and fourth months of pregnancy. Accordingly, exposure to DES during this critical period often adversely affects development of the upper vagina, cervix, uterus, fallopian tubes, and male sperm ducts. This could explain why the severity of reproductive abnormalities caused by prenatal DES exposure varies dependent upon the exact time and duration of exposure during the first half of pregnancy. For example, it is highly unlikely that the offspring of women who ingested DES for a brief period of time during early pregnancy would have severe developmental abnormalities of the reproductive tract, while the offspring of women who were exposed to DES for an extended period of time extending through the third and fourth months of pregnancy would be very likely to be affected.

DES was prescribed in the late '50s and early '60s for the purpose of preventing miscarriages. Some women with a history of previous miscarriages were prescribed DES in the hope of preventing spontaneous abortion from occurring in the current pregnancy. In a number of such cases (the minority), the administration of DES was continued beyond the second and third month of pregnancy (i.e., the critical period of Mullerian development). The offspring of these women were highly likely to develop serious DES-related complications. Fortunately, in the majority of cases DES was only prescribed for a brief period of time during the second month of pregnancy while the woman was experiencing vaginal bleeding (a threatened miscarriage) and was discontinued when bleeding stopped. These women usually did not ingest DES during the critical phase of Mullerian development and accordingly the reproductive function of their offspring was left unaffected. This probably explains why most DES exposed individuals do not experience reproductive failure.

Women who experience reproductive failure due to DES exposure often exhibit characteristic abnormalities of their reproductive tracts. These include structural deformities of the upper vagina and cervix, as well as the presence of glandular tissue (normally absent in the vagina and outer cervix) referred to as vaginal adenosis. The cervical canal, which connects the vagina to the uterine cavity, is often long and distorted in DES-affected women whose uterine cavities are often disproportionately short and distorted. Moreover, the walls of the DES uterus tend to be more fibrous. Perhaps this results in reduced ability of the DES uterus to stretch and is responsible for the high incidence of premature births.

The abnormal uterine cavity associated with DES exposure can be readily demonstrated through the performance of a dye X-ray (a hysterosalpingogram) which often reveals a T- or butterfly-shape rather than a normal rounded pear-shaped appearance.

The fallopian tubes of the DES daughter are also often deformed. They tend to be shorter than normal and have an abnormal inner structure. The typical longitudinal folds of the inner lining of the normal fallopian tube are often absent, irregular, or distorted, a possible explanation for the high ectopic (tubular) pregnancy rate associated with DES anomalies.

It is important to emphasize that the ovaries are not of Mullerian origin and are accordingly unaffected by prenatal DES exposure. DES daughters usually ovulate normally; have normal blood hormone levels, and perfectly normal temperature charts. It is probably for this reason that the cause of reproductive failure sometimes goes undetected in such cases.

The above-mentioned structural abnormalities explain most of the serious reproductive complications that occur in women who were exposed to DES prenatally. However, these anomalies do not completely explain the relatively high incidence of early and recurrent spontaneous miscarriages that so commonly occur in association with DES uterine anomalies. Recent research has demonstrated that prenatal DES exposure at the critical period of Mullerian development might permanently alter the structure and function of estrogen receptors, rendering them permanently incapable of responding appropriately to natural estrogen in later life. This could explain why the uterine lining (endometrium) and cervical lining of DES daughters often fail to respond appropriately to estrogen. Our own research has confirmed that women with obvious Mullerian anomalies secondary to prenatal DES exposure commonly present with cervical mucus insufficiency and a thin endometrial lining in spite of normal blood estrogen concentrations around the time of ovulation. The poor quality cervical mucus and thin uterine linings might explain the high incidence of infertility associated with DES anomalies. The thin uterine lining is likely responsible for the relatively high incidence of early miscarriages. Perhaps the poor thickness and quality of the uterine lining compromises healthy implantation and development of the placenta (placentation) that is essential for early fetal development and growth.

The close structural similarity between DES and clomiphene citrate could explain why the administration of clomiphene to DES daughters is more likely to result in an inadequate uterine lining and abnormal quality cervical mucus than in non-DES affected women and probably explains the low pregnancy rate associated with such therapy in these cases. We have demonstrated in non-DES exposed women, that prolonged usage of clomiphene citrate for more than three months in a row (back-to-back) almost invariably results in progressive and often profound thinning of the uterine lining as well as cervical mucus insufficiency, thereby producing a relative "contraceptive effect." We have further observed that this tendency is far more profound when clomiphene is administered to women with DES Mullerian anomalies and accordingly rarely recommend the administration of clomiphene citrate in such cases.

And so it is that "ill-conceived" administration of DES to women more than forty years ago, without clear evidence of potential benefit, resulted in serious reproductive consequences to their offspring. Perhaps we will learn an important lesson from this tragedy, one that calls upon the medical profession to resist the temptation of administering medications to patients simply on anecdotal grounds. We should insist upon concrete evidence of benefit before recommending the administration of untried therapeutic regimens if we are to avoid a repetition of the DES disaster.

The thin uterine lining associated with DES uterine abnormalities can sometimes be successfully treated with vaginal Viagra suppositories. In fact, the first woman ever to conceive with IVF following such treatment had experienced a restoration of her uterine lining with vaginal Viagra therapy.

Ectopic Pregnancy

By definition, an ectopic pregnancy is a gestation that occurs outside of the uterine cavity. The most common site is in the fallopian tube, but sometimes it can also occur in the ovary, the cervix, or even the abdominal cavity. Estimates put the incidence of ectopic pregnancy at about 1 in 200 pregnancies; but it has been reported to occur in about one out of 30 pregnancies resulting from in vitro fertilization. Ectopic pregnancy is one of the most dangerous complications of pregnancy. If undetected, the ectopic pregnancy will continue to grow and will ultimately burst through the wall of the fallopian tube, often resulting in catastrophic intra-abdominal bleeding, which can even be fatal.

The introduction of sophisticated ultrasonographic and hormonal monitoring technology now makes it possible to detect an ectopic pregnancy much earlier than previously, usually well in advance of it rupturing. A decade or two ago, the diagnosis of an ectopic pregnancy, ruptured or not, was an indication for immediate laparotomy to avoid the risk of catastrophic hemorrhagic shock. This often resulted in the affected fallopian tube having to be completely removed, sometimes along with the adjacent ovary.

In the late 1980s, early conservative surgical intervention by laparoscopy began replacing laparotomy (a wide incision made in the abdominal wall) for the treatment of ectopic pregnancy, often allowing the affected fallopian tube to be preserved and shortening the period of post-surgical convalescence. In the '90s, early detection combined with the advent of medical management with methotrexate (MTX) has all but eliminated the need for surgical intervention in the majority of patients. If administered early enough, MTX will allow spontaneous resorbtion of the pregnancy and a dramatic reduction in the incidence of catastrophic bleeding. This was especially true in ectopic pregnancies arising from in vitro fertilization, where the early progress of pregnancy is usually carefully monitored with hormone levels and ultrasound.

Causes of Ectopic Pregnancy. The fertilization of the human egg normally takes place in the fallopian tube. The embryo then travels into the uterus, where it implants into the endometrial lining 6–7 days after ovulation. Anything that delays the passage of the embryo down the fallopian tube can result in the embryo hatching and sending its "root system" into the wall of the fallopian tube and initiating growth within the tube. One of the most common predisposing factors is pelvic inflammatory disease (PID) in which microorganisms, such as chlamydia and gonorrhea, damage the inner lining (endosalpinx) and eventually also the muscular walls of the tube(s) by the formation of scar tissue. The endosalpinx has a very complex and delicate internal architecture, with small hairs and secretions that help to propel the embryo toward the uterine cavity. Once damaged, this lining can never regenerate. This is one of the reasons why women who manage to conceive following surgery to unblock fallopian tubes severely damaged by PID have about a 1:4 chance of a subsequent pregnancy developing within the fallopian tube (ectopic).

Congenital malformations of the fallopian tube, associated with shortening of, or small pockets and side channels within, the tube are capable of interrupting the smooth passage of the embryo down the fallopian tube, are another cause of an ectopic pregnancy.

A woman who has had one ectopic pregnancy has almost four times as great a risk of an ectopic in a future pregnancy and with every subsequent ectopic this risk increases dramatically.

Since the lining of the fallopian tube does not represent an optimal site for healthy implantation, a large percentage of pregnancies that gain early attachment to its inner lining will usually be absorbed before the woman even knows that she is pregnant. This is often referred to as a tubal abortion.

Clinical presentation. Classically, women with an ectopic pregnancy present with the following symptoms:

1. *Missed menstrual period(s).* Although some patients will have spotting or other abnormal bleeding. The pregnancy test will be positive in such cases.

2. *Vaginal bleeding.* When a pregnancy inadvertently implants in the fallopian tube, the lining of the uterus undergoes profound hormonal changes associated with pregnancy (primarily associated with the hormone progesterone). When the embryo dies, the lining of the uterus separates. Initially, vaginal bleeding is dark and usually is quite scanty, even less than with a normal menstrual period. In some cases of ectopic pregnancy bleeding is more severe, similar to that experienced in association with a miscarriage. This sometimes leads to an ectopic pregnancy initially being misdiagnosed as a miscarriage and is the reason to examine the material that is passed vaginally, for evidence of products of conception.

3. *Pain.* In the early stages this is typically cramp-like in nature, located on one or another side of the lower abdomen. It is caused by spasm of the muscular wall of the fallopian tube(s). When a tubal pregnancy ruptures the woman will usually experience an abrupt onset of severe abdominal pain followed by light-headedness, coldness, and clamminess and will often collapse due to shock. Her pulse will become rapid and thready (weak and rapid) and her blood pressure will drop. Sometimes the woman will experience pain in the right shoulder. The reason for this is that blood along the side of the abdominal cavity finds its way to the area immediately below the diaphragm, above the liver (on the patient's right side), irritates the endings of the phrenic nerve, which supplies that part of the diaphragm. This results in the referral of the pain to the neck and the right shoulder. The clinical picture is often so typical that making the diagnosis usually presents no difficulty at all. However, with less typical presentations the most important conditions to differentiate from an ectopic pregnancy are a ruptured ovarian cyst, appendicitis, acute pelvic inflammatory disease (PID), or an inevitable miscarriage.

4. *Diagnosis.* The easiest and most common method of diagnosing an ectopic pregnancy is by tracking the rate of rise in the blood

levels of hCG. With a normal intrauterine pregnancy, these usually double every two days throughout the first few weeks. While a slow rate of increase in blood hCG usually suggests an impending miscarriage, it might also point to an ectopic pregnancy. Thus the hCG blood levels should be followed serially until a clear pattern emerges.

A vaginal ultrasound examination usually will clinch the diagnosis by showing the ectopic pregnancy within a fallopian tube and if the tube has already ruptured or internal bleeding has occurred, ultrasound examination will inevitably detect the presence of free fluid in the abdominal cavity.

If there has been a significant amount of intra-abdominal bleeding, irritation of the peritoneal membrane will cause the abdominal wall to become hard, tense, and, depending on the amount of internal bleeding, abdominal distention will be evident. Palpation of the abdominal wall will evoke significant pain and when a vaginal examination is done, movement of the cervix will produce excruciating pain, especially on the side of the affected fallopian tube.

Surgical Treatment. In questionable situations laparoscopy is usually performed for diagnostic purposes. If an ectopic pregnancy is in fact detected, a small longitudinal incision over the tubal pregnancy will allow its removal, without necessitating removal of the tube (linear salpingotomy). Bleeding points on the fallopian tube can usually be accessed directly and appropriately ligated (tied) via the laparoscope. Sometimes the damage to the fallopian tube has been so extensive that the entire tube will require removal.

On occasions where very severe intra-abdominal bleeding heralds a potential catastrophe, a laparotomy (an incision made to open the abdominal cavity) is performed to stop the bleeding post haste. In such cases a blood transfusion is usually required and may be life saving.

Medical Treatment. The introduction of Methotrexate (MTX) therapy for the treatment of ectopic pregnancy has profoundly reduced the need for surgery in most patients. MTX is a chemotherapeutic that kills rapidly dividing cells, such as those present in the "root system" of the conceptus. Extremely low doses of MTX are used to treat ectopic pregnancy. Accordingly the side effects that are often associated with such chemotherapy used for the treatment of other conditions are seldom seen. It is important to confirm that the ectopic pregnancy has not yet ruptured prior to administering MTX.

MTX is given by intramuscular injection. Prior to its administration, blood is drawn to get a baseline blood hCG level. After the injection of MTX the patient is allowed to return home with strict instructions that she should always have someone with her and never be alone in the ensuing week. The concern is that were the patient to be on her own and an intra-abdominal bleed were to occur, she might not readily be able to access someone who could get her to the hospital immediately. Instructions are also given to look for early signs that might point towards severe intra-abdominal bleeding, such as the sudden onset of severe pain, light-headedness, or fainting.

The patient returns to the doctor's office four days later to check the blood hCG level. Three days later (7 days after MTX), the level is checked again. By this time the hCG level should have dropped at least 15% from the value on day 4. If not, a second MTX injection is given and the blood levels are tested twice weekly until hCG level is undetectable. Once this occurs, vaginal bleeding will usually ensue within a week or two.

It is important to note, especially in cases where more than one embryo or blastocyst has been transferred to the uterine cavity, that implantation may occur in two sites simultaneously (i.e., in the fallopian tube as well as inside the uterine cavity). This is referred to as a heterotopic pregnancy. It is therefore important that before administering MTX, which will cause the death and absorption of any early pregnancy, that the physician makes certain that he/she is not dealing with a heterotopic pregnancy. In such cases, surgery is required to treat the tubal ectopic, while every precaution is taken to protect the pregnancy growing within the uterine cavity.

Recent advances in the field of ultrasound diagnosis along with the introduction of MTX therapy have revolutionized the treatment of ectopic pregnancy and have significantly reduced both the high morbidity and mortality rates previously associated with this condition.

When an ectopic pregnancy occurs following infertility treatment, there is the added advantage that the physician will be on the lookout for the earliest possible signs of trouble. The performance of a vaginal ultrasound within two weeks of a positive blood pregnancy (hCG) test following IVF allows for early detection of the unruptured pregnancy and timely intervention with MTX and/or laparoscopy.

Thrombophilias

Thrombophilia is the inherited tendency to develop blood clots. Thrombophilias are due to either the presence of too much of certain blood-clotting factors or too little of anti-clotting proteins in the blood. As many as one in five people in the United States has a thrombophilia.

Most women with a thrombophilia have healthy pregnancies. However, the thrombophilias can contribute to a number of pregnancy complications, including pregnancy loss (that most commonly occurs in the second or third trimester), placental abruption (when the placenta separates from the uterine wall, partially or completely, before delivery), and poor fetal growth. The thrombophilias also may cause preeclampsia, a pregnancy-related disorder characterized by high blood pressure and protein in the urine that can pose serious risks for mother and baby. Several of these problems are believed to result from blood clots in placental blood vessels that lead to changes in the placenta and reduced blood flow to the fetus.

Pregnant women in general are more likely than non-pregnant women to develop a venous thrombotic episode (VTE), or development of a blood clot in a vein. This is due to normal pregnancy-related changes in blood clotting in order to limit blood loss during labor and delivery. And pregnant women with a thrombophilia are at a higher risk than other pregnant women of developing a VTE. Studies suggest that more than half of pregnant women who develop a VTE have an underlying thrombophilia.

All pregnant women who have had a blood clot should be offered testing for hereditary thrombophilias. In addition, women with a family history of blood clots, pulmonary embolism (blood clot in the lung), or strokes that occurred prior to age 60; or a history of pregnancy complications, including stillbirth, early or severe preeclampsia, placental abruption, or poor fetal growth due to undetermined causes may be considered for testing.

Some pregnant women with thrombophilia are treated with one or more daily injections of low dose heparin, a blood-thinning drug, which does not cross the placenta and is safe for the baby. In some cases, physicians may recommend low doses of aspirin along with heparin. Low-dose aspirin with the B vitamins folic acid, B6, and B12 can be given to women who have one of the milder thrombophilias and a history of pregnancy complications, but not a history of blood clots.

Not all pregnant women with a thrombophilia need heparin treatment during pregnancy. Regular heparin can be supplanted with a newer form of heparin, called low-molecular-weight heparin (Lovenox and Clexane), that appears to pose a lower risk of side effects such as bone loss and can be injected once instead of twice daily (as with regular heparin) and which reduces the risk of local bruising, significantly.

Generally, treatment is not recommended for most pregnant women with one of the less severe thrombophilias (such as factor V Leiden or prothrombin mutation) and no history of blood clots or pregnancy complications. This is because the risk of blood clots or pregnancy complications due to thrombophilia appears to be less than 1 percent in these women. However, treatment may be recommended for about six weeks after birth, when the risk of blood clots may be highest, if the woman has a strong family history of blood clots or if she has had a cesarean delivery.

Heparinoid (heparin, Lovenox, Clexane) treatment is recommended throughout pregnancy and the postpartum period for women who have one of the more severe thrombophilias (e.g., homozygous MTHFR mutation, Protein C deficiency and Factor 11 G20210A), even if they have not experienced any blood clots or pregnancy complications. Women with a thrombophilia (regardless of severity) who have a past history of blood clots are usually treated with heparin during pregnancy and the postpartum period. *Warfarin* (also a blood-thinning drug) may be used safely in addition to, or instead of, heparin in the post-partum period and during breastfeeding. However, it is not recommended during pregnancy because it can cause birth defects.

As yet, no proven cause and effect relationship has been shown to exist between thrombophilia and failed embryo implantation, poor IVF outcome, and/or early recurrent miscarriages.

Polycystic Ovarian Syndrome (PCOS)

Polycystic ovarian syndrome (PCOS) occurs in 5-10% of women of reproductive age. The condition is characterized by abnormal ovarian function (irregular or absent periods, abnormal or absent ovulation and infertility), androgenicity (increased body hair or hirsutism, acne), and increased body weight–body mass index or BMI. The ovaries of women with PCOS characteristically contain multiple micro-cysts often arranged like a "string of pearls" immediately below the ovarian surface (capsule) interspersed by an overgrowth of ovarian connective tissue (stroma). PCOS women often have a family history of diabetes and demonstrable insulin resistance (evidenced by high blood insulin levels and an abnormal 2-hour glucose tolerance test). This underlying Diabetes mellitus tendency could play a role in the development of PCOS and contribute to the development of obesity, an abnormal blood lipid profile, and a predisposition to coronary vascular disease. Women with PCOS are slightly more at risk of developing uterine, ovarian, and possibly also breast cancer in later life and accordingly should be evaluated for these conditions on a more frequent basis than would ordinarily be recommended to non-PCOS women.

Most women with PCOS either do not ovulate at all or they ovulate infrequently and irregularly. As a consequence they usually experience delayed, absent, or irregular menstruation. In addition, an inordinate percentage of the eggs produced by PCOS women following ovulation induction tend to be chromosomally abnormal (aneuploid). Rather than being due to an intrinsic egg defect inherent in PCOS women, the poor egg quality is more than likely the result of over-exposure to male hormones (predominantly testosterone) produced by the ovarian stroma. These two factors (ovulation dysfunction and poor egg quality) are the main reasons for the poor reproductive performance (infertility and an increased miscarriage rate) in PCOS women.

PCOS patients are at an inordinate risk of severely over-responding to fertility drugs, both oral varieties (e.g., Clomid, Serophene & Femara) and especially the injectables (e.g., Follistim, Puregon, Gonal F, Menopur, and Bravelle) by forming large numbers of ovarian follicles. This can lead to life-endangering complications associated with severe ovarian hyperstimulation (OHSS). In addition PCOS women receiving fertility drugs often experience multiple ovulations, putting them at severe risk (40%+) of high-order multiple pregnancy with often devastating consequences.

Types of Polycystic Ovarian Syndrome:

1. *Hypothalamic-pituitary PCOS.* This is the most common form of PCOS and is often genetically transmitted and is characteristically associated with a blood concentration of Luteinizing Hormone (LH) that is uncharacteristically much higher than the Follicle Stimulating Hormone (FSH) level (FSH is normally higher than the LH concentration) as well as high-normal or blood androgen (male) hormone concentrations (e.g., androstenedione, testosterone, and dehydroepiandrosterone (DHEA)). Hypothalamic-pituitary-ovarian PCOS is also associated with insulin resistance in about 40%-50% of the cases.

2. *Adrenal PCOS.* Here the excess of male hormones are derived from overactive adrenal glands rather than from the ovaries. Blood levels of testosterone and/or androstenedione is raised but here, the blood level of dehydroepiandrosterone (DHEAS) is also raised, clinching the diagnosis.

3. *Severe pelvic adhesive disease, secondary to severe endometriosis, chronic pelvic inflammatory disease, and/or extensive pelvic surgery.* Women who have this type of PCOS tend to be less likely to hyperstimulate in response to ovulation induction. Here DHEAS is also not raised.

Treatment

Hypothalamic-pituitary-ovarian PCOS: *Ovulation induction* with fertility drugs such as clomiphene citrate, Letrozole (Femara) or gonadotropins, with or without intrauterine insemination (IUI) is often highly successful in establishing pregnancies in PCOS women. However, IVF is fast becoming a treatment of choice (see below). In about 40% of cases, 3–6 months of oral *Metformin* (Glucophage) treatment results in a significant reduction of insulin resistance, lowering of blood androgen levels, an improvement in ovulatory function, and/or some amelioration of androgenous symptoms and signs.

Surgical treatment by "ovarian drilling" of the many small ovarian cysts lying immediately below the envelopment (capsule) of the ovaries, is often used, but is by and large unsuccessful. At best, it is merely temporarily effective. The older form of surgical treatment, using ovarian wedge resection is rarely used any longer as it can produce severe pelvic adhesion formation.

Adrenal PCOS is treated with steroids such as prednisone or dexamethasone, which over a period of several weeks will suppress adrenal androgen production, allowing regular ovulation to take place spontaneously. This is often combined with clomiphene, Letrozole and/or gonadotropin therapy to initiate ovulation.

PCOS attributable to Pelvic Adhesive Disease is often associated with decreased ovarian reserve (DOR). In many such cases, high dosage of gonadotropins (FSH-dominant) with "estrogen priming" will often elicit an ovarian response necessary for successful ovulation induction and/or IVF. Neither steroids nor Metformin are helpful in the vast majority of such cases.

TUBAL SURGERY VERSUS IVF: AN "APPLES AND ORANGES" COMPARISON

Blockage of the fallopian tubes is one of the most common causes of infertility. As explained earlier in this chapter, tubal damage is often caused by PID, endometriosis, previous abdominal surgery (especially due to a

Note: PCOS women undergoing ovulation induction usually release multiple eggs following the hCG trigger and are thus at inordinate risk of twin or higher-order multiple pregnancies. They are also at risk of developing OHSS. Many now believe that IVF should be regarded as a primary and preferential treatment for PCOS. The reason is that it is only through this approach that the number of embryos reaching the uterus can be controlled and in this manner the risk of high-order multiples can be minimized and it is only in the course of IVF treatment that a novel treatment method known as "prolonged coasting" (see below) which prevents OHSS, can be implemented.

ruptured appendix or ruptured ovarian cyst), or ectopic pregnancy.

Even if procedures such as laparoscopy or HSG determine that the tubes are patent, with a history of PID there is likely to be damage within the tube that destroys its normal functions. PID is one of the most common causes of tubal damage that almost always affects both tubes, and even if one tube is open it is still highly likely to be functionally compromised. While surgery can open tubes, it cannot restore normal function. Tubal disease, especially if it is due to PID, is best treated by IVF.

In the case of hydrosalpynx (the fallopian tubes are distended with fluid), tubes so affected must be ligated at the junction with the uterus or removed lest they compromise IVF outcome. Removal (salpingectomy) is preferable to ligation because it is the only sure way to avert pain and complications in the long run.

In my opinion, given the high success rates in good IVF programs, surgery to repair damaged tubes, with few exceptions, can no longer be justified financially or ethically. Other than tubal reanastomosis (surgical reconnection of the fallopian tubes, usually performed after a previous tubal ligation), the only time that tubal surgery would occasionally enhance the ability to conceive is when the fimbriated ends of the fallopian tubes are normal. Without functional fimbriae, it is highly unlikely that an egg would find its way from the ovary into the fallopian tube. For example, surgically reopening the end of a blocked fallopian tube (often eliminating the fimbriae) provides relatively little hope for the infertile couple. In such cases, the woman often stands less than a 20 percent chance of having a baby within two years of tubal surgery, whereas the same woman would have better than double the chance after a single attempt at IVF performed in an optimal IVF program. In addition, such major surgery carries with it prolonged hospitalization, the risk of complications, increased cost, and lost time away from work, incapacitation, and significantly greater discomfort.

A reasonable birthrate of about 40 percent can be expected within two to three years of reproductive surgery to remove adhesions surrounding the fallopian tubes as long as the fimbriae and the insides of the tubes are otherwise normal. Women under 35 under such circumstances still may choose surgery over IVF in such cases, provided they are willing to allow two to three years for the surgery to have a good chance to work. It is, however, a reality that more than 80 percent of women who undergo tubal surgery for the treatment of infertility will ultimately require IVF.

As long as insurance companies in the United States reimburse for about 80 percent of the costs of tubal surgery but are often unwilling to fund IVF, and as long as consumers remain uninformed about the benefits of IVF, most couples will still select tubal surgery over IVF for financial reasons. Two-thirds of all tubal surgeries performed in the United States are still being done in cases where for all practical purposes the fallopian tubes have been irreparably damaged. In the remaining one-third, tubal surgery is more appropriately performed to free adhesions around the fallopian tubes and ovaries, remove fibroid tumors, and treat endometriosis.

Actually, comparing tubal surgery with IVF is a futile exercise. How can a procedure such as IVF, where success rates are determined on the basis of a single menstrual cycle of treatment, be compared with tubal surgery, in which evaluation of the success rate per procedure requires a wait-and-see approach that often spans two or more years? Three or four attempts at IVF, performed even in the average IVF setting, are likely to result in a higher success rate than any form of tubal surgery.

The insurance environment surrounding IVF in the United States can be expected to ultimately change if current legislative and judicial trends continue (see chapter 15). As more lawmakers and courts direct insurance carriers to fund IVF, the popularity of IVF will inevitably surpass that of most forms of tubal surgery. We predict that when the financial burden is eliminated, virtually all women would choose IVF in preference to undergoing major tubal surgery.

Table 9-1 Tubal Surgery vs. IVF

	Tubal Surgery	IVF
Risk of complications	+	-
Cost (out-of-pocket)	+	++
Risk of ectopic pregnancy	++	-

+ = moderate

- = almost absent

++ = great

Another point to be considered is that a 3 percent tubal or ectopic pregnancy rate occurs following IVF pregnancy, as compared with approximately a 20% risk following the performance of tubal reconstructive surgery.

10

IS IVF THE MOST APPROPRIATE OPTION?

WHEN DOES THE MAN'S FERTILITY STATUS DEMAND CONSIDERATION FOR IVF?

Evaluation of male fertility revolves around assessing the quality of the sperm, which must be thoroughly evaluated by all possible methods before the couple resort to IVF. This interactive process, which requires cooperation among the urologist, the reproductive endocrinologist or gynecologist, the laboratory, and the couple, has three stages: (1) The urologist seeks specific pathological causes for poor semen quality so therapy can be directed at improving it, (2) the laboratory performs tests that evaluate sperm function and often can enhance the sperms' ability to fertilize an egg, and (3) IVF/ICSI can be used if necessary to achieve fertilization.

Male infertility can be treated by surgically repairing anatomical defects in the reproductive tract or by administering hormones to stimulate the testicles. In rare situations, a disease outside the reproductive tract that hinders sperm production may be corrected medically or surgically. In other cases, there may be very severe structural problems within the sperm ducts brought about by infection, trauma, or even surgery, such as a vasectomy. In cases of total absence of sperm production due to improperly developed testes, usually very little can be done to improve male fertility. When the sperm ducts are blocked, surgical methods can sometimes restore patency; but this does not necessarily mean even if the man can subsequently produce an adequate amount of sperm that he will be able to initiate pregnancy. If the cause of the man's infertility is not correctable through minor surgery or administration of hormones, IVF/ICSI becomes the option of choice.

The probability of successful fertilization occurring either within the petri dish or within the fallopian tube is lower when male-factor infertility is present because as the total number of normal, motile sperm decreases, the fertilization rate also declines. However, the introduction of ICSI has changed all that. Without question, ICSI has made IVF the treatment of choice for moderate or severe male infertility that is unresponsive to simple medical or surgical correction. Now it is possible to achieve the same fertilization and birthrates in cases of male infertility as with indications for IVF. Furthermore, even men who produce no sperm at all in their ejaculates can produce sperm by means of testicular sperm extraction (TESE) or testicular sperm aspiration (TESA), followed by ICSI on their partner's eggs, and still father their own children.

We state categorically that because of dismal success rates in cases of moderate or severe male infertility, intrauterine insemination (IUI) is inadvisable in such cases.

Many of the tests that the male partner of a couple considering IVF should undergo for the purpose of assessment and possible treatment of sperm function are discussed below.

Semen Analysis

The sperm's morphology (percentage of normally shaped sperm), configuration, motility (ability to travel through the reproductive tract and fertilize an egg), and count (number produced in a semen specimen) can be determined under the laboratory microscope in a standard semen analysis or, as is now much more commonly the case, by computerized evaluation. Sperm that appear to be normally shaped are more likely to fertilize an egg, while those with obvious structural abnormalities are less likely or perhaps cannot do so at all. Sophisticated testing may be necessary if the problem cannot be readily identified. However, it is possible for the man to be fertile even when the percentage of normal sperm is low.

Varicocele

The urologist looks for anatomical abnormalities, evidence of obstruction in the scrotum, and physical signs of infection. One anatomical abnormality would be a varicocele, an enlargement of veins in the scrotum, which results in elevated temperatures around the testes that may harm sperm production. In carefully selected cases, tying off or occluding these veins under X-ray visualization may improve semen quality.

A varicocele is a collection of dilated veins in the scrotum. It can surround one testicle or be or present around testes. To the touch, a varicocele feels like a "bag of worms." Varicoceles do in some cases compromise sperm function. This is believed to be due to increased blood flow that increases the local temperature to the point of compromising sperm motility and compromising sperm maturation. Contrary to popular belief, varicoceles seldom reduce sperm count. In fact in cases of low-sperm count, treatment of the varicocele rarely results an improvement in sperm production. It is important to recognize that the majority of men who have varicoceles will have NO evidence of sperm dysfunction.

As stated, when a varicocele causes sperm dysfunction, this most commonly manifests as reduced motility and/or sperm progression as well as a high percentage of "immature sperm forms ("a stress pattern"). Often, a Sperm Chromatin Structure Assay (SCSA) will show an increase in the DNA Fragmentation Index (DFI). In such cases the likelihood of a viable pregnancy occurring naturally or following intracytoplasmic sperm injection (ICSI) will be reduced.

Traditional treatment is surgical (varicocelectomy) aimed at occluding dilated blood vessels by tying off one or both spermatic veins. While surgery is usually curative, the post-surgical recurrence is quite common. Another approach is interventional radiological obliteration of the spermatic vein(s). This is a less costly, less traumatic outpatient procedure that is also less likely to result in recurrence. In my view it in fact represents the preferred method of treatment.

Regardless of whether surgery or interventional radiology is contemplated, it is always advisable for the patient to take a male fertility blend that is rich in antioxidants. This will often result in an improvement in the DFI within 3-6 months. An example of such a regime can be found in products such as Proceptin or ProXeed, which should be taken for at least 12 weeks whereupon the SDIA should be repeated.

It is important to bear in mind that surgical or radiological treatment will only be likely to improve sperm function in about 35% of men who have varicocele. Understandably, it is tempting to attribute a cause and effect relationship to fertility problems and a varicocele. But, the truth is that the existence of a varicocele is often coincidental (unrelated) to the underlying cause of the infertility.

The following, in my opinion, represent situations where treatment of a varicocele (whether surgical or radiologic) is unlikely to resolve the male fertility issue:

1. When the man has an elevated blood FSH level (greater than 12 MIU/ml)
2. In cases where there is a persistently low sperm count (<20million/ml)
3. When the SCSA shows a DFI of below 30%. In such cases ICSI is the best approach.

Obstruction of the Vas Deferens or Epididymis

When the sperm count is zero and the FSH is normal, the cause may be due to obstruction of the vas deferens or epididymis. If so, TESE/TESA addresses the problem (see below).

Hormonal Problems

If the sperm count or motility initially appears to be abnormal, the physician should determine whether hormonal problems are the cause. This might require extensive blood testing to evaluate the function of the thyroid gland, the output of the pituitary gland, and the secretion of sex hormones by the testicles into the man's blood. In cases of absent sperm in the ejaculate (azoospermia), measurement of blood FSH levels will usually permit distinguishing between testicular failure and obstruction of sperm ducts. If the FSH is elevated, it points to the former, while if the FSH is normal, it is suggestive of the latter (i.e., obstruction). Similarly, in cases of oligospermia (low sperm count), the detection of an elevated FSH suggests intractable testicular failure, while a low FSH level is suggestive of potentially reversible (using clomiphene gonadotropins) under-production of sperm by the testes.

The Zona-Free Hamster-Egg Penetration Test—Sperm Penetration Assay (SPA)

An older, somewhat outmoded technique known as the zona-free hamster-egg penetration test sometimes can help determine whether the sperm are likely to fertilize healthy eggs. In this test, the sperm are placed in a laboratory dish along with hamster eggs from which the eggshell-like zona pellucida has been removed. Then the number of sperm that penetrate the eggs are counted and evaluated. Failure to penetrate a sufficient percentage of eggs may indicate severe male infertility. (Although hamster eggs can be penetrated by human sperm, they will not cleave and develop into viable embryos.)

One of the drawbacks of the zona-free hamster-egg penetration test is that it may produce misleading results. For example, a small percentage of women whose partners failed the hamster test subsequently get pregnant. In other cases, the test results will appear to be normal although the man's fertility is severely impaired. Because this test has a high potential for error, various laboratories may interpret it differently, with conflicting results.

Testicular Sperm Extraction (TESE) or Testicular Sperm Aspiration (TESA)

TESE/TESA enables men with sperm duct blockage due to trauma, inflammation, a previous vasectomy, or *azoospermia* (no sperm in the ejaculate due to poor testicular sperm production) to father a child through IVF almost as if there were no obstruction to sperm passage at all. The procedures have rendered surgical vasectomy reversal in men with long-standing vasectomies (10 years or more) totally unnecessary. TESE and TESA are both simple, low-cost, safe, and relatively pain-free. Most men can literally take off a few hours for the procedure and return to normal activity soon thereafter. And unlike vasectomy reversal, the procedure allows the man to retain his vasectomy for future contraception purposes.

TESE involves the introduction of a needle through the skin of the scrotum directly into the testicle(s), a 15- to 30-minute procedure usually under local anesthesia. Hair-thin specimens of testicular tissue are removed, sperm is extracted from the tissue, and a single sperm is injected into each egg using ICSI. TESA involves direct aspiration of sperm via the needle inserted into a sperm duct. Following successful TESE/TESA the fertilization rate is 70 percent when ICSI is performed in centers of excellence. The IVF birthrate per TESE procedure performed on women under 40 in these centers is better than 40 percent (i.e., no different than conventional IVF birthrates in women of comparable age). When TESE is performed on men with azoospermia, pregnancy rates are halved.

Microsurgical Epididymal Aspiration (MESA)

MESA involves making an incision in the scrotum and exposing the small sperm-collecting ducts on the surface of the testicles. Sperm is aspirated through a needle inserted into these ducts. The method is much more traumatic and invasive than are either TESE or TESA and only has a place in cases where it is intended to collect enough sperm to perform IVF/ICI with some sperm left over for freezing.

An Abnormal SCSA

An abnormal SCSA (see Chapter 8) augers poorly for but does not totally preclude a successful IVF/ICSI pregnancy. However, the prognosis worsens progressively as the age of the egg provider advances beyond 35 years. Selective surgical or medical treatment can sometimes cause the SCSA to revert to normal, such as antioxidant therapy taken for 10 to 12 weeks. Men who have varicoceles associated with an abnormal SCSA may experience a reversion of the SCSA to normal from three to six months following surgical or radiological excision of the varico-cele. In rare cases, abnormal SCSA results revert to normal spontane-ously. Upon reversion of the SCSA to normal, sperm is collected and cryopreserved for later use. If, in spite of treatment (which presently should be regarded as being in the experimental realm) a grossly abnor-mal SCSA fails to revert to normal, the use of donor sperm becomes an option, especially where the egg provider is over 35.

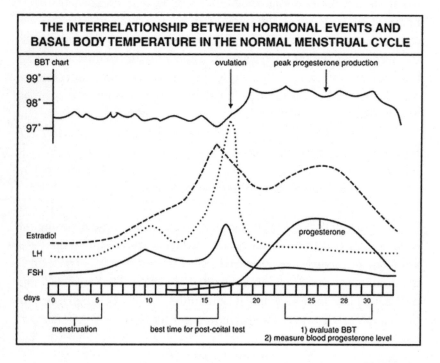

Figure 10-1

WHEN IS THE WOMAN READY FOR IVF?

As with the man, defining the cause of a woman's infertility requires careful analysis of her history and a clinical examination by a fertility specialist. Three areas need to be carefully assessed: (1) the pattern of ovulation, (2) the anatomical integrity of the reproductive tract, and (3) the status of the cervical mucus.

The Pattern of Ovulation

As explained in Chapter 2, a woman is unlikely to conceive unless she ovulates at the right time in the proper hormonal environment. Reliable evidence of ovulation can only be obtained by examining the woman's ovaries through a laparoscope, by repeated ultrasound examinations around the time of presumed ovulation (to detect a collapsed follicle and/or some follicular fluid pooled in the abdominal cavity), or—the only really reliable way—by confirming a pregnancy with ultrasound.

It is important to remember that the purpose of assessing ovulation is not simply to determine whether the woman ovulated but whether she ovulated at the proper time, within the proper hormonal setting, and if the lining of the uterus is properly prepared. While the following tests will not provide conclusive evidence that the woman has ovulated, they will help the physician determine how well synchronized these vital components are during the luteal phase (second half) of the menstrual cycle. These tests are valuable indicators of the appropriateness of ovulation and the hormonal environment when their results are considered together.

The BBT chart. One way to assess the pattern of ovulation is by compiling a daily body temperature chart. The woman does this by taking her oral temperature each morning before she gets out of bed and before she has anything to drink. She then charts her temperature on a basal body temperature (BBT) chart. The pattern on the chart will mirror the output of the hormone progesterone by the corpus luteum in the ovary. A woman's temperature begins rising about 12 to 24 hours following ovulation, and this rise will be sustained through the rest of the menstrual cycle (when the ovaries are producing hormones to prepare the endometrium). In other words, the woman's temperature goes up when progesterone is produced and stays up until its levels drop with the demise of the corpus luteum. This phenomenon occurs because progesterone acts on the biological thermostat in the brain that regulates body temperature, setting it one notch higher when progesterone is being produced and lowering it at or just before the beginning of the menstrual period. As long as the temperature is up, it can be assumed that progesterone is present.

Because ovulation usually occurs 14 days before the expected menstrual period, the woman's temperature will usually be about 0.5°–1°F higher during the last two weeks of her cycle. A biphasic pattern such as this (the first phase is lower than the second phase) suggests ovulation. It is not important whether the increase is sudden or gradual.

Figure 10-1 shows how the biphasic BBT pattern is synchronized with hormone production, ovulation, and other aspects of the menstrual cycle. Estrogen levels in the blood (including estradiol, as shown in figure 10-1) peak at the time of ovulation. This triggers the LH surge and to a lesser extent a synchronous rapid rise and fall in the FSH levels. The woman ovulates eight to 36 hours after LH is first detected in the urine by home ovulation testing. About a day later the temperature rises. The estrogen level falls progressively immediately prior to and for a few hours following ovulation and then rises again, only to drop precipitously immediately prior to menstruation. Measurable amounts of progesterone first appear in the bloodstream around the time of ovulation and then escalate during the second half of the menstrual cycle and, as with estrogen levels, also drop sharply preceding the onset of menstruation.

All of these hormonal interrelationships are orchestrated by the follicle, which contains the developing egg and produces estrogen. Immediately after ovulation, the follicle collapses and forms the corpus luteum, which during the second half of the menstrual cycle produces both estrogen and progesterone. The corpus luteum has a natural life span of about 12 to 14 days, whereupon its failure causes the abrupt fall in estrogen and progesterone levels cited above. This results in a withdrawal of the hormonal support of the endometrium, thereby precipitating menstruation. Should pregnancy occur, the corpus luteum's survival is prolonged, estrogen and progesterone levels continue to rise, and menstruation is deferred (see Chapter 2).

The BBT chart, therefore, (1) indicates that the hormonal events associated with ovulation have occurred and that the woman presumably released an egg from her ovary and (2) provides a rough idea about when ovulation occurred and the length of the second half of the cycle. Nothing more should be read into the chart, however. It is a misconception that the BBT chart can precisely pinpoint the ideal time for intercourse.

The cervical mucus begins to thicken rapidly a few hours following ovulation and becomes almost impenetrable to sperm within 24 to 48 hours after ovulation. As the temperature rises around the same time, the likelihood that pregnancy will occur when natural intercourse is timed with the temperature rise is remote. Therefore, the thinking behind the old scenario of the woman saying, "Hurry home, honey, my temperature has risen and we should try and have a baby!" is without foundation. By that time, it will already be too late to get pregnant. It is far better to time intercourse with the onset of the LH surge as determined by urine testing as the detection of LH in the urine precedes ovulation by eight to 36 hours, a time when the condition of the cervical mucus should be optimal.

Regular menstrual periods. Regular menstrual periods associated with breast tenderness and, often, mood changes preceding the onset of the periods, and some discomfort (cramping) during menstruation are all clinical indications that the woman is likely to be ovulating.

Urine Ovulation Tests. Since the surge of the hormone LH triggers ovulation, detection of LH in the urine suggests that ovulation has probably occurred. The woman can easily take this urine test at home around the time of ovulation by performing one of the commercially available home ovulation tests on a sample of her urine. The actual time of ovulation can be predicted by daily, twice daily, or even more frequent performance of the test and charting of the results. It should be kept in mind that there is a two- to four-hour lag before the urine test will reflect the surge of LH in the bloodstream (see figure 10-1).

LH blood-hormone test. An LH blood-hormone test done several times daily around the time of presumed ovulation (at least 14 days prior to the menstrual period, or when the temperature goes up) is a relatively sophisticated indicator of likely ovulation. This is related to the fact that the LH surge in the middle of the cycle precedes ovulation.

When women used to undergo IVF in natural, unstimulated cycles or when they were given clomiphene citrate without hCG (which acts like an artificial surge of LH), it was necessary to measure LH by repeated blood tests. This series of tests was necessary in order to pinpoint the time of expected ovulation so the eggs could be retrieved before they were ovulated into the fallopian tube or abdominal cavity. Today, the dipstick urine tests that measure the excretion of LH are accurate enough. Serial LH blood testing, which is expensive, time-consuming, and painful, has been virtually supplanted by serial urine LH testing to pinpoint ovulation.

Endometrial biopsy.   An endometrial biopsy, which can be performed in a doctor's office, evaluates the condition of the lining of the uterus. In this relatively painless procedure the physician inserts a small curette or suction apparatus into the uterus a few days prior to expected menstruation and removes a sliver of the endometrium for examination under the microscope. If the endometrium is secretory, indicating the effect of the progesterone, it is likely that the woman has already ovulated. A pathologist is frequently able to pinpoint almost to the day when ovulation is likely to have occurred by microscopically examining the secretory endometrium.

It is also possible to determine whether the endometrial sample is appropriately developed for the stage of the menstrual cycle at which it was taken, thus providing yet another parameter of whether ovulation is occurring in the proper hormonal environment. It is important to remember that although estrogen is not measured in this test, progesterone can act only on a lining that has been stimulated by estrogen. So if microscopic examination shows that the endometrium development is in sync in the middle of the luteal phase, it can be assumed that estrogen stimulation was adequate as well. By combining the endometrial biopsy with measurement of blood or urine hormone levels, it is possible to further refine the evaluation of ovulation.

Progesterone blood-hormone test.   The most common indicator of presumed ovulation is the level of the blood hormone progesterone in the woman's blood, as measured a few days before her anticipated menstrual period. This test usually will indicate whether or not the woman is likely to have ovulated, again because progesterone is typically only present in significant amounts in the bloodstream after ovulation.

Analysis of both the LH and progesterone values measures not only whether these hormones are present but also the appropriateness of their levels in the blood relative to the time of the cycle (see figure 10-1).

The bottom line. It is important to view all these tests in context. For example, (1) the blood progesterone level of a week or so prior to menstruation may suggest that ovulation has occurred, (2) a microscopic examination of an endometrial biopsy done a few days prior to menstruation might show that the endometrium has responded appropriately to progesterone, and (3) the length of the luteal phase (as gauged from the urine dipstick test or temperature rise on the BBT chart to the onset of menstruation) was 13 to 14 days. This would indicate a good luteal phase (proper length, enough progesterone, and a normal uterine lining).

The opposite situation might be, on day 25 of the cycle: (1) an endometrium typical of day 19, (2) a significantly lower-than-normal progesterone level a week before menstruation, and (3) a luteal phase of about nine days. This would suggest possible corpus luteum insufficiency and/or insufficient stimulation of the endometrium. In this case the luteal phase is too short, the endometrial response is inappropriate for the timing of the cycle, or the hormonal environment is inadequate. The presence of any of these parameters will lead to the diagnosis of an abnormal hormonal environment. Administration of fertility drugs such as clomiphene, hMG gonadotropins, and hCG will often regulate the pattern of ovulation so that most women with such problems can have a reasonable chance of conceiving. Therefore, ovulation problems alone do not require IVF as a solution.

Evaluating the Anatomical Integrity of the Female Reproductive Tract

Since pregnancy can occur only when the reproductive system does not inhibit the passage of sperm, eggs, and embryos, an abnormality within the tract is likely to interfere with the woman's ability to conceive. Careful analysis of her medical history, including any previous venereal diseases, infections following the use of an IUD, and the results of previous fertility tests may suggest the presence of an abnormality such as damaged fallopian tubes, endometriosis, or fibroid tumors. However, defects in the reproductive system can only be confirmed through tests such as those outlined below.

Hysterosalpingogram (HSG).   The hysterosalpingogram tests the patency of the fallopian tubes and the shape of the uterus. During the HSG procedure the physician injects a dye into the uterus via the vagina and cervix. The dye shows up as a shadow on an X-ray. The HSG can identify a blockage in the fallopian tubes and may also point out some obvious abnormalities inside the uterus. These could include fibroid tumors, scarring, and abnormalities of uterine development that might occur spontaneously or as a result of DES exposure during the woman's own prenatal development.

The major shortcoming of the HSG is that its usefulness is limited to assessing the shape of the uterine cavity and the patency of the fallopian tubes. It is not a reliable method for detecting small surface lesions in the uterine cavity (e.g., polyps, scarring, and small uterine fibroids that protrude into the cavity). Nor does the HSG yield any information about the ovaries. In other words, fertility problems in which the inside of the fallopian tubes and uterus may appear perfectly normal but where the fallopian tubes are unable to retrieve the eggs from the ovaries because of surrounding scar tissue or ovarian tumors cannot be diagnosed by an HSG. Also, an HSG cannot diagnose endometriosis, in which case the fallopian tubes are usually open.

Women who undergo an HSG should be aware that the procedure is relatively painful, often causing severe cramping. In addition, there is about a 2 percent risk that the dye could convert a dormant infection into a full-blown pelvic inflammation. Women should also be aware that infection can be introduced if the procedure is not performed using the proper sterile technique. Finally, because non-water-soluble dyes tend to collect in damaged tubes and produce infection and complications, there has been a move away from using such dyes. However, the iodine solution in both water-soluble and non-water-soluble dyes can also cause reactions.

Laparoscopy.   One way to both assess the patency of the fallopian tubes and examine the pelvic cavity is by inserting a laparoscope through a small incision in the abdomen. It enables the physician to look inside the abdominal cavity and perform surgery at the same time. The physician can directly visualize the patency of the fallopian tubes during laparoscopy by injecting a colored, water-soluble (non-iodine) solution into the uterus through the vagina and cervix, and observing the fluid's passage through the fallopian tubes. It is also possible to microscopically examine the ends of the fallopian tubes through the laparoscope. Conditions such as endometriosis and pelvic adhesions can be diagnosed with confidence only by laparoscopy or laparotomy, which often afford the opportunity for the physician to treat the problem surgically at the same time. Laparoscopy is usually performed as an outpatient procedure with the patient under general anesthesia. Laparoscopy has largely replaced the HSG as the most popular method of assessing the anatomical integrity of the reproductive tract.

Hysteroscopy. *Hysteroscopy* is a procedure where a telescope-like instrument is inserted via the vagina through the cervical canal into the uterine cavity for evaluation of the interior of the uterus. It is an important procedure because it allows for diagnosis and treatment of surface lesions inside the uterine cavity that adversely affect the ability of an embryo to attach to the uterine lining. Such lesions are often missed in the performance of an HSG.

Surgical procedures to correct defects can be done hysteroscopically. This usually requires prior distension of the uterus with a fluid. Laser-directed procedures can also be performed through the hysteroscope, thereby reducing the chance of bleeding. Therapeutic hysteroscopy has eliminated much of the need for major abdominal surgery, along with its incumbent risks.

Diagnostic hysteroscopy is performed in the office under intravenous sedation, general anesthesia, or paracervical block, with minimal discomfort to the patient. This procedure involves the insertion of a thin, lighted, telescope-like instrument known as a hysteroscope through the vagina and cervix into the uterus in order to fully examine the uterine cavity. The uterus is first distended with a sterile clear solution (usually physiologic saline) or with carbon dioxide gas, which is passed through a sleeve adjacent to the hysteroscope.

The diagnostic hysteroscopy facilitates examination of the cervical canal and the inside of the uterus under direct vision for defects that might interfere with implantation. Conditions such as fibroid tumors, polyps, bands of scar tissue, or congenital abnormalities can readily be detected. Because we have observed that approximately one in eight candidates for IVF has lesions that require attention prior to undergoing IVF in order to optimize the chances of a successful outcome, we strongly recommend that all patients undergo hysteroscopy or the performance of an FUS exam (see below) so that any lesions so detected can be treated surgically before initiating ART.

Therapeutic hysteroscopy requires general anesthesia and should be performed in an outpatient surgical facility or conventional operating room where facilities are available for laparotomy, a procedure in which an incision is made in the abdomen to expose the abdominal contents for diagnosis. Therapeutic hysteroscopy is usually combined with laparoscopy.

Fluid ultrasonography-FUS (Sonohysterogram). *Fluid ultrasonography* (FUS), or *sonohysterogram*, is a simple and relatively painless procedure whereby a sterile solution of saline is injected via a catheter through the cervix and into the uterine cavity. The fluid-distended cavity is examined by vaginal ultrasound for any irregularities that might point to surface lesions such as polyps, fibroid tumors, scarring, or a uterine septum. FUS is highly effective in identifying even the smallest intrauterine lesions and can supplant diagnostic hysteroscopy in the preparation of women for IVF. Moreover, FUS is much less expensive than, less traumatic than, and equally as effective as diagnostic hysteroscopy. The only disadvantage lies in the fact that if a lesion is detected, treatment of the problem may require the subsequent performance of hysteroscopy anyway.

When Should One Consider Surgery to Correct Anatomical Defects?

In most cases, the physician would first attempt to correct defects in the reproductive tract by the least traumatic form of surgery, probably through the laparoscope or hysteroscope. Today almost all pathologic conditions of the uterus, fallopian tubes, or surrounding structures that compromise fertility are accessible to laparoscopic or hysteroscopic surgical treatment. Except for women under 35 who have had a tubal ligation for sterilization purposes, any anatomical defect that cannot be corrected using the laparoscope or hysteroscope probably requires IVF. Laparotomy for tubal disease is fast becoming a thing of the past.

The advisability of corrective surgery on the fallopian tubes depends on the situation. If a young woman has had a tubal ligation for the purpose of sterilization and now wants her fallopian tubes reconnected, tubal microsurgery may be her best option, depending on whether (1) the entire tube was destroyed in the process, (2) there is enough of the tube remaining on either end to allow reconnection, (3) the fimbriated ends of the fallopian tubes are intact, and (4) previous surgery has caused scarring around the tube that inhibits normal egg pickup by the fimbriae.

Condition of the Cervical Mucus

Cervical mucus insufficiency causes about 5 percent of all infertility problems. Some of the causes of cervical mucus problems include previous surgery for cervical cancer, which sometimes destroys the mucus-producing glands of the cervix, and excessive freezing (cryocautery) of the cervix because of lesions, early cancer, or exposure to drugs such as DES while the woman was inside her mother's womb. Women with DES exposure will likewise also be unable to produce a lush endometrial lining in spite of normal ovulation and normal blood estrogen levels prior to ovulation.

Cervical mucus evaluation at ovulation. The simplest way to evaluate the cervical mucus is to examine the woman around the time of presumed ovulation. At the appropriate time the physician inserts a speculum in the woman's vagina, retrieves some cervical mucus, and evaluates the physical-chemical properties that normally occur in the mucus at ovulation. Healthy cervical mucus should be clear, stringy (stretchy), and should form a fernlike pattern when dry.

Postcoital test (PCT), or Hühner test. At the same time the physician may conduct a postcoital test (PCT), or Hühner test, to assess the interaction of the mucus and sperm. The woman should have inter-course from six to 18 hours before her appointment. Then the physician will take a mucus sample from her cervical canal via a catheter and examine the mucus on a slide under the microscope.

The PCT assesses the number of sperm in the mucus and evaluates their motility. The presence of a large number of sperm moving in a linear and purposeful fashion usually indicates that the mucus is healthy. The PCT is a good screening test because it provides a rough evaluation of the quality of the sperm as well as of the cervical mucus. At the same time, a less favorable postcoital test does not necessarily indicate a cervical-mucus deficiency because the sperm could be at fault. It should be borne in mind that the most common causes of a poor postcoital test are the following:

1. Poor timing of the test. If the test is performed more than 12 hours after ovulation has occurred, the cervical mucus may have become thick and tenacious, thereby preventing the invasion of sperm. Accordingly, the postcoital test should be performed immediately prior to or at the time of ovulation. The best method of ensuring that the timing is correct is by performing daily home ovulation urine testing, which will show a color change eight to 36 hours prior to the occurrence of ovulation.

2. Male infertility because the male partner has a low sperm count

3. Inflammation of the cervix (cervicitis)—often due to ureaplasma, chlamydia, gonorrhea, or other organisms

4. The presence of sperm antibodies in the woman's or the man's reproductive secretions

5. Destruction or absence of the cervical glands because of surgery or infection, which will limit the amount of cervical mucus produced and also adversely affect its quality, thereby yielding a poor postcoital test

6. The prior use of clomiphene citrate for more than three consecutive months. In the case of clomiphene citrate being used in women over 40, a hostile cervical mucus is often observed in the very first cycle of stimulation.

7. A DES abnormality of the reproductive tract (see Chapter 9), which is commonly associated with poor mucus production

Tests of the cervical mucus and blood for antibodies. If analysis of the cervical mucus at ovulation and a postcoital test are not sufficient, the physician may look for sperm antibodies in the cervical mucus and blood. In such cases it may be necessary to culture the mucus or analyze the blood for various microorganisms that might have destroyed the cervical glands' ability to produce the proper mucus.

IVF SHOULD BE CAREFULLY WEIGHED AGAINST ALL OTHER OPTIONS

Factors that should be considered when deciding between alternative procedures and IVF include (1) success rates of the various procedures, (2) financial considerations, (3) physical toll, (4) emotional investment, and (5) the insistent ticking of the biological clock, which may mandate quick action if ovarian failure for the woman is imminent.

With alternatives to IVF, especially surgical options, a woman is usually given long-range hope: "Now that you've had your operation, let's see how you do in the next two to three years." There is always the possibility that during those 24 to 36 months she will not conceive. And gradually coming to terms with failure in such circumstances is an easier, slower adjustment than it would be with IVF. With IVF, the time frame is compressed into one month; and when a couple fails to conceive during one treatment cycle, they know immediately they have nothing to show for their efforts. The emotional impact is far greater with IVF. It is abrupt and painfully traumatic. Accordingly, couples should decide whether other alternatives that require a lengthy period of anticipation might be more appropriate for them before embarking on IVF. But when couples choose IVF over other assisted reproductive technologies, the rewards can be great.

The following comments from two first-time parents in their mid-forties describe how repeated failures at pregnancy shaped their attitude toward IVF:

> ***Husband:*** *We started trying to have a baby when there wasn't anything like IVF available. We went through all the different*

fertility tests, and sometimes we gave up temporarily and then decided to try again. We had a lot of disappointments.

   Wife: *If it hadn't been for my husband I would never have tried IVF, because I was so tired of being let down. But he said if you don't try you have nothing. It was hard emotionally to go through IVF, to relive those hopes and risk getting hurt again, but I'm so glad I did. We have a three-month-old daughter now who has dramatically changed our lives.*

Procreation—and with it the ability to achieve immortality by living on through one's children—is an inalienable right as well as one of the most insatiable human needs. This strong natural urge exerts tremendous pressure on couples unable to have a baby. And the pressure to reproduce becomes increasingly acute as couples grow older and become more aware of their own mortality.

Although IVF offers hope to many infertile couples who until recently had no way of conceiving, it is not a panacea for every couple who want a baby. In addition, every IVF procedure exacts an emotional, physical, and financial price from both partners. No one gets through the process without paying the toll. All couples considering IVF should learn what they can reasonably expect from it before they commit to the procedure. Once they have shaped realistic expectations about their probable experiences, they are ready to decide whether IVF is truly for them.

11

SHAPING REALISTIC EXPECTATIONS ABOUT IVF

WHAT ARE A COUPLE'S REALISTIC CHANCES OF SUCCESS?

The following profile fits the ideal candidate/couple for IVF:

1. The woman is under 40.
2. The egg provider has at least one healthy ovary capable of responding normally to fertility agents (a low FSH and a normal Inhibin B on the third day of the cycle).
3. The uterus and endometrial lining of the embryo recipient are normal and capable of sustaining a healthy pregnancy.
4. The egg provider has been pregnant in the past, thereby proving that her eggs can fertilize.
5. There are no alloimmune impediments to implantation.
6. The sperm provider has motile sperm and a normal SCSA.

These criteria are not absolute, however. For example, in many cases the adverse effect of advancing age on egg and hence embryo quality could in part be offset by transferring a greater number of embryos to the woman's uterus, thereby permitting natural selection to determine which embryos are healthy enough to implant. Alternatively, the application of advanced technologies such as assisted fertilization through ICSI might promote fertilization in cases associated with sperm dysfunction, or assisted hatching might possibly improve implantation potential in cases where the zona pellucida enveloping the embryo is too thick or resistant, as is now believed to occur with advancing age.

Here is a practical example. Let's say a woman is 34 years old, her partner has normal sperm function, and following stimulation with fertility drugs eight eggs are retrieved from her ovaries. She has a normal uterine cavity, as assessed by FUS, and an excellent endometrial lining, as evaluated by ultrasound. Such a woman would, in an optimal IVF setting, have about a 50 percent chance of conceiving following a single IVF cycle of treatment.

Now, if the same woman had a male partner with sperm dysfunction, but by employing ICSI the physician was able to transfer two good quality embryos to her uterus, she could be expected to have the same chance of getting pregnant regardless of male infertility. High technology, by improving the chances of fertilization, has offset the adverse effect of sperm dysfunction on outcome.

Here is another example. Let's say the woman is 40 years old with (apart from her age) exactly the same optimal circumstances as the younger woman described above. Her chances of pregnancy would be significantly reduced because of the adverse effect of age on egg and embryo quality. Her chances of having an IVF baby after one attempt in the same setting would be about 25 percent if two good-quality blastocysts are transferred. Here, an age-related embryo-quality deficiency has been partly offset by transferring a greater number of embryos. It could be argued that she might have a strong chance of a multiple pregnancy if so many embryos were put into her uterus. But this is not necessarily the case because most of her embryos would likely be rendered aneuploid and thus "incompetent" by age and thus would not propagate a viable pregnancy. Effectively, only one out of the eight cleaved embryos or about 1 in 4-5 blastocysts might be healthy enough to produce a baby. Therefore, couples who are contemplating IVF should initially base their realistic expectations for success on those criteria that have the potential to predict outcome, and then temper their expectations with the realization that many of the adverse factors can be partially overcome. However, it is not always possible to overcome severe deficiencies. For example, embryos may never be able to implant into a uterus with surface lesions, such as fibroid polyps that protrude into the uterine cavity, or severe scarring in the uterine cavity due to previous infection. Such conditions would interfere with implantation.

Each couple and their physician, then, must assess these criteria, given their own unique set of circumstances and the environment of the IVF program they have selected, to determine their own realistic expectations of getting pregnant.

THE COUPLE MUST BE SURE THEY ARE TRYING TO CONCEIVE FOR THE RIGHT REASONS

Both partners owe it to themselves, each other, and their unborn child to examine what they expect to achieve from parenthood and what they are willing to contribute before they get on the IVF roller coaster. Successful parenting is usually rooted in a stable relationship and a sincere desire for children. An infertile couple that embarks on the IVF journey without first considering their motivation can end up with problems even worse than the infertility problem that brought them into IVF in the first place. The addition of a baby to a troubled relationship will compound existing problems as well as create new ones.

Some childless women/couples get caught up in the pursuit of pregnancy because they have an idealized picture of what it would be like to have a baby. They are so intent on proving they can conceive that they lose sight of how their lives will change when a baby becomes part of the family. They may not fully consider whether they are willing to adapt their lifestyle to accommodate a child's demands on their time, energy, mobility, an d financial situation—from babyhood on. They must be sure they are not trying to have a child to please someone else—a mother who has always wanted a grandchild, for example. Each partner should feel comfortable knowing that it is okay not to have children at all if either or both prefer to be child-free. Granted, it is often difficult to come to terms with family and societal pressures, but it can be done.

But when a woman/couple want(s) a baby for the right reasons, family and friends are likely to share in the joy over the baby's birth. As one new IVF mother reported:

We've had nothing but total support from our entire family. They call Caryn the "miracle baby." Friends I went to high school with have called or sent cards, and people I don't even know have sent gifts. We're very proud that we went through IVF and that she's here.

The woman's mother expressed her feelings about her daughter's IVF experience with these words:

My daughter tried for seven years to get pregnant. I was beginning to feel I was never going to have a grandchild, and I worried through the whole nine months of her pregnancy. But IVF was marvelous for all of us. It was very exciting, very satisfying.

The woman's father, who was concerned about the procedure's effect on his daughter, was won over after the baby's birth:

My daughter had undergone tubal surgery and laparoscopies and so much pain that I thought if IVF failed it would be so defeating for her. I wondered if it was going to be worth it. Of course now I can see that it was well worth it. I just didn't want to see her undergo any more traumas.

And the new mother's best friend told us:

When you have friends who have had infertility problems for years, you suffer with them. You feel guilty about the pleasure you're having from your own family every time they come to visit. So we all feel like Caryn is our baby. She's theirs, but they still have to share her because we've shared all the pain with them.

Couples who choose IVF for the right reasons are likely to reap the greatest rewards from parenthood. They are often the most committed of all parents because they are making the greatest sacrifice to have a baby.

IVF IS AN EMOTIONAL, PHYSICAL, AND FINANCIAL ROLLER-COASTER RIDE

The biggest decision an infertile couple will ever make in regard to IVF is whether or not they really want to become parents. Once they agree that they are committed to parenthood, they must next decide whether they are ready to deal with the emotional, physical, and financial consequences of their actions.

Both Partners Must Share in the Emotional Cost

An IVF procedure requires an enormous emotional commitment at each level of the program, whether or not IVF is successful. This has a permanent impact on the couple. Because the toll can be so great, both partners must be committed to supporting each other from the very beginning.

Based on the statistics reported by our program at the time of this writing, approximately 50 percent of women under the age of 39 who undergo IVF at our program will likely conceive and about 40% are likely to have a baby following a first attempt at embryo transfer. For women between 39 and 42, the comparable rate is about 30 and 20 percent. The success rate falls sharply after age 43 (to single digits) that these women would probably be best advised not to undergo IVF with their own eggs and to resort to ovum donation instead.

The comparable chance of a baby being born following one cycle of IVF performed in an optimal setting using donor eggs (provided the donor is younger than 35 and the recipient has a normal uterine cavity) is about 55–60 percent, regardless of the birth mother's age. The success rate for the second attempt is about the same as for the first. Success rates tend to decline after the third failed attempt.

Only twenty years ago the existence of sperm dysfunction roughly halved the anticipated success rates in all age categories and circumstances. However, since the introduction of ICSI, good IVF programs are achieving almost the same success with IVF performed in cases associated with sperm dysfunction as when the procedure is undertaken using normal sperm. ICSI has virtually (but not completely) leveled the playing field.

Some women who fail on the first three tries do in fact get pregnant after four or more attempts. Therefore, it is realistic to be cautiously optimistic. But the couple should also be realistic enough to prepare themselves emotionally so that they are not overwhelmed by failure in case IVF does not succeed.

The IVF Procedure Is Stressful

Both partners should be prepared to respond to a variety of emotionally stressful demands as they undergo IVF:

1. Dealing with the general stress "baggage" (shame, guilt, anxiety, depression, anger) they bring into the program because of their long-standing battle with infertility.
2. Following new procedures; interacting with a strange and sometimes impersonal clinical staff, perhaps with a constantly changing cast of characters.
3. Living in an unfamiliar environment: different state or country (many couples travel from another state or country to undergo IVF in a good program), different daily schedule, time-zone changes, separation from their normal support network.
4. Coping with the unpredictable emotions that the fertility drugs trigger in the woman.
5. Reacting to family and marital stress, which may be heightened by the constant need for mutual support.
6. Managing the financial aspects of the procedure.

Couples react to the demands of IVF in strikingly different ways. One expectant mother thought the stimulation phase of her second IVF treatment cycle (her first cycle had ended in an ectopic pregnancy) was the most stressful:

> One of the most difficult things I went through was the roller-coaster ride waiting for the estradiol level. Would it be

*high enough? Would I have enough eggs? Would I have to be on
another day of fertility injections? It was really the most exhausting part of the entire process.*

Fortunately, she produced three eggs and had two embryos transferred (as opposed to five during the first attempt), and she since went
on to deliver a healthy little girl.

The mother of a one-month-old IVF son also found the waiting to
be most trying:

*The expectation between each step was difficult for me. But
waiting for the pregnancy test—that was the hardest part!*

In contrast, the mother of IVF triplets said:

*I was at the point of giving up, and then found new hope
through IVF. I was so excited—exhilarated—through the whole
process that the time just flew by.*

IVF-related stress cannot be entirely avoided, but it can be mitigated
by a staff that helps normalize or demystify the experience as much
as possible. The creation of an environment where all the couples are
"like me" can be encouraging to the anxious IVF couple. In addition,
the opportunity to talk with other couples undergoing the procedure
or with representatives of a support group may be helpful. Finally, the
services of an in-house counselor can be particularly beneficial.

A Realistic Attitude toward Miscarriage (See Chapter 14 for Information on Recurrent Pregnancy Loss (RPL))

It is important to remember that the miscarriage rate after IVF is
probably no higher than in nature. The reason the IVF miscarriage rate
sometimes appears to be higher is that an IVF pregnancy is diagnosed
long before it normally would be in the case of a natural pregnancy.
Most women who conceive on their own do not test themselves for

pregnancy until they have missed their period, whereas with IVF the diagnosis of pregnancy is made before the woman misses a period. One should remember, however, that a pregnancy is not confirmed until the presence of a gestational sac has been diagnosed by ultrasound. If this criterion is used to verify pregnancy, then the miscarriage rate with IVF is no greater than that of the population at large.

Painful as it is to the couple, miscarriage can have a positive side. It is reasonable to expect that although a successful pregnancy was not possible on the first try, the fact that they proved they could initiate a pregnancy means that their overall chances of having a baby will increase on subsequent IVF attempts.

A Realistic Attitude toward Ectopic Pregnancy

When an ectopic pregnancy occurs following infertility treatment, the physician should be on the lookout for the earliest possible signs of trouble (see Chapter 9). The performance of a vaginal ultrasound within two weeks of a positive blood pregnancy (hCG) test following IVF allows for early detection of the unruptured pregnancy and timely intervention with MTX (methotrexate) and/or laparoscopy.

Ectopic pregnancies sometimes occur after IVF when the fluid in which the embryos are ejected from the catheter during embryo transfer drains into a fallopian tube, carrying the embryos with it. The risk of ectopic pregnancy following IVF is only about 3 percent.

A Realistic Attitude toward IVF Success

Couples must realize that no matter how hard they try to become pregnant, they cannot control the outcome of IVF. There is nothing they can do to influence whether they succeed or fail. When couples become so intent on trying to conceive that they lose sight of the other aspects of their relationship, one clinical coordinator reminds her patients to "lighten up" a bit by writing them prescriptions for candlelight and wine.

The father of triplets, meeting with a group of other IVF couples, commented:

All of us have one thing in common—we've been through the highs and lows of I VF. My wife and I represent the high! But it wasn't always easy for us. I can't emphasize enough how important it is for everyone to keep their chin up through the whole procedure.

Another man, holding his one-month-old son in his arms, added:

I would encourage everyone definitely to maintain a positive attitude. The hardest part of the whole procedure is dealing with failures. It's inevitable that when the first IVF attempt fails you just stop wanting to try because you don't want to fail again. If you could just keep it in perspective and know IVF is a trial-and-error scientific procedure and sometimes you just have to expect problems, that will help a great deal.

A Realistic Attitude toward IVF Failure

It is important for couples to realize that there is little the woman can do to influence outcome following IVF in either a positive or negative way. Women often tend to blame themselves when they get a negative result. This is almost always unfounded and counterproductive, but it is also unfortunately relatively inevitable. Appropriate counseling and a good emotional support system can go a long way toward minimizing this misperception.

Coping with IVF's Physical Demands

The physical demands of IVF range from the annoyance of hormone shots and blood tests to the discomfort of egg retrieval for the woman and the need for the man to produce a semen specimen on demand. The couple probably will have undergone a variety of diagnostic procedures to determine the reason for their infertility and thus may already be familiar with some of these demands.

Certainly when compared with tubal surgery, the process of ultrasound egg retrieval presents a minimal degree of risk, discomfort, and complications. However, it is still an emotionally and physically draining experience. In addition, if the woman has selected a program in another state or country, she may undergo additional physical discomfort as a result of the stress of travel, including jet lag and the general disorientation caused by temporarily living in unfamiliar surroundings.

Proper emotional preparation and mutual support throughout the treatment cycle will help both partners cope more effectively with the physical demands on the woman. And they should keep in mind that once the pregnancy is confirmed, the remainder of the gestational period will probably vary little from pregnancies experienced by all other expectant women.

IVF Requires a Significant Financial Commitment

Until IVF is universally funded by medical insurance in the United States, it will continue to be a program for the haves, not the have-nots. This is true even though its cost only really becomes significant when the woman is wheeled into the operating room for egg retrieval. That is when the fees for anesthesiology, surgery, processing and fertilizing the eggs and sperm, and transferring the embryos mount into thousands of dollars within a few days. Until the egg retrieval, the couple only has to pay relatively minimal costs.

However, the cost of attempting to conceive is not usually limited to the IVF procedure. Many couples have learned how high the overall expenses of attempting to conceive can be. As one newly expectant IVF patient said:

> So far we've spent about $80,000 trying to get pregnant, so the IVF portion was really a minor part of the total cost. I first went through reconstructive surgery, then five or six laparoscopies. I shudder to think of the money we spent on airfare to consult with doctors in other cities, plus hotel rooms and meals, to say nothing of all the income we lost by taking so much time away from work. Had we known that my tubes were permanently blocked, we could have saved a lot of money by going directly to IVF. But out

of that $80,000 our insurance company has paid about $35,000,
so we have been pretty lucky financially.

Although this woman considered herself lucky to have paid "only" $45,000 out of her own pocket, a similar outlay would be prohibitive for most other couples. That is why couples contemplating IVF should first determine whether their budget can accommodate all the direct and indirect expenses that IVF entails.

A Realistic Attitude toward Budgeting for IVF

When inquiring about costs at a particular IVF program, the couple should always ask for written quotations that cover all the charges they will incur. This is to avoid any distressing surprises that might be caused, for example, if the program omitted a hefty charge for multiple tests from its price quotation. The couple should not be afraid to ask about items they do not understand.

In addition to the total fee quoted by the program, the couple who must travel from their locality to a program elsewhere should budget generously for the kinds of expenses mentioned above: air or ground transportation, meals, hotels, other travel expenses, allowances for lost income, even babysitters or house sitters while they are on the road. If they plan to visit several IVF programs before selecting one, they should also allow for the expenses they will incur during each site inspection.

In many cases, the couple will have to pay up front for the entire procedure. IVF programs usually request payment in advance in order to avoid problems collecting from the couples who do not get pregnant. Most programs will advise the couple how to bill the insurance company for the reimbursable components of the procedure but will not bill the company directly.

A Realistic Attitude toward Insurance Coverage

Couples should not automatically assume that their insurance will cover the IVF expenses. Reimbursement practices vary from company to company and from state to state. Currently, insurers in less than one-third of the states in the United States offer varying degrees of coverage for IVF. As we have mentioned throughout this book, the attitude of insurance companies with regard to IVF could improve. As one new mother said vehemently:

> We're still waiting for our insurance to pay. It's been over a year since we went through the IVF program, and they just keep making excuses. So far we've only received $670!

The father of triplets expressed his concern about the unfairness of insurance companies that refuse to fund IVF but cover other surgical procedures without question:

> Through all of our infertility treatments, including artificial insemination and surgeries, the insurance companies argued and refused to pay. Then our triplets were born seven weeks premature, and the hospital bill for them and my wife was $188,000! The insurance company said that was no problem and they were going to pay the whole thing.

The financial risk in IVF is great, but the return can be priceless. That is why it is so important for each couple to be absolutely sure of their willingness and financial ability to make such an investment before they attempt IVF. Yet more and more couples are willing to make the financial commitment. Why? When asked if he and his wife had difficulty deciding whether to undergo IVF given its cost and uncertain outcome, one new IVF father responded:

> Well, when you really want children you set your priorities. We think babies are more important than fancy vacations or a sailboat. We were able to budget for IVF. But we're sorry that insurance doesn't usually cover it because a lot of people just can't spend $12,000 to $25,000 or so to go through these procedures.

In Chapter 16 we explain in more detail why most insurance companies still do not reimburse for IVF.

HOW MANY TIMES SHOULD A COUPLE ATTEMPT IVF?

Because of the emotional, physical, and financial toll exacted by IVF, it is preferable that no one undertake a one-shot attempt. If a couple can only afford one treatment cycle, IVF is probably not the right procedure for them. After all, in good programs there is still only about a two-in-five chance that IVF will be successful—and there's a tremendous letdown if it fails.

We believe it is unreasonable to undergo IVF with the attitude that "if it doesn't work the first time, we're giving up." IVF is a gamble even in the best of circumstances. But on average, the ideal IVF candidate (using their own eggs) selecting a premier IVF program is likely to have better than an 80 percent chance within three IVF egg retrievals with fresh embryo transfers and as many FETs as available frozen embryos would allow.

If conventional IVF using own eggs fails, it is important not to proceed further without doing whatever is needed to ascertain the reason for the failure. Then, if in spite of thorough investigation, no definitive cause for failure can be determined, the patient/couple might try one or two additional attempts (certainly not more than 4 in number) and thereupon other options, such as embryo banking IVF egg donation, use of donor sperm, embryo adoption, IVF surrogacy, or adoption need to be considered. However, in my experience, many IVF failures, rather than being "unexplained" are simply "undiagnosed." Here are two examples that illustrate this:

1. A few years ago I treated an Australian woman of 42 years who had undergone 22 prior failed attempts at IVF (using her own eggs). Upon thorough investigation for a cause, I determined that she had an immunologic implantation dysfunction (IID) associated with activation of her uterine natural killer cells (NKa). We treated her for this with (short term) intravenous gamma globulin (IVIg) and corticosteroids. She immediately conceived and went on to deliver a healthy full-term male infant.

2. Another case involved a 37-year-old British patient who had failed three (3) IVF attempts using her own eggs and two (2) attempts using donor eggs, in London, England. We evaluated her and found her also to have IID, and went on to treat this and to perform IVF on her, using her own eggs. Not only did she promptly conceive and deliver a healthy baby, but she returned 18 months later to do another IVF with SIRM and gave birth to another healthy baby. In my opinion, therefore, the time to stop doing IVF would not simply be based upon the number of prior failed attempts. Rather, it should hinge upon whether a potentially treatable reason for the prior IVF failures can be identified and whether the cause is amenable to treatment.

One woman, who eventually adopted a newborn boy, described her disappointment over three failed procedures:

> *It's very difficult to deal with. You go into any of these procedures with the expectation they will work. Somehow we are raised in our society to think that it's not whether you are going to have children, but how many do you want? We plan for our car, and we plan for our house—and assume that the children are going to come. And when they don't, it's devastating. You are basically out of control of your own body.*

Couples who choose to undergo IVF should realize from the outset that the inability to become pregnant should never be considered a reflection on them as individuals. They should view the entire procedure with guarded optimism but nevertheless must be emotionally prepared to deal with the ever-present possibility of failure.

IVF PATIENTS/COUPLES MUST CONSIDER THE POSSIBILITY OF A MULTIPLE PREGNANCY

As we mentioned earlier, patients who are unwilling to settle for a low pregnancy rate must be prepared for the possibility of multiple offspring. With IVF, twins are born in 25 percent of pregnancies and triplets in 3 percent. Compare this to twins once every 80 births and triplets once every 6,000 in natural spontaneous conceptions. It is important to distinguish between the number of multiple births (being discussed here) and the number of multiple pregnancies. This is because most women who are carrying more than twins will opt for pregnancy reduction. Also, many multiple pregnancies reduce spontaneously.

Because the incidence of larger, more hazardous multiple pregnancies is higher with IVF, the couple should be familiar with the concept of selective pregnancy reduction. This trade-off between pregnancy rate and the possibility of multiple births is one of the most important issues involving realistic expectations that couples must resolve.

Selective Reduction of Pregnancy

Some women, because of uterine pathology (e.g., multiple fibroids), surgery, congenital abnormalities, or prenatal exposure to DES, are at risk of premature labor even with a singleton pregnancy. For many such women, carrying twins would likely present an unacceptable risk. However, most women undergoing IVF can usually tolerate and many even covet a twin pregnancy.

A high-order multiple pregnancy (triplets or greater) is another matter altogether, since the increased incidence of prematurity poses an inordinate threat to the well-being of the mother and her babies. What is more, the higher the multiple, the greater the hazard. For the mother, risks include: high blood pressure, uterine bleeding, and surgical complications associated with a cesarean section. For the babies, the risks relate primarily to premature birth; and the higher the multiple, the more premature the birth is likely to be.

It has been determined that in about 40 percent of high-order multiple pregnancies, at least one of the babies is likely to expire or suffer permanently from physical and/or neurologic complications associated with premature birth. For this reason, most IVF programs limit the number of embryos/blastocysts transferred to two or (maybe) three. In cases where a high-order multiple pregnancy occurs, many programs counsel the couple with regard to selectively reducing the multiple pregnancy down to twins and in certain cases, to a singleton. In such circumstances, selective pregnancy reduction could be regarded as a morally justifiable decision aimed at optimizing the quality of life after birth. Furthermore, given the heart-rending nature of the decision, selective pregnancy reduction might even be considered to be laudable.

Selective reduction of pregnancy is usually performed prior to completion of the third month of gestation. It involves the injection of a chemical, under guidance by ultrasound, directly into one or more developing concepti so as to reduce the total number (usually to twins). This is soon followed by absorption of the products of conception by the body. Properly performed by an expert, selective reduction of pregnancy, rarely (2–7 percent of cases) results in total loss of the pregnancy.

SOME COUPLES HAVE MORAL/ETHICAL/RELIGIOUS OBJECTIONS TO IVF

While a discussion of the moral, ethical, and religious dilemmas created by IVF is not within the scope of this book, we would encourage all couples to come to terms with their concerns in this regard before entering an IVF program. No one should be excluded from an IVF program because of religion any more than because of age, race, marital status, or sexual preference. Every case should be assessed on its own merit. The couple should be willing to discuss concerns openly with their physician; the IVF program staff; and their minister, priest, rabbi, or mullah. Sometimes, by working together, it is possible to find approaches that will satisfactorily resolve everyone's concerns.

MATCHING REALISTIC EXPECTATIONS WITH THE RIGHT PROGRAM

Once the couple have realistic expectations about IVF and have decided to undergo the procedure, it is time to select a program. When evaluating potential programs, the couple should expect an IVF provider to meet three basic criteria: (1) provide the highest quality of medical care, (2) ensure that the couple will have the best possible opportunity of conceiving within the guidelines of sound medical practice, and (3) deal with the couple in a manner consistent with the emotional, physical, and financial investment they will make. The following chapter explains how consumers can evaluate IVF programs on the basis of these characteristics.

The infertile couple (or woman) should begin their search for the right IVF program by talking with their own physician and/or a local fertility support group. If there are no fertility support groups in the area, the couple should contact the national headquarters of one of these organizations. They may also wish to talk to couples who have already undergone IVF, as these couples tend to develop a close network and will probably be happy to share their experiences. Contacts made through such networking will likely lead to even more sources of information.

We wish to stress that no matter how strongly the couple feels that time is closing in, it is important to devote a few months to diligent research rather than rushing arbitrarily into the most convenient program.

12

HOW TO FIND THE RIGHT IVF PROGRAM

HOW SHOULD THE SUCCESS OF AN IVF PROGRAM BE EVALUATED?

The process of selecting an IVF program is significantly different from that of choosing a physician, whose credentials alone assure the couple of his or her competence and expertise. First, there is currently no accrediting agency that provides audited, fully verifiable outcome-based information to consumers about an IVF program's competence and success.

The couple should evaluate more than the expertise of just one person. They should also take into account the success rate of all the individuals who operate as a team. For example, a laboratory that is not very successful at fertilization would be a drawback in a program that has a friendly, supportive staff and otherwise presents a reliable, innovative image.

How does one gauge the success of an IVF program? In the broadest terms an IVF program's success can be measured by its:

1. **results** (a track record that is consistent with currently accepted rates for successful IVF procedures)
2. **caring** (the degree to which the couple perceive an attitude of caring manifested by the staff)
3. **staff interaction** (whether there seems to be open, harmonious interaction among the staff involved in the program, and whether the couple feel comfortable dealing with the staff)

4. **reputation** (how the program is regarded by those who have undergone IVF, by the community in which it is situated, by other physicians—and don't forget the program's financial stability).

The only basis for judgment the couple will have when trying to select the most appropriate IVF program is observation of the way the program operates—from initial contact until patient discharge. In order to properly research individual IVF programs, they will first have to learn to understand and interpret the terms and statistics they will probably encounter.

HOW DOES THE PROGRAM DEFINE PREGNANCY?

The word *pregnancy* often means different things to different people. For example, the terms *chemical pregnancy* and *clinical pregnancy* are frequently used interchangeably although they have completely different meanings. It's necessary to understand both of these definitions in order to avoid misinterpreting the statistics that may be quoted.

Chemical Pregnancy

Chemical pregnancy refers to biochemical evidence of a possible developing pregnancy. A positive blood or urine pregnancy test confirms a chemical pregnancy provided that the woman has not received the hormone hCG recently and does not have a tumor that releases hCG into her blood. (See Chapter 7 for a discussion of the quantitative beta hCG blood pregnancy test.)

About 20% of early elevations in blood beta hCG levels following embryo transfer turn out to be chemical pregnancies that subsequently are lost before being clinically confirmed. It is likely that the frequency with which this happens is the same following natural conceptions as with IVF. However, because blood pregnancy tests are rarely performed as early following natural conception as with IVF, the diagnosis is often missed. So what are the causes of chemical pregnancy and post-ultrasound confirmed, early pregnancy loss?

Embryo abnormalities: It is important to recognize that most (>75%) early pregnancy losses are due to embryo "incompetence." This is in large part due to embryo aneuploidy (irregular number of chromosomes). But embryo aneuploidy is by no means the only cause of embryo "incompetence." Certain structural chromosomal, epigenetic, and metabolic factors can (albeit infrequently) lead to chemical pregnancy/early pregnancy loss. It is important to recognize that embryo aneuploidy usually results from egg (rather than sperm) aneuploidy and that the incidence of the latter increases progressively with advancing maternal age. Egg aneuploidy is also more common following ovarian stimulation in women with diminished ovarian reserve (DOR) and women who have polycystic ovarian syndrome (PCOS), especially when, in such patients, high-LH output ovarian protocols (e.g., "flare protocols" with clomiphene and Letrozole or high doses of hCG/LH containing gonadotropins such as Menopur) are used.

Implantation Dysfunction: About 25% of early pregnancy loss results from implantation dysfunction. Here, a non-receptive endometrial environment thwarts optimal permeation of the uterine lining by the embryo's root system (i.e., trophoblast) such that growth is arrested, implantation fails, and the embryo is rejected. Causes include anatomical defects (e.g., endometrial polyps, fibroids, and post inflammatory/surgical scarring), b) poor estrogen-induced endometrial thickening (<8mm), and c) IID.

The first thing to understand is that since embryo aneuploidy is mostly unavoidable and the rate of aneuploidy increases with the age of the egg provider, the best way to identify "competent embryos" is through full embryo karyotyping (e.g., CGH).

However, the selective transfer of CGH-normal embryos, especially when IVF is conducted in women who are the greatest at risk of egg/embryo aneuploidy (i.e., older women, women with DOR, and those with PCOS), can and does minimize the risk of early pregnancy loss, reduce chromosomal birth defects, and can optimize IVF outcome. This is especially apparent in women who because of DOR and/or advancing age produce fewer eggs/embryos. Such women will benefit significantly through "banking" CGH-normal embryos over several

IVF cycles (in advance of embryo transfer) such that once a sufficient number of "competent" embryos have been cryobanked (vitrified) and stockpiled, they can be transferred one or two at a time with a high expectation of a successful IVF birth. Only through such "embryo banking" can the ravages of the biological clock be partially offset.

Failed IVF (negative pregnancy test, chemical pregnancy, and early pregnancy loss) that is due to implantation dysfunction is more amenable to successful preventive treatment than when the cause of failure is due to "embryo incompetence." Here surgical correction of uterine surface lesions, the use of vaginal sildenafil (Viagra) to improve the uterine lining, and selective immunotherapy with heparinoids, corticosteroids and intralipid to treat uterine NK/T-cell activation, often corrects the problem. And in those few cases where all else fails, the use of a gestational surrogate will, by providing a more friendly environment for healthy implantation, ultimately provide a last-resort solution.

The only difference between IVF failure where the blood pregnancy test is negative from the onset and chemical pregnancy/early pregnancy loss where the blood hCG level at first rises and then declines, is chronology. The former occurs before implantation begins while the latter occurs later. However, the causes are often the same and so should be the approach to treatment.

Clinical Pregnancy

A clinical pregnancy is one that is *confirmed rather than merely presumed*, as with a chemical pregnancy. A pregnancy can be confirmed when evidence of gestation either in the uterus or fallopian tube is detected by ultrasound and/or when pathological evidence of placental or fetal tissue is obtained following miscarriage or surgery. A blood or urine test alone is not sufficient to confirm a clinical pregnancy.

Chemical vs. Clinical Pregnancy

The couple should keep in mind that on average, only about 20 percent of all naturally conceived pregnancies survive long enough to postpone the menstrual period and thus create the suspicion that the woman is pregnant. This means that most chemical pregnancies never become clinical pregnancies.

Verifying a chemical pregnancy when a woman has undergone IVF is complicated by the fact that she will almost invariably have received an injection of hCG at least 11 to 12 days prior to the first beta hCG blood pregnancy test. Depending upon her body's absorption and excretion rates, small amounts of the hCG may still be present in her blood at the time of the test and could result in the false suggestion of a pregnancy.

Therefore, the term *chemical pregnancy* when applied to IVF rates might mean one of three things: (1) a true chemical pregnancy is present but will not progress to a clinical pregnancy (the most likely scenario), (2) a chemical pregnancy is in the process of developing into a clinical pregnancy, or (3) the result was a false indication of a chemical pregnancy caused by residual hCG.

If the terms *chemical pregnancy* and *clinical pregnancy* are used interchangeably, a quoted pregnancy rate could be falsely inflated, per-haps by as much as 100 percent, by citing the percentage of chemical pregnancies for that particular program. For this reason most reputable IVF programs will not report chemical pregnancies in their statistics.

Consumers should be aware that some programs report "inclusive pregnancy rates," which are clinical and chemical pregnancy rates combined. However, since it is not always possible to determine which terms are actually being quoted when this reporting method is used, couples should not be afraid to ask the proper questions to clarify and distinguish between these two terms.

HOW SHOULD IVF SUCCESS BE EXPRESSED?

A.R.T. programs have in the past reported IVF success rates in a number of categories:

- Number of IVF cycles initiated in a given year
- Number of single and multiple pregnancies that occurred
- Number of cycles that resulted in live births

In addition, a variety of denominators are used to express outcome. These include:

- Pregnancies per cycle of IVF initiated
- Pregnancies per egg retrieval procedure
- Pregnancies per embryo transfer

The data is then further sub-classified by fresh or frozen embryo cycles, and by whether the woman's own eggs or donor eggs were used.

The current method of defining success is both flawed and, regardless of methodology, subject to manipulation and bias. There are two good reasons why the time has come to completely restructure the way in which IVF outcome statistics are expressed:

1. **The relatively recent introduction of ultrarapid embryo cryopreservation (vitrification):** This has been a "game changer" in the IVF arena because, by using this embryo freezing method, the vast majority of embryos survive both the freeze and the thaw, while retaining the viability they had before being frozen. Indeed, there is now strong evidence that thawed, pre-vitrified embryos have at least the same ability to propagate a viable pregnancy as do their freshly transferred counterparts. In fact, several recent studies even suggest that when it comes to birthrate, frozen/thawed embryos may have a slight edge.

2. **The introduction of "competent" embryo selection by full karyotyping:** The growing popularity of full embryo karyotyping using methods such as comparative genomic hybridization (CGH) for selecting "competent" embryos, by and large, requires that biopsied embryos be vitrified while awaiting the result of genetic testing. This, in most cases, requires that the embryos be cryostored and that a frozen embryo transfer (FET) be performed in a subsequent cycle. The deliberate performance of an FET is fast replacing fresh ETs and becoming the norm, rather than the exception.

What all this means is that the time has come for us to alter the way in which we express IVF success rate. Rather than being based on the number of egg retrievals performed, success should be based on the number of embryos transferred, whether fresh or by FET. This would not only make sense, but it would also create a more meaningful yardstick of expertise. It is also becoming more the rule than the exception to transfer few embryos at a time. In fact, IVF success should be reported as "live births per embryo transferred," subcategorized into different age categories, regardless of the type of IVF (fresh vs. frozen cycles, a patient's own eggs vs. donor eggs, etc.). Not only would this allow for uniform, simple, and reliable interpretation, but, by removing the incentive to transfer multiple embryos at a time, it would likely reduce the alarmingly high incidence of IVF multiple births. All that would be needed to put the IVF house in order would be to implement an enforceable and verifiable system. This would likely also have the added benefit of leveling the playing field while at the same time serving as a disincentive for physicians to transfer several embryos at a time, solely for the purpose of being able report higher success rates.

COUPLES HAVE THE RIGHT TO EXPECT COMPETENT, CARING TREATMENT

Another barometer of an IVF clinic's success is the way it treats its patients. A reputable IVF program should help each couple establish rational expectations right from the beginning and then follow through with a professional, understanding, organized program that meets the needs of both partners.

Consumers should look for a program that says, in effect: "We cannot guarantee that you will get pregnant, but we can promise you professionalism, the highest quality of care and expertise, a reasonable chance of getting pregnant, and that you will be treated all along the line with courtesy, understanding, and compassion."

Couples should look for a dedicated, committed team trained to deal with the emotional consequences of an IVF procedure and should avoid a program that is so preoccupied with the technical side of IVF that it loses sight of the human aspects of the procedure. No couple should feel they have to settle for a program that offers poor support and lacks compassion because they have nowhere else to go.

The morale and enthusiasm of the staff are good indicators of the kind of treatment the couple can expect. Morale in clinics that consistently report pregnancies is likely to be higher because staff members feel that they are part of a successful program. One program reinforces this enthusiasm by contacting patients who have a positive pregnancy test via speakerphone or Skype. This enables everyone to share the joy and excitement with the couple.

Consumers might want to look for a program that offers a professional counselor to deal with both partners' emotional needs. The counselor, who is pivotal to any IVF program, usually acts as a buffer between the couple and the clinical team. Counseling can help a couple become positively involved in an IVF program and also steer them away from false hopes.

It is wise to inquire about the size of the staff and verify that the program has enough people to respond to the couple's needs at all times. No one wants to have to reschedule egg retrieval because the doctor in an understaffed clinic was called away unexpectedly.

Care and caring go together in the truly successful IVF program. If the perception of caring truly indicates a successful program, then the program that elicited the following comment from this woman (who adopted a baby after her IVF pregnancy ended in miscarriage) must indeed be successful:

> I don't think I'd try IVF again in the very near future because I have a six-week-old at home, but thanks to the staff at the clinic I have a positive attitude and outlook about IVF, and would seriously consider trying again later.

WHAT IS THE BEST WAY TO ACCESS INFORMATION?

The most rational approach to assessing the IVF situation is by first becoming aware of the facts and statistics, asking pertinent questions according to one's own needs, and then actually visiting the site. A reputable program should be willing to answer questions and give the couple access to the facility.

When seeking information about a program, the couple should look for staff who are willing to take the time to talk and to respond to questions frankly and openly. Some consumer-oriented staffs will even send literature about the program on request, as well as copies of articles from accredited professional journals, videotapes, stories about the program from newspapers and magazines, and sometimes names of previous patients who are willing to discuss their experiences.

If the clinic does not volunteer information, the couple/patient might have to be assertive. At a minimum, they should expect to receive literature about how the program operates. The lack of such information for potential patients is a sign of poor organization. The couple should be wary of any program that refuses to provide information and statistics in writing or insists they come into the office. If the couple feel that they have to pry answers from an evasive staff, they should think twice about that program.

Finally, I recommend that when asking for success rates the researching couple should hold IVF programs accountable by requesting that they provide all statistics in written form. It is also helpful to ask for long-term statistics (two to three years' worth) to account for the turnover in key staff members that frequently occurs in many IVF programs.

Preliminary Information Can Be Obtained by Telephone/Skype

The only way to ferret out success rates is by talking directly to someone at the clinic. We recommend that before calling a prospective program the couple should reread "How Does the Program Define Pregancy?" and "How Should IVF Success Be Expressed?" in this chapter. Then they should be prepared to ask the following questions:

1. How long has your program been established?
2. How many patients have you treated?
3. How many babies have been born?
4. How many egg retrievals have you performed?
5. How many embryo transfers have you done?
6. How many embryos do you transfer at a time?

7. What is the baby (birth) rate per embryo that you transfer?
8. Do you perform ultrarapid embryo freezing (vitrification) and how successful has this been?
9. Do you offer egg donation and IVF surrogacy in your program?
10. Do you offer egg freezing, Fertility Preservation (FP), at your program?
11. Do you turn away women over a certain age? If so, what age? (This is to be asked if age cut-off is a concern for the couple.)
12. Does your program offer embryo selection through CGH testing?
13. How do you prefer to transfer cleaved embryos or blastocysts?
14. Do you arbitrarily cancel an IVF cycle if there are "few" mature follicles, or do you include the couple in this decision-making process?

In order to form the most rational expectations about each program, the couple should attempt to learn how the prognostic indicators for IVF might impact on their personal chance of pregnancy in each particular program. One way to do this would be to direct the conversation to their personal situation after having obtained general statistics about the program. The couple might first offer some information about themselves, including their ages, how long they have been infertile, what has been diagnosed as the cause of their infertility, the status of the man's fertility, and previous surgeries the woman may have undergone to correct her infertility. They should also be willing to supply other information the staff may request in order to become more familiar with the case.

Then the couple might ask:

1. In your program per embryo transferred, what would be the chance of conceiving a clinical pregnancy?
2. What would you say are our chances of actually having a baby per embryo transferred?

Once again, couples should request the answers to the questions in writing. Thereupon, after narrowing down the list of prospective clinics to those that responded most satisfactorily to these questions, the couple are ready for the next step—the pre-enrollment interview.

A Pre-Enrollment Interview Is Worth the Time and Expense

Just as few people would select a college without first visiting its campus, consumers also should visit each prospective program if at all possible. A program that refuses to grant a pre-enrollment interview should be dropped from further consideration.

A pre-enrollment interview will give the couple a chance to meet some of the staff and see what kind of people they will be dealing with. Is there an air of camaraderie, or do the staff seem disgruntled and unhappy? If the staff obviously regard their positions as nine-to-five drudgery, the couple most likely is in the wrong place.

The couple should try to meet a nurse coordinator during their visit because he or she is the person they will deal with daily. They should be sure the coordinator is in control of the program on a daily basis and will be congenial to work with.

Sometimes it is not possible to visit the IVF center in person. For example, many of my patients journey from out of state or from abroad to me for treatment in Las Vegas, NV, or St. Louis, MO. Thus it is often not possible for them to visit our center for an in-person pre-enrollment interview. So it is that most of the communication I and my nurse coordinator have with such patients is by phone or by Skype. In such cases the initial consultation as well as follow-up interactions with me and my team are done by phone or via Skype. Both I and my patients find the latter to be very agreeable. I also provide all my patients with my personal cell phone number so they can reach me at any time.

If it is not possible to meet the doctor and his/her team in person or via videoconference, it is often helpful to investigate how the doctor and program are viewed outside the clinic. Do he or she and the staff get along well with people? IVF is a popular topic for discussion these days, and many people have strong opinions about the doctors who practice in this specialty. The couple might be surprised at how easy it is to get that information. Another great way to make such contact is to access the center's website. Our website, www.haveababy.com, the SIRM Facebook site, https://www.facebook.com/HaveABaby, and my blog, www.IVFauthority.com, are accessible to anyone, and all provide uncensored forums which allow interaction between doctors and visitors as well as between visitors who wish to communicate with one another, independently. This makes it easy to get a feel about how the practice is regarded.

If a pre-enrollment interview cannot be arranged, other approaches can be used to gather more information about a specific program. Phone calls to previous patients will be invaluable. The chapter of an infertility support group in the city where the program is located probably would be willing to help. The couple might even retain someone living near the clinic to conduct research for them. Perhaps the couple's own doctor knows a local physician who can provide information. The couple may even decide to randomly telephone some gynecologists who practice in that community and ask them about the program.

While such research about a program can be helpful, in most cases nothing can really replace the information gained during a site inspection. A pre-enrollment trip is well worth the time and expense.

Consumers should expect to do a lot of homework when searching for an IVF program. Unfortunately, we do not believe that it will get any easier in the near future. As an IVF father told us:

> We have a library at home of all kinds of clippings, and virtually every book, magazine, and periodical you can imagine about IVF. We also are on Google all the time, visiting the websites of different IVF centers. My wife did a tremendous amount of research on which clinics are the most highly rated, what kinds of procedures were being used, what the latest technology was. Her training as a nurse certainly gave her a better handle on those strange-sounding hormones that are used as part of the process. Really, it was a matter of doing a lot of research for us before we were able to locate the right IVF program.

Helpful as it would be when selecting an IVF program, it is not necessary for every couple to have access to an RN to use the guidelines suggested in this chapter. When consumers know what to look for and what questions to ask, they will be prepared to make an informed choice—a decision that should always be based on rational expectations, not false hopes.

What about the SART/CDC Report?

At the time of writing this book, IVF outcome statistics reported annually by the Society for Assisted Reproductive Technology (SART), in my opinion, still lack both reliability and credibility. The reason is that to date, in spite of public demands and congressional decrees spanning a period of more than three decades, SART has failed to institute a fully verifiable reporting process by IVF programs. Instead, the IVF outcome data reported annually on the SART report comprises outcome data that is largely self-generated by member programs with little oversight by SART. For this reason, while the SART Report could be used as a guideline, I do not recommend using it as the primary determinant for selecting an IVF program.

13

IUI, GIFT, AND OTHER ALTERNATIVES TO IVF

ARTIFICIAL INSEMINATION

This chapter outlines some of the therapeutic gamete-related technologies available to the infertile couple. The term *therapeutic gamete-related technologies* refers to those procedures that involve enhancement, insemination, or transfer of eggs and/or sperm into the woman's uterus, fallopian tubes, or peritoneal cavity in the hope that in vivo (inside the body) fertilization and the subsequent birth of one or more healthy babies will follow. In contrast, IVF involves fertilization in the laboratory and transfer into the uterus of embryos/blastocysts rather than gametes.

The procedures mentioned in this section are directed mostly but not exclusively to situations in which infertility is due to problems other than female organic pelvic disease and male-factor infertility. Indications for artificial insemination include cervical mucus insufficiency unrelated to sperm antibodies in the woman's secretions, unexplained infertility, and donor-sperm insemination. It is relatively contraindicated in situations of male-factor infertility, female immunologic infertility (due to sperm antibodies), tubal disease, chronic pelvic adhesions, and for women in their 40s where the chance of having a baby would be less than 4 percent per cycle. Couples for whom artificial insemination is indicated might consider the following alternatives before electing to undergo IVF. IVF would be performed if insemination procedures fail to achieve a pregnancy in spite of repeated attempts.

Intrauterine Insemination (IUI)

Intrauterine insemination (IUI), the injection of sperm into the uterus by means of a catheter directed through the cervix, has been practiced for many years. The premise of this procedure is that sperm can reach and fertilize the egg more easily if placed directly into the uterine cavity.

Up until the 1980s, physicians were injecting small quantities of raw, untreated semen (sperm plus the seminal plasma) directly into the uterus at the time of expected ovulation. However, when more than 0.2 ml of semen was injected into the uterus, serious and sometimes life-endangering shock-like reactions often occurred. It was subsequently determined that such reactions were related to the presence of prostaglandins within the seminal plasma. This led to the practice of injecting small amounts (less than 0.2 ml) of raw semen into the uterus. However, the pregnancy rates were dismal; and side effects, such as severe cramping and infection, were rampant. (Women are protected against the reaction during intercourse because the semen pools in the vagina; the sperm are then safely filtered through the cervical mucus, thereby preventing seminal plasma from reaching the uterine cavity.)

As far back as 1982, I began to recognize the potential advantage of washing and centrifuging raw semen so as to separate sperm from the seminal fluid, and thereby remove the prostaglandins that cause most of the problems. We subsequently introduced and, thereupon, became the first to publish on IUI in the prestigious journal *Fertility and Sterility* (April 1984).

Indications for IUI

1. *Artificial insemination with cryopreserved donor sperm.* The recognition of HIV and Hepatitis C infection as sexually transmitted diseases, coupled with the fact that the HIV virus is present in semen months before it can, in most cases, be

detected in the blood, mandates that all sperm donors have their semen cryopreserved (frozen) and stored for at least six months, whereupon they will be retested for HIV infection. Ideally, only upon confirmation of a negative test should the cryopreserved semen specimen be thawed and used for insemination. Since cryopreservation inevitably reduces sperm motility and function, it is not adequate to simply thaw the frozen specimen and then inseminate the raw semen into the vagina. Rather, the semen specimen should be processed for IUI. Provided that the recipient is ovulating normally, there is no need to administer fertility drugs, such as clomiphene citrate.

The introduction of tests that can accurately detect HIV without the need to wait for the development of antibodies could change the situation and might in the future again permit the use of fresh sperm.

2. *Artificial insemination with partner's sperm.*   In cases of sexual dysfunction (impotence, retrograde ejaculation, etc.) or timing issues, the partner's sperm may need to be collected and processed in preparation for IUI.

3. *Cervical mucus hostility.*   Sometimes the cervical mucus acts as a barrier to the activation and passage of sperm as it passes through the cervical canal. This may be due to poor physical qualities of the mucus, cervical infection, or the presence of anti-sperm antibodies. In all but the latter case, IUI can readily be performed during natural cycles unless the woman has ovulation dysfunction. However, when infertility results from the presence of antibodies in the cervical mucus, IUI will likely be ineffectual and should be replaced by IVF.

4. *Abnormal ovulation.*   In some cases where the woman requires the use of fertility drugs to induce normal ovulation, the concomitant performance of IUI could optimize pregnancy rates.

5. *Clomiphene citrate (Serophene).*   A recent study confirmed that normally ovulating women taking clomiphene citrate experience a reduced chance of achieving pregnancy when compared with fertile women who are not taking clomiphene. Furthermore,

additional studies have reported very few viable clomiphene-induced pregnancies in women over the age of 40. The reason is clomiphene's anti-estrogen effect on the lining of the uterus and the production of cervical mucus. The only advantage to clomiphene therapy lies in its simplicity of administration, low incidence of side effects, and relatively low cost. It should also be recognized that clomiphene should not be used for more than three consecutive months without taking a full month's break before starting a fourth cycle of treatment. This is because after the third consecutive month of clomiphene therapy there is a progressive decline in fertility, to the point that following six or more back-to-back cycles of treatment the drug exerts a strong contraceptive influence. This results from a buildup of the anti-estrogenic properties of clomiphene. The good news is that upon discontinuation of clomiphene for six weeks, all of these adverse effects disappear.

6. *Letrozole.*   Letrozole, a relatively new oral fertility agent (see Chapter 5), works similarly to clomiphene but does not exhibit the same local anti-estrogenic effects on the uterine lining and the cervical glands. Accordingly, the selective use of Letrozole might prove to be useful in the performance of IUI.

7. *Gonadotropins.*   Women with absent or abnormal ovulation who require fertility drugs in preparation for IUI should receive gonadotropins (e.g., Menopur, Gonal F, Follistim, Bravelle). Granted, these agents are relatively expensive, but they have no anti-estrogenic properties, and in the hands of the experienced physician the pregnancy rate is nearly double that which can be achieved with clomiphene. Side effects can be either prevented or readily managed.

IUI Success Rates

Success rates with IUI are contingent upon (1) indication for which it is being performed, (2) whether the woman is ovulating normally on her own, and (3) the age of the woman. By and large, birthrates per cycle of IUI performed for the correct indications are reported to be about 15% for women less than 30 years of age, 12% for women 30 to 35 years, 7%–8% for women 35 to 39 years, and less than 4% for women over 40.

Contraindications to IUI

1. *Moderate to severe male infertility.* Contrary to popular belief, the performance of IUI in cases of moderate or severe male infertility hardly improves success rates over regular and well-timed intercourse alone. IVF with intracytoplasmic sperm injection (IVF/ICSI) is the only method to optimize pregnancy rates in association with male refractory infertility.

2. *Tubal disease.* Since pelvic inflammatory disease (PID) inevitably damages the intricate and sophisticated inner lining of the fallopian tubes, no surgery to the outside of the tube(s) will remedy damage done to the inner lining. As such, the pregnancy rate can be expected to be at least 10 times lower than average when fertility drugs and/or IUI are used in such cases. Moreover, the incidence of ectopic pregnancy is about one in six. Bypassing the "damaged plumbing" with IVF is the only rational treatment is such cases.

3. *Age.* Women over 40 do not have the time to waste on IUI since the success rate is less than 3 percent birthrate per month of trying.

4. *Endometriosis.* While the exact cause of endometriosis remains an enigma, it is now apparent that a toxic environment exists in the pelvis (surrounding the tubes and ovaries) in patients with this condition. As a consequence, ovulation, whether spontaneous or induced by fertility drugs, commits the egg to pass through a toxic pelvic environment in order to reach the sperm waiting in the fallopian tube. This significantly reduces the egg's fertilization potential. Furthermore, once the fertilized egg reaches the uterus, immunologic factors present in about one-third of cases of endometriosis (regardless of its severity) increase the risk of the embryo being rejected before pregnancy can be diagnosed.

Such women may experience repeated "mini-miscarriages." In spite of these anti-fertility influences, many women with mild endometriosis in fact do conceive on their own or following ovarian stimulation with fertility drugs. However, for reasons already referred to, the chances of conception are significantly reduced, and if the women are ovulating normally on their own, the addition of fertility drugs will afford no additional benefit. Simply put, women in their late 20s to mid-30s, who have the time and inclination to wait, can anticipate about a 30 percent chance of conceiving on their own within three years, contingent upon their ovulating normally and having fertile male partners. The occurrence of pregnancy in the latter cases occurs in spite of, rather than due to, such treatment. Such women should consider deferring all invasive treatments in favor of a "wait-and-see" attitude. Conversely, for women over the age of 35 whose egg quality is inevitably on the decline, IVF offers the only rational approach.

Fertility Drugs and Multiple Births with IUI

Women who ovulate normally do not experience much of an increase in multiple birthrates following ovulation induction, while those with absent or abnormal ovulation have a higher success rate as well as a much greater multiple pregnancy rate. In an attempt to explain this observation, we compared and reported on differences in ovarian response to gonadotropin stimulation between women who ovulate normally and those who have dysfunctional ovulation or do not ovulate at all. Serial ultrasound examinations around the time of induced ovulation were performed on women undergoing ovarian stimulation with gonadotropins in preparation for IUI. We observed that normally ovulating women presented with one and sometimes two follicles significantly larger than the rest (dominant follicles), while the absent/abnormal ovulators often had numerous large follicles of a similar size. Following the hCG trigger in the normal ovulating group, the one (and sometimes two) dominant follicle(s) would ovulate while the remaining follicles did not. Conversely, in absent/abnormal ovulators, the numerous follicles ovulated. We concluded that in normally ovulating women, once the dominant follicle(s) released the egg(s), the ovulation of the remaining follicles was blocked.

Thus, the belief that administration of gonadotropins to normally ovulating women will trigger the release of multiple eggs and thereby significantly increase the pregnancy rate is, to say the least, vastly over-stated. Neither the multiple pregnancy rate nor the overall pregnancy rate per cycle is substantially increased in this manner. In contrast, when gonadotropins are administered to non-ovulating women and/or women with dysfunctional ovulation, such as women with polycystic ovarian syndrome (or PCOS, where the ability to select one or more dominant follicle(s) is absent or compromised, and multiple eggs may be released), the pregnancy rate per cycle as well as the incidence of multiple pregnancy is markedly increased.

It follows that only those women with absent or abnormal ovulation are at real risk of having high-order multiple pregnancies. They, there-fore, need to be counseled regarding the consequences of premature birth and the availability of selective pregnancy reduction toward the end of the third month of pregnancy. Another alternative is to avoid the issue completely by choosing IVF, where the number of potential babies can be limited by the number of embryos transferred to the uterus.

It is indeed unfortunate that fertility treatment has become so regi-mented that most patients find themselves being ushered through a "scripted treatment process," one that almost mandates surgery if the fallopian tubes are damaged or blocked, and clomiphene/IUI for all other cases, even including male infertility. For the majority of couples, who require an individualized strategic plan of action at an early stage, such an approach is emotionally, physically, and financially draining, leaving them both suspicious and critical of the intent of the medical profession.

IUI, like any other form of fertility treatment, can be of great value if used appropriately and selectively for the correct indications. The use of fertility drugs should not be regarded as a necessary adjunct in all cases of IUI, which in turn should not be considered as a required preliminary to

IVF. Some women are better off with fertility drugs alone, some women require IUI alone, some require IUI with fertility drugs, while others should go directly to IVF.

Intravaginal Insemination (IVI) with Partner's Semen

Intravaginal insemination (IVI) using the partner's semen involves the injection of semen into the vagina in proximity to the cervix rather than into the uterus, as is the case with IUI. Intravaginal insemination is most often employed to assist a woman with a subfertile partner to conceive naturally at the time of ovulation. However, IVI usually offers no advantage over normal coital ejaculation that occurs during intercourse. The only cases when IVI might be advantageous would be certain forms of male impotence in which the man cannot produce semen with intercourse.

Artificial Insemination by Donor (AID)

Artificial insemination by donor (AID) is the most common form of insemination in cases in which donor sperm is required because the woman's partner is infertile. Artificial insemination by donor can be done via IVI or IUI.

As mentioned under IUI above, the use of cryopreserved donor sperm is the safest method of performing donor insemination, given the significant risk of HIV/Hepatitis C. After the donor has been tested for HIV/Hepatitis, the sperm are cryopreserved for at least six months, following which the donor is retested. If HIV/hepatitis is not present, the likelihood that the original specimen is infected is remote, and the specimen is then released. Again, since cryopreservation inevitably reduces sperm motility and function, it is not adequate to simply thaw the frozen specimen and then inseminate the raw semen into the vagina. Rather, the semen specimen should be processed for AID. Provided that the recipient is ovulating normally, there is no need to administer fertility drugs, such as clomiphene citrate.

GAMETE INTRAFALLOPIAN TRANSFER (GIFT)

In 1984, Dr. Ricardo Asch introduced a therapeutic gamete-related technique that in the '80s and '90s gained widespread popularity in the United States. It involved the injection of one or more eggs mixed with washed, capacitated, and incubated sperm directly into the fallopian tubes.

Because GIFT as currently performed requires laparoscopy, it is also significantly more expensive and physically demanding than most other techniques described in this chapter. The cost of GIFT approaches that of IVF because, in addition to laparoscopy, it also requires general anesthesia.

The intensive care provided by the IVF laboratory maximizes the chances for fertilization. GIFT, in contrast, simply places a large number of sperm in the fallopian tube near an otherwise unprepared egg. Hence, fertilization is much more of a hit-or-miss situation. With perhaps one notable exception, I do not believe that GIFT is a good choice for treatment of unexplained or male infertility. The exception applies to devout Catholics who refuse IVF because this treatment is prohibited by the Catholic church on the grounds that it separates the "unitive" (sex act) from the "generative" (the procreative act). The Church does not disallow GIFT.

Note: GIFT is an outmoded procedure that has no advantage and as such it should finally be relegated to the history books.

ZYGOTE INTRAFALLOPIAN TRANSFER (ZIFT) OR TUBAL EMBRYO TRANSFER (TET)

Another option which has largely been relegated to being of historic interest only is *zygote intrafallopian transfer* (ZIFT), or *tubal embryo transfer* (TET). This procedure involes transferring the fertilized egg(s) directly into the fallopian tube(s) and as such was only suited to cases where infertility is unrelated to female tubal disease. As with routine IVF, ZIFT/TET requires initial egg retrieval through transvaginal needle-aspiration and fertilization of the eggs in the laboratory. One or two days later, the fertilized eggs or embryos are loaded into a thin catheter and injected into the outer third of one or both fallopian tubes during laparoscopy.

In the past, proponents of ZIFT/TET argued that enabling the embryo to reach the uterus via its natural route (the fallopian tube) rather than by embryo transfer through the cervix increases the likelihood of implantation and a successful pregnancy.

It must be emphasized that older studies that previously reported encouraging and even superior results with ZIFT/TET were all poorly controlled. Subsequent well-conducted studies have shown that the pregnancy rate per embryo transferred with ZIFT/TET is in fact lower than that which is achievable through IVF. Accordingly, there is no longer a justifiable indication for the performance of ZIFT/TET in preference to IVF.

NATURAL-CYCLE IVF

Natural-cycle (NC) IVF involves accessing one and sometimes two follicles that might develop in a woman during a normal cycle (without the use of fertility drugs) for the purpose of fertilizing the eggs in vitro and transferring them to the uterus. Several advantages of this method have cited, that (1) since fertility drugs are not used, the woman's eggs are not adversely influenced by induced hormonal changes in the ovary and thus are more likely to be of good quality, (2) that the absence of fertility drugs also favors an optimum environment into which to place the embryos, and (3) by avoiding fertility drugs, the cost is considerably less than with conventional IVF.

But an objective look at these arguments finds considerable evidence to the contrary. First, the amount of monitoring in a natural cycle often significantly exceeds that which has to be done in a conventional IVF cycle. The eggs must still be harvested, the sperm prepared in the laboratory, the embryo or embryos transferred, and an increased amount of blood testing is required in order to accurately monitor the woman's progress. Additionally, since far fewer eggs are harvested than with conventional IVF, pregnancy rates are three times lower with NC-IVF. This is particularly problematic when it comes to women over 35 years where the rising prevalence of egg aneuploidy translates into a very much reduced likelihood of transferring even one "competent" embryo to the uterus per NC-IVF attempt. Rather than being a function of the cost of an IVF procedure, the real consideration should be the cost of having a baby. Furthermore, it involves an emotional and physical as well as a financial component. Accordingly it can be concluded that the performance of NC-IVF in fact does not really lower the overall cost of the procedure much. Finally, given the very low success rate with NC-IVF in older women who also face an ever-accelerating "biological clock," to recommend this approach in such cases is unjustified and even borders on being disingenuous.

14

RECURRENT PREGNANCY LOSS (RPL)

When it comes to reproduction, humans are the poorest performers of all mammals. In fact we are so inefficient that up to 75% of fertilized eggs do not produce live births, and up to 30% of pregnancies end up being lost within 10 weeks of conception (in the 1st trimester).

RPL is defined as two (2) or more failed pregnancies. Less than 5% of women will experience two (2) consecutive miscarriages, and only 1% experience three or more.

Pregnancy loss can be classified by the stage of pregnancy when the loss occurs:

1. Early pregnancy loss (1st trimester)
2. Late pregnancy loss (after the 1st trimester)
3. Occult "hidden" and not clinically recognized, (chemical) pregnancy loss (occurs prior to ultrasound confirmation of pregnancy)

Early pregnancy losses usually occur sporadically (are not repetitive). In more than 70% of cases the loss is due to embryo aneuploidy (where there are more or less than the normal quota of 46 chromosomes). Conversely, repeated losses (RPL), with isolated exceptions where the cause is structural (e.g., unbalanced translocations), are seldom attributable to numerical chromosomal abnormalities (aneuploidy). In fact, the vast majority of cases of RPL are attributable to non-chromosomal causes such as anatomical uterine abnormalities (see below) or *Immunologic Implantation Dysfunction* (IID).

Since most early pregnancy losses are induced by chromosomal factors and thus are non-repetitive, having had a single miscarriage the likelihood of a second one occurring is no greater than average. However, once having had two losses the chance of a third one occurring is double (35-40%) and after having had three losses the chance of a fourth miscarriage increases to about 60%. The reason for this reason is that the more miscarriages a woman has, the greater is the likelihood of this being due to a non-chromosomal (repetitive) cause such as IID. It follows that if chromosomal analysis (karyotyping) of embryonic/fetal products derived from a miscarriage tests karyotypically normal, then by a process of elimination, there would be a strong likelihood of a miscarriage repeating in subsequent pregnancies and one would not have to wait for the disaster to recur before taking action. This is precisely why I strongly advocate that all miscarriage specimens be karyotyped. There is however one caveat to be taken into consideration. That is that the laboratory performing the karyotyping might unwittingly be testing the mother's cells rather than that of the conceptus. That is why it is not possible to confidently exclude aneuploidy in cases where karyotyping of products suggests a "chromosomally normal" (euploid) female.

Late pregnancy losses (occuring after completion of the 1st trimester/12th week) occur far less frequently (1%) than early pregnancy losses. They are most commonly due to anatomical abnormalities of the uterus and/or cervix. Weakness of the neck of the cervix rendering it able to act as an effective valve that retains the pregnancy (i.e., cervical incompetence) is in fact one of the commonest causes of late pregnancy loss. So also are developmental (congenital) abnormalities of the uterus (e.g., a uterine septum) and uterine fibroid tumors. In some cases intrauterine growth retardation, premature separation of the placenta (placental abruption), premature rupture of the membranes and premature labor can also causes of late pregnancy loss.

Much progress has been made in understanding the mechanisms involved in RPL. There are two broad categories:

1. *Problems involving the uterine environment* in which a normal embryo is prohibited from properly implanting and developing. Possible causes include:

a) Inadequate thickening of the uterine lining.

b) Irregularity in the contour of the uterine cavity (polyps, fibroid tumors in the uterine wall, intra-uterine scarring and adenomyosis).

c) Hormonal imbalances (Progesterone deficiency or Luteal phase defects). This most commonly results in occult RPL.

d) Deficient blood flow to the uterine lining (thin uterine lining).

e) Immunologic implantation dysfunction (IID). A major cause of RPL. Plays a role in 75% of cases where chromosomally normal preimplantation embryos fail to implant.

f) Interference of blood supply to the developing conceptus can occur due to a hereditary clotting disorder known as Thrombophilia.

2. *Genetic and/or structural chromosomal abnormality of the embryo.* Genetic abnormalities are rare causes of RPL. Structural chromosomal abnormalities are slightly more common but are also occur infrequently (1%). These are referred to as unbalanced translocation and they result from part of one chromosome detaching and then fusing with another chromosome. Additionally, a number of studies suggest the existence of paternal (sperm derived) effect on human embryo quality and pregnancy outcome that are not reflected as a chromosomal abnormality. Damaged sperm DNA can have a negative impact on fetal development and present clinically as occult or early clinical miscarriage. The Sperm Chromatin Structure Assay (SCSA) which measures the same endpoints are newer and possibly improved methods for evaluating.

Furthermore there is developing research into the immunologic causes of pregnancy loss. These instances are known as Immunologic Implantation Dysfunction (IID) and have two basic categories:

1. *Alloimmune IID* (see Chapter 8), i.e., where antibodies are formed against antigens derived from another member of the same species, is believed to be a relatively common immunologic cause of recurrent pregnancy loss. A pregnancy must be recognized as foreign to trigger the appropriate immunologic mechanisms.

Sometimes when a male partner transmits (via his sperm contribution to the embryo) certain genes that are similar to the mother's, then the embryo becomes regarded as being "too similar" to the mother's genetic make-up and is duly rejected. Such rejection usually takes the form of an early miscarriage but sometimes (rarely) the rejection can be so abrupt as to completely prevent recognition of a pregnancy. In such cases the couple might present with "unexplained infertility" or "unexplained IVF failure." Alloimmune implantation dysfunction, while being an relatively uncommon cause of immunologic IVF implantation failure (<10%), is believed to be a very common immunologic cause of recurrent pregnancy loss. Testing for alloimmune similarities is thus a very important part of the evaluation of non-chromosomal recurrent pregnancy loss. It requires comparing the mother's and father's HLA and DQ alpha status (see below).

2. *Autoimmune ID*: Here an immunologic reaction is produced by the individual to his/her body's own cellular components. The most common antibodies that form in such situations are antiphospholipid antibodies (APA), antithyroid antibodies (ATA), and anti-ovarian antibodies (AOA).

But it is only when specialized immune cells in the uterine lining, known as cytotoxic lymphocytes (CTL) and natural killer (NK) cells, become activated (CTLa/NKa) and start to release an excessive/disproportionate amount of TH-1 cytokines that attack the root system of the embryo, that implantation potential is jeopardized. Diagnosis of such activation requires highly specialized blood tests and/or endometrial evaluation for cytokine activity that can only be performed by a handful of reproductive immunology reference laboratories in the United States.

Autoimmune IID is often genetically transmitted. Thus it should not be surprising to learn that it is more likely to exist in women who have a family (or personal) history of primary autoimmune diseases such as Lupus Erythematosus (LE), Scleroderma or hypothyroidism, Rheumatoid Arthritis, etc. Reactionary (secondary) autoimmunity can occur in conjunction with any medical condition associated with widespread tissue damage. One such gynecologic condition is endometriosis.

Since autoimmune IID is usually associated with activated NK and T-cells from the outset, it usually results in such very early destruction of the embryo's root system that the patient does not even recognize that she is pregnant. Accordingly the condition usually presents as "unexplained infertility" or "unexplained IVF failure" rather than as a miscarriage. Alloimmune IID, on the other hand, usually starts off presenting as unexplained miscarriages (often manifesting as RPL). Over time as NK/T cell activation builds and eventually becomes permanently established the patient often goes from RPL to "infertility" due to failed implantation.

In reality, regardless of whether miscarriage is due to autoimmune or alloimmune IID, the final blow to the pregnancy is the result of activated NK and T-cells in the uterine lining that damage the developing embryo's "root system" (trophoblast) so that it can no longer sustain the growing conceptus. This having been said, it is important to note that autoimmune IID is readily amenable to reversal through timely, appropriately administered, selective immunotherapy, and alloimmune IID is not. It is much more difficult to treat successfully, even with the use of immunotherapy. In fact, in some cases the only solution will be to revert to selective immunotherapy plus using donor sperm (provided there is no "match" between the donor's DQa profile and that of the female recipient) or alternatively to resort to gestational surrogacy.

DIAGNOSING THE CAUSE OF RPL

In the past, women who miscarried were not evaluated thoroughly until they had lost several pregnancies in a row. This was because sporadic miscarriages are most commonly the result of embryo numerical chromosomal irregularities (aneuploidy) and thus not treatable. However, a series of miscarriages in a row, pointed to a repetitive cause that was non-chromosomal and potentially remediable. Since RPL is most commonly due to a uterine pathology or immunologic causes that are potentially treatable, it follows that early chromosomal evaluation of products of conception could point to a potentially treatable situation. Thus I strongly recommend that such testing be done in most cases of miscarriage. Doing so will avoid a great deal of unnecessary heartache for many patients.

Establishing the correct diagnosis is the first step in determining effective treatment for couples with recurrent pregnancy loss, also referred to as recurrent miscarriage or repeat pregnancy loss. RPL results from a problem within the pregnancy itself or within the uterine environment where the pregnancy implants and grows. Diagnostic tests useful in identifying individuals at greater risk for a problem within the pregnancy itself include:

1. Karyotyping (chromosome analysis) both prospective parents
2. Assessment of the karyotype of products of conception derived from previous miscarriage specimens
3. Ultrasound examination of the uterine cavity after sterile water is injected or hysterosonography (saline ultrasound, sonohysterogram, fluid ultrasound, etc.)
4. Hysterosalpingogram (dye X-ray test)
5. Hysteroscopic evaluation of the uterine cavity
6. Full hormonal evaluation (estrogen, progesterone, adrenal steroid hormones, thyroid hormones, FSH/LH, etc.)
7. Immunologic testing to include:
   a) Antiphospholipid antibody (APA) panel
   b) Antinuclear antibody (ANA) panel
   c) Antithyroid antibody panel (i.e., antithyroglobulin and antimicrosomal antibodies)
   d) Reproductive immunophenotype
   e) natural killer cell activity (NKa) assay (i.e., K562 target cell test)
   f) CTL by an immunophenotype
   g) Alloimmune testing of both the male and female partners (DQ alpha and HLA)
   h) Thrombophilia Mutation Panel

TREATMENT OF RPL

Treatment for anatomic abnormalities of the uterus involves restoration through removal of local lesions such as fibroids, scar tissue, and endometrial polyps or timely insertion of a cervical cerclage (a stitch placed around the neck of the weakened cervix) or the excision of a uterine septum when indicated.

A thin endometrial lining has been shown to correlate with compromised pregnancy outcome. Often this will be associated with reduced resistance to blood flow to the endometrium. Such decreased blood flow to the uterus can be improved through treatment with sildenafil and, possibly, aspirin.

Sildenafil (Viagra) Therapy. Viagra has been used successfully to increase uterine blood flow. However, to be effective it must be administered starting as soon as the period stops up until the day of ovulation and it must be administered vaginally (not orally). Viagra in the form of vaginal suppositories given in the dosage of 25 mg four times a day has been shown to increase uterine blood flow as well as thickness of the uterine lining. To date, we have seen significant improvement of the thickness of the uterine lining in about 70% of women treated. Successful pregnancy resulted in 42% of women who responded to the Viagra. It should be remembered that most of these women had previously experienced repeated IVF failures.

Aspirin. This is an anti-prostaglandin that improves blood flow to the endometrium. It is administered at a dosage of 81 mg orally, daily from the beginning of the cycle until ovulation.

Selective Immunotherapy

Intralipid (IL), immunoglobulin (IVIg), heparin (Lovenox/Clexane), and corticosteroids (dexamethasone, prednisone, prednisolone). Many causes of pregnancy loss or failure can be treated with immunotherapy comprising combinations of heparin and corticosteroids, IL (and/or IVIg), aspirin, and folic acid.

Use of IVF

In the following circumstances, IVF is the preferred option:

1. When in addition to a history of RPL, another standard indication for IVF (e.g., tubal factor, endometriosis, and male factor infertility) is superimposed.
2. In cases where selective immunotherapy (see above) is needed to treat an immunologic implantation dysfunction.

The reason for IVF being a preferred approach in such cases is that in order to be effective, the immunotherapy needs to be initiated well before spontaneous or induced ovulation. Given the fact that the anticipated birthrate per cycle of COS with or without IUI is at best about 15% it follows that short of IVF, to have even a reasonable chance of a live birth, most women with immunologic causes of RPL would need to undergo immunotherapy repeatedly, over consecutive cycles. Conversely, with IVF, the chance of a successful outcome in a single cycle of treatment is several times greater and, because of the attenuated and concentrated time period required for treatment, IVF is far safer and thus represents a more practicable alternative

Since embryo aneuploidy is a common cause of miscarriage, the use of preimplantation genetic diagnosis (PGD), with tests such as CGH, can provide a valuable diagnostic and therapeutic advantage in cases of RPL. PGD requires IVF to provide access to embryos for testing.

There are a few cases of intractable alloimmune dysfunction due to absolute DQ alpha matching (Chapter 8) where *Gestational Surrogacy* (Chapter 15) or use of donor sperm could represent the only viable recourse, other than abandoning treatment altogether and/or resorting to adoption. Other non-immunologic factors such as an intractably thin uterine lining or severe uterine pathology might also warrant that last resort consideration be given to gestational surrogacy.

The good news is that if a couple with RPL is open to all of the diagnostic and treatment options referred to above, a live birthrate of 70%–80% is ultimately achievable.

CHAPTER

15

OTHER OPTIONS FOR COUPLES WITH INTRACTABLE INFERTILITY

For many couples who are unable to achieve pregnancy through conventional treatments, third-party parenting offers tremendous hope for success. Third-party parenting is a collective term for egg donation, embryo adoption, gestational surrogacy, donor sperm insemination, and adoption of a child. These procedures are options for the infertile couple to consider when the woman, for some reason, cannot produce healthy eggs or the proper gestational environment for a pregnancy, or when the man cannot produce healthy sperm.

Only a few years ago, women who did not have a healthy uterus and those who could not produce healthy eggs had the lowest chance of having their own baby. Now, quite paradoxically, through the advent of egg donation and IVF/surrogacy (IVF third-party parenting) these women have the greatest chance by far of conceiving, greater than with any other cause of infertility.

For some infertile women, disease and/or the onset of ovarian failure precludes their ability to produce a fertilizable egg. But if they have a healthy uterus and are otherwise able to bear a child, egg donation offers a realistic opportunity for pregnancy. Egg donation involves stimulating the donor with fertility drugs, retrieving the eggs from the donor, fertilizing them in the laboratory with sperm from the recipient's partner, and transferring the resulting embryos into the uterus of the recipient, who will carry the baby to term.

Some women are born without a uterus, while others undergo surgical removal of the uterus in later life. Sometimes uterine disease renders the woman incapable of bearing a child, and, in a minority of cases chronic ill health, such as severe diabetes, makes pregnancy inadvisable. For these couples, the option exists of having another woman—a third party or surrogate—bear a child for them. Surrogate parenting can be divided into two categories: classic surrogacy and IVF surrogacy.

In *classic surrogacy*, a healthy young woman (usually under 35) agrees with an infertile couple to be artificially inseminated with the male partner's sperm, carry the baby to term, and then turn the baby over to the couple shortly after birth. Classic surrogacy has brightened the lives of many desperate infertile couples, but it also brings with it many ethical, moral, and medico-legal dilemmas. There is no getting around the fact that because the classic surrogate provides both the egg and the womb, she is biologically the child's mother. This is the primary cause of surrogates' last-minute decisions not to give up the child. Who can ignore the intense media coverage that often erupts when a surrogate decides against giving up the baby to the infertile couple? Situations like this cause wrenching emotional turmoil for the parents, for the surrogate, and (sooner or later) for the child. Classic surrogacy currently is, nevertheless, still a widely employed method of surrogate parenting. Since we do not offer classic surrogacy in our programs at the present time, we will not discuss it further here.

EGG DONATION (ED)

For many women, disease and/or diminished ovarian reserve precludes achieving a pregnancy with their own eggs. Since the vast majority of such women are otherwise quite healthy and physically capable of bearing a child, egg donation (ED) provides them with a realistic opportunity of going from infertility to parenthood.

Egg donation is associated with definite benefits. Firstly, in many instances, more eggs are retrieved from a young donor than would ordinarily be needed to complete a single IVF cycle. As a result, there are often supernumerary (leftover) embryos for cryopreservation and storage. Secondly, since eggs derived from a young woman are less likely than their older counterparts to produce aneuploid (chromosomally abnormal) embryos, the risk of miscarriage and birth defects such as Down syndrome is considerably reduced.

Egg donation-related fresh and frozen embryo transfer cycles account for 10%-15% of IVF performed in the United States. The vast majority of egg donation procedures performed in the U.S. involve women with declining ovarian reserve. While some of these are done for premature ovarian failure, the majority are undertaken in women over 40 years of age. Recurrent IVF failure due to "poor quality" eggs or embryos is also a relatively common indication for ED in the U.S. A growing indication for ED is in cases of same-sex relationships (predominantly female) where both partners wish to share in the parenting experience by one serving as egg provider and the other as the recipient.

Ninety percent of egg donation in the U.S. is done through the solicitation of anonymous donors who are recruited through a state-licensed egg donor agency. It is less common for recipients to solicit known donors through the services of a donor agency, although this does happen on occasion. It is also not easy to find donors who are willing to enter into such an open arrangement. Accordingly, in the vast majority of cases where the services of a known donor are solicited, it is by virtue of a private arrangement. While the services of non-family members are sometimes sought, it is much more common for recipients to approach close family members to serve as their egg donor.

Some recipients feel the compulsion to know or at least to have met their egg donor, so as to gain firsthand familiarity with her physical characteristics, intellect, and character. This having been said, in the U.S. it is much more common to seek the services of anonymous donors. In terms of disclosure to their family, friends, and child(ren), recipients using anonymous donors tend to be far more open than those of known donors about the nature of the child's conception. Most, if not all, egg donor agencies provide a detailed profile, photos, medical and family history of each prospective donor for the benefit and information of the recipient. Agencies generally have a website through which recipients can access donor profiles in the privacy of their own homes in order to select the ideal donor.

Interaction between the recipient and the egg donor program may be conducted in-person, by telephone, via Skype, or online in the initial stages. Once the choice of a donor has been narrowed down to two or three, the recipient is asked to forward all relevant medical records to their chosen IVF physician. Upon receipt of her records, a detailed medical consultation will subsequently be held and a physical examination by the treating physician or by a designated alternative qualified counterpart is scheduled. This entire process is usually overseen, facilitated and orchestrated by one of the donor program's nurse coordinators who, in concert with the treating physician, will address all clinical, financial, and logistical issues, as well as answering any questions. At the same time, the final process of donor selection and donor-recipient matching is completed.

Egg donor agencies usually limit the age of egg donors to women under 35 years with normal ovarian reserve in an attempt to minimize the risk of ovarian resistance and negate adverse influence of the "biological clock" (donor age) on egg quality.

No single factor instills more confidence regarding the reproductive potential of a prospective egg donor than a history of her having previously achieved a pregnancy on her own, or one or more recipients of her eggs having achieved a live birth. Moreover, such a track record makes it far more likely that such an ED will have "good quality eggs." Furthermore, the fact that an ED readily conceived on her own lessens the likelihood that she herself has tubal or organic infertility. This having been said, the current shortage in the supply of egg donors makes it both impractical and unfeasible to confine donor recruitment to those women who could fulfill such stringent criteria for qualification.

It is not unheard of for a donor who, at some point after donating eggs, finds herself unable to conceive on her own due to pelvic adhesions or tubal disease, to blame her infertility on complications caused by the prior surgical egg retrieval process. She may even embark upon legal proceedings against the IVF physician and program. It should therefore come as no surprise that it provides a measurable degree of comfort to ED programs when a prospective donor is able to provide evidence of having experienced a relatively recent, trouble-free spontaneous pregnancy.

Screening Egg Donors

Genetic Screening: The vast majority of IVF programs in the U.S. follow the recommendations and guidelines of the American Society of Reproductive Medicine (ASRM) for selective genetic screening of prospective egg donors for conditions such as sickle cell trait or disease, Thalassemia, cystic fibrosis and Tay Sachs disease, when medically indicated. Consultation with a geneticist is available through about 90% of programs.

Most recipient couples place a great deal of importance on emotional, physical, ethnic, cultural, and religious compatibility with their chosen egg donor. In fact they often will insist that the egg donor be heterosexual.

Psychological Screening: Americans tend to place great emphasis on psychological screening of egg donors. Since most donors are "anonymous," it is incumbent upon the ED agency or the IVF program to determine the donor's degree of commitment as well as her motivation for deciding to provide this service. I have on occasion encountered donors who have buckled under the stress and defaulted midstream during their cycle of stimulation with gonadotropins. In one case, a donor knowingly stopped administering gonadotropins without informing anyone. She simply awaited cancellation, which was effected when follicles stopped growing and her plasma E2 concentration failed to rise.

Such concerns mandate that assessment of donor motivation and commitment be given appropriate priority. Most recipients in the U.S. tend to be very much influenced by the "character" of the prospective egg donor, believing that a flawed character is likely to be carried over genetically to the offspring. In reality, unlike certain psychoses such as schizophrenia or bipolar disorders, character flaws are usually neuroses and are most likely to be determined by environmental factors associated with upbringing. They are unlikely to be genetically transmitted. Nevertheless, egg donors should be subjected to counseling and screening and should be selectively tested by a qualified psychologists. When in doubt, they should be referred to a psychiatrist for more definitive testing. Selective use of tests such as the MMPI, Meyers-Briggs and NEO-Personality Indicator are used to assess for personality disorders. Significant abnormalities, once detected, should lead to the automatic disqualification of such prospective donors.

When it comes to choosing a known egg donor, it is equally important to make sure that she was not coerced into participating. We try to caution recipients who are considering having a close friend or family member serve as their designated egg donor, that in doing so, the potential always exists that the donor might become a permanent and an unwanted participant in the lives of their new family.

Drug Screening: Because of the prevalence of substance abuse in our society, we selectively call for urine and/or serum drug testing of our egg donors.

Screening for Sexually Transmittable Diseases (STDs): FDA and ASRM guidelines recommend that all egg donors be tested for sexually transmittable diseases before entering into a cycle of IVF. While it is highly improbable that DNA and RNA viruses could be transmitted to an egg or an embryo through sexual intercourse or IVF, women infected with viruses such as hepatitis B, C, HTLV, HIV, etc., must be disqualified from participating in IVF with egg donation due to the (albeit remote) possibility of transmission, as well as the potential legal consequences of the egg donation process being blamed for their occurrence.

In addition, evidence of prior or existing infection with chlamydia or gonorrhea introduces the possibility that the egg donor might have pelvic adhesions or even irreparably damaged fallopian tubes that might have rendered her infertile. As previously stated, such infertility, subsequently detected, might be blamed on infection that occurred during the process of egg retrieval, exposing the caregivers to litigation. Even if an egg donor or a recipient who carries a sexually transmittable viral or bacterial agent is willing to waive all rights of legal recourse, a potential risk still exists that a subsequently affected offspring might in later in life sue for wrongful birth.

Screening of Recipient(s)

Medical Screening: While advancing age, beyond 40 years, is indeed associated with an escalating incidence of pregnancy complications, such risks are largely predictable through careful medical assessment prior to pregnancy. The fundamental question, namely: "Is the woman capable of safely engaging a pregnancy that would culminate in the safe birth of a healthy baby?" must be answered in the affirmative, before any infertility treatment is initiated. For this reason, a thorough cardiovascular, hepatorenal, metabolic, and anatomical reproductive evaluation must be done prior to initiating IVF in all cases.

Infectious Screening: The need for careful infectious screening for embryo recipients cannot be overemphasized. Aside from tests for debilitating sexually transmittable diseases, some physicians recommend that both cervical mucus and semen be free of infection with ureaplasma urealyticum. This organism which rarely causes symptoms frequents the cervical glands of 15-20% of women in the U.S. The introduction of an embryo transfer catheter via a so-infected cervix might transmit the organism into an otherwise sterile uterine cavity leading to early implantation failure and/or first trimester miscarriage.

Immunologic Screening: Certain autoimmune and alloimmune disorders (see elsewhere) can be associated with immunologic implantation dysfunction (IID). In order to prevent otherwise avoidable treatment failure, it is advisable to evaluate the recipient for autoimmune IDD and also to test both the recipient and the sperm provider for alloimmune similarities that could compromise implantation.

DISCLOSURE AND CONSENT

Preparation for egg donation requires full disclosure to all participants regarding what each step of the process involves from start to finish, as well as potential medical and psychological risks. This necessitates that significant time be devoted to this task and that there be a willingness to painstakingly address all questions and concerns posed by all parties involved in the process. An important component of full disclosure involves clear interpretation of the medical and psychological components assessed during the evaluation process. All parties should be advised to seek independent legal counsel so as to avoid conflicts of interest that might arise from legal advice given by the same attorney. Appropriate consent forms are then reviewed and signed independently by the donor and the recipient couple.

Most embryo recipients fully anticipate that their chosen donor will yield a large number of mature, good quality eggs, sufficient to provide enough embryos to afford a good chance of pregnancy as well as several for cryopreservation (freezing) and storage. While such expectations are often met, this is not always the case. Accordingly, to minimize the trauma of unexpected and usually unavoidable disappointment, it is essential that in the process of counseling and of consummating agreements, the respective parties be fully informed that by making their best efforts to provide the highest standards of care, the caregivers can only assure optimal intent and performance in keeping with accepted standards of care. *No one can ever promise an optimal outcome.* All parties should be made aware that no definitive representation can or will be made as to the number or quality of eggs and embryos that will or are likely to become available, the number of supernumerary embryos that will be available for cryopreservation, or the subsequent outcome of the IVF donor process.

Types of Egg Donation

Conventional Egg Donation: This is the basic format used for conducting the process of egg donor IVF. It involves synchronizing the menstrual cycles of both the recipient and the donor by placing the donor and the recipient on a birth control pill so that both parties start stimulation with fertility drugs simultaneously. This ultimately allows for precise timing of the fresh embryo transfer. Using this approach, the anticipated egg donation birthrate is >50% per cycle.

CGH-Egg Donation: The recent introduction of CGH and Staggered IVF has the potential to change the manner in which egg donation is likely to be performed in the future. CGH allows full egg/embryo chromosome analysis providing a 70–80% assurance that the embryo(s) so selected for transfer are highly likely to be "competent" (i.e., capable of producing a healthy baby). Such CGH-embryo selection provides about a >60% chance of a baby per blastocyst transferred. This is at least double that reported when conventional egg donation is used. As a result, CGH-Egg Donation allows for excellent results when one or two embryos are transferred, virtually eliminating the risk of high-order multiple pregnancies (triplets or greater). Moreover, since numerical chromosomal irregularities (aneuploidy) are responsible for most sporadic miscarriages, the use of CGH also significantly reduces this dreaded complication. CGH embryo selection of necessity mandates the use of St-IVF. Here the egg donor cycle is divided into two parts. The first involves the egg retrieval, fertilization, embryo biopsy for CGH analysis, and embryo cryostorage. The second part involving warming or thawing of the frozen embryo(s) and the subsequent transfer of "competent" embryo(s) to the recipient's uterus is conducted electively at least several weeks later once the results of CGH testing are available. Since with St-IVF the egg retrieval and embryo transfer are separated in time, the retrieval can be performed without first having to synchronize the menstrual cycles of the recipient and the egg the donor. In fact, the recipient does not even have to be available when the egg donor is going through cycle. All that is needed is for designated sperm to be available (fresh or frozen) on the day of egg retrieval. This avoids unnecessary travel and inconvenience, and minimizes stress and cost.

Donor Egg Banking

Another imminent advance is the introduction of egg banking. Being able to freeze and bank donor eggs would solve most of these challenges. By using CGH in combination with a vitrification, we are now capable of improving the birthrate per warmed/thawed egg by a factor of

7 (from a previous average of <5% per egg to almost 30%). Through an electronic catalogue, recipients will be able to select and purchase 1-3 CGH-normal eggs from the comfort of their homes. Thereupon, the selective transfer of 1 or 2 embryos derived from such chromosomally normal eggs could achieve a >70% pregnancy rate without the risk of initiating high-order multiple pregnancies in the process. Through this process, the cost, inconvenience, and risks associated with "conventional" fresh egg donor cycles would also be reduced significantly.

Financial Considerations

In the United States, the fee paid to the egg donor agency per cycle usually ranges between $2,000 and $8,000. This does not include the cost associated with psychological and clinical pre-testing, fertility drugs, and donor insurance, which commonly range between $3,000 and $6,000. The medical service costs of the IVF treatment cycle ranges between $8,000 and $14,000. The donor stipend can range from $5,000 to as high $50,000 depending upon the exotic requirements of the recipient couple as well as supply and demand. Thus the total out of pocket expenses for an egg donor cycle in the United States range between $15,000 and $80,000, putting egg donation outside the financial capability of most couples needing this service.

The growing gap between need and affordability has spawned a number of creative ways to try and make IVF with egg donation more affordable. Here are a few examples:

1. Egg banking (see above).
2. Egg Donor Sharing, where one comprehensive fee is shared between two recipients and the eggs are then divided between them. The downside is that fewer eggs are available for transfer and/or cryopreservation.
3. Egg Bartering, where in the course of conventional IVF, a woman undergoing IVF remits some of her eggs to the clinic (which in turn provides it to a recipient patient) in exchange for a deferment of some or all of the IVF fee. In my opinion, such an arrangement can be fraught with problems. For example, in the

event that the woman donating some of her eggs fails to conceive while the recipient of her eggs does, it is very possible that she might suffer emotional despair and even go so far as to seek out her genetic offspring. Such action could be very damaging to her and the recipient, as well as the child.

4. Financial Risk Sharing. Certain IVF programs offer financial risk sharing (FRS), which most recipient couples favor greatly. FRS offers qualifying candidates a refund of fees paid if egg donation is unsuccessful. FRS is designed to spread the risk between the providers and the recipient couple.

Moral, Ethical, Religious, and Legal Considerations

The "Uniform Parentage Act," which has been adopted by most states in the United States, declares that the woman who gives birth to the child will be regarded as the rightful mother. Accordingly, there have to date not been any grounds for legal dispute when it comes to maternal custody of a child born through IVF with egg donation in the majority of states. In a few states, such as Mississippi and Arizona, the law is less clear but nevertheless, as yet, has not been contested.

The moral, ethical, and religious implications of egg donation are diverse and have a profound effect on cultural acceptance of this process. The widely held view that everyone is entitled to their own opinion and has the right to have such opinions respected, governs much of the attitude towards this process in the U.S. The extreme views on each end of the spectrum hold the gentle central swing of the pendulum in place. This attitude is a reflection of the general acceptance in the United States of diverse views and opinions and the willingness to allow free expression of such views and beliefs provided that they don't infringe on the rights of others.

EMBRYO BANKING

An ever increasing number of couples are choosing to delay having children because of financial and career-related reasons. For a woman, such a decision carries with it an ever present risk that when she ultimately decides to have a baby, she might find herself unable to conceive.

It is an undeniable fact that a woman's fecundity (the ability to conceive per month of trying) declines in her mid-30s and then falls off precipitously after 40. Unfortunately, most women/couples do not realize that there could be a price to pay for delaying starting a family. Clearly, aspiring parents need to understand this reality so that they can make informed choices when it comes to planning their family.

Upon becoming aware of the impact of the biological clock, many women/couples become desperate and look to in vitro fertilization as a solution. For women approaching or entering their 40s, achieving a pregnancy without help or through the use of fertility drugs and/or intrauterine insemination offers less than a 5% per month chance of having a baby. Given such relatively poor odds many such women, for good reason, turn to IVF as it can significantly improve the chance of becoming pregnant before time runs out. However IVF is certainly not a panacea.

Regardless of the method used to achieve a pregnancy, older women inevitably will have to confront the following hurdles:
- A progressive and accelerated decline in egg quality
- A progressive decline in the number of eggs they will be able to produce in response to fertility drugs (as evidenced by rising FSH and declining AMH levels)
- A marked increase in the miscarriage rate, which could be as high as 70% by age 45
- An increased risk of chromosomal birth defects such as Down syndrome, which reaches 1 in 30 by age 45

Another factor to be considered is the fact that many women trying to start a family at an older age would often like to have more than one baby. In such cases, they will need to come to terms with the fact that by the time they have had their first child and have breastfed for a year or so, 2-3 critical years will have been lost, making the likelihood of having another baby (even through IVF) much less probable.

It is important to recognize that the main reason for declining fertility with age relates to a progressive and inevitable decline in the chromosomal integrity of a woman's eggs as she advances beyond her mid-30s and into her 40s. The simple fact is that there is no medical remedy for this problem. As an example: At 30–35 years about 40% of a woman's eggs are chromosomally normal. At 40, less than 20% are likely to be normal, while by age 45, well under 10% are chromosomally intact. The good news is that a chromosomally normal egg is just as likely to propagate a healthy embryo/baby regardless of the age of the egg provider. A chromosomally normal egg from a woman of 45 probably has close to the same chance of producing a healthy baby as does a normal egg taken from a 25-year-old.

The introduction of CGH enables us to identify chromosomally "competent" eggs or embryos. Such normal embryos transferred to the uterus of a healthy woman would propagate a healthy baby about 60% of the time, regardless of the age of the "egg provider."

What is embryo banking/stockpiling all about? We recently began offering women the opportunity to freeze/store and then stockpile/bank their CGH-normal embryos for future dispensation. To do this, they undergo multiple IVF procedures that each proceed through fertilization of their eggs. The resulting embryos are then biopsied and allowed to progress to the blastocyst stage (the most advanced preimplantation stage of embryo development), whereupon they are vitrified (ultra-rapidly frozen) and then banked.

Several such cycles are conducted in the hope of stockpiling a number of advanced embryos (blastocysts) for later use. Once the last cycle of embryo banking is completed, the biopsied samples derived from all surviving blastocysts are subjected to genetic (CGH) testing only once, thereby minimizing cost that otherwise would have had to be incurred were CGH testing to be performed after each procedure.

Selective banking of genetically tested embryos in women for whom the end of their reproductive career is in sight dramatically expands reproductive choices available to them. First, it allows them to have more than one baby without the ever-present fear that by the time they have had the first one they might not be able to have another. Second, for women who are only interested in having one baby, it establishes realistic and rational expectations of success versus failure, and thus will help them decide when it is time to stop doing IVF, adopt, or go to egg donation. Simply stated, it establishes either a favorable resolution or closure.

It behooves all individuals/couples who are intent upon having a family to be aware of the fact that a woman's biological clock cannot be reset. It is relentless, merciless, and unforgiving. It is also well to bear in mind that a woman's fertility potential can suddenly decline over a few years – both due to, or independent of, advancing age. While the threat of declining fertility is greatest in the late 30s and early 40s, it could just as easily occur in younger women. Because of this reality, women of reproductive age are well advised to undergo hormonal and physical assessments of their fertility potential every few years and to increase the frequency in their mid-30s.

EMBRYO ADOPTION

Embryo adoption refers to the situation in which a woman receives embryos to which she and her partner have not contributed biologically. When both partners are infertile, both donor sperm and donor eggs must be used if the woman is to become pregnant. Previously, adoption of a child would have been such a couple's only option. Now, however, prenatal embryo adoption can be an alternative to adoption of a baby or child. We perform these adoptive procedures because we believe that apart from the fact that embryo adoption occurs far earlier than baby adoption, there is otherwise little difference between the two processes.

Donor embryos can come from several sources. For example, a woman who cannot produce her own eggs might choose to adopt one or more embryos from a donor and have them transferred into her uterus. An additional source of embryos would be couples who, finding they have more embryos than they wish to transfer after IVF, donate the extras to another couple.

The aspiring parents undergo a thorough clinical, psychological, and laboratory assessment prior to adopting embryos for transfer into the woman's uterus.

IVF (GESTATIONAL) SURROGACY

IVF surrogacy involves the transfer of one or more embryos derived from the woman's eggs and from sperm of her partner (or a sperm donor) into the uterus of a surrogate. In this case, the surrogate provides a host womb but does not contribute genetically to the baby. While ethical, moral, and medico-legal issues still apply, IVF surrogacy appears to have gained more social acceptance than classic surrogacy. We offer IVF surrogacy as an option in most of our programs.

Candidates for IVF Gestational Surrogacy

Candidates for IVF surrogacy can be divided into two groups: (1) women born without a uterus or who because of uterine surgery or disease are not capable of carrying a pregnancy to full term and (2) women who have been advised against undertaking a pregnancy because of systemic illnesses, such as diabetes, heart disease, hypertension, or certain malignant conditions.

As in preparation for other assisted reproductive techniques, the biological parents undergo a thorough clinical, psychological, and laboratory assessment prior to selecting a surrogate. The purpose is to exclude sexually transmitted diseases that might be carried to the surrogate at the time of embryo transfer. They are also counseled on issues faced by all IVF aspiring parents, such as the possibility of multiple births, ectopic pregnancy, and miscarriage.

All legal issues pertaining to custody and the rights of the biological parents and the surrogate should be discussed in detail and the appropriate consent forms completed following full disclosure. We recommend that the surrogate and biological parents get separate legal counsel to avoid the conflict of interest that would arise were one attorney to counsel both parties.

Selecting a Surrogate

Many infertile couples who qualify for IVF surrogate parenting solicit the assistance of empathic friends or family members to act as surrogates.

Other couples seek surrogates by advertising in the media. Many couples with the necessary financial resources retain a surrogacy agency to find a suitable candidate. We direct our patients to a reputable surrogacy agency with access to many surrogates. Because the surrogate gives birth, it is rarely realistic or even possible for her to remain anonymous.

Screening a Surrogate

Once the surrogate has been selected, she will undergo thorough medical and psychological evaluations, including:

1. A cervical culture and/or DNA test to screen for infection with chlamydia, ureaplasma, gonococcus, and other infective organisms that might interfere with a successful outcome.

2. Blood tests (as appropriate) for HIV, hepatitis, and other sexually transmitted diseases. She will also have a blood test performed to ensure that she is immune to the development of rubella (German measles) and will have a variety of blood-hormone tests, such as the measurement of plasma prolactin and thyroid-stimulating hormone (TSH).

Whether recruited from an agency, family members, or through personal solicitation, the surrogate should be carefully evaluated psychologically as well as physically. This is especially important in cases where a relatively young surrogate or family member is recruited. In such cases, it is important to ensure that the surrogate has not been subjected to any pressure or coercion.

The surrogate should also be counseled on issues faced by all IVF aspiring parents, such as multiple births. She should also visit with the clinical coordinator, who will outline the exact process step by step. She should be informed that she has full right of access to the clinic staff and that her concerns will be addressed promptly at all times. And she should be aware that if pregnancy occurs, she will be referred to an obstetrician for prenatal care and delivery.

After the evaluations and counseling of both the couple and the surrogate have been completed, the three of them will meet. And once all the evaluations have been completed, the couple will select a date to begin treatment.

Controlled Ovarian Stimulation and Monitoring of the Female Partner (Egg Provider)

The procedure used to stimulate the female partner of the infertile couple with fertility drugs and monitor her condition strongly resembles that used for an egg donor. In order to stimulate ovulation of enough eggs to increase the chances of a viable pregnancy, the female partner will be stimulated with gonadotropins. Approximately seven days after ovulation occurs (as assessed by a BBT chart or a urine home-ovulation test kit), GnRHa is administered daily to prepare the ovaries. With the onset of menstruation approximately seven to 12 days later, the female partner is given a blood test and baseline ultrasound examination to confirm that the ovaries are prepared and to exclude the presence of ovarian cysts. The decision is made then about when gonadotropin therapy should commence.

On the eighth day of gonadotropin injections, the program would likely begin intensive daily monitoring by means of blood hormone measurements and ultrasound examinations. Usually, one to three additional days of gonadotropin therapy will be required. Once monitoring confirms that the female partner's ovarian follicles have developed optimally, she is given an injection of the ovulatory trigger hCG. Then, in order to capture the eggs prior to ovulation, they are harvested 36 hours after the hCG injection by transvaginal ultrasound needle-guided aspiration.

Synchronizing the Cycles of the Surrogate and the Aspiring Mother

The surrogate will receive estrogen orally, by skin patches, or by injections (estradiol valerate/delestrogen), and then progesterone to help prepare her uterine lining for implantation. As with preparing the recipient for IVF/ovum donation, we use biweekly estradiol valerate injections in our programs. GnRHa is administered for a period of seven to 12 days in order to prepare the ovaries prior to administration of estradiol valerate. The duration of GnRHa therapy is adjusted to synchronize the cycle of the woman undergoing follicular stimulation with that of the surrogate. Once the prospective mother commences follic-ular stimulation, the surrogate will be given estradiol injections while continuing GnRHa therapy.

Building the Surrogate's Uterine Lining with Hormonal Injections

At SIRM the surrogate receives estradiol valerate injections on Tues-days and Fridays, and her blood is drawn on Mondays and Thursdays to measure estradiol concentrations so the physician can determine the subsequent hormonal dosage. She also undergoes ultrasound examina-tions 10 days to two weeks after the first estradiol valerate injection to evaluate development of her uterine lining. Approximately four days prior to the expected day of embryo transfer, the recipient is given daily injections of progesterone to optimize endometrial development. In the uncommon event of poor endometrial development, the couple will be given the choice of having the aspiring mother's eggs harvested, fertil-ized, and frozen for transfer to a surrogate's uterus in a subsequent cycle, or canceling the procedure.

Transferring Embryos to the Surrogate's Uterus

After the egg provider (woman partner) has undergone transvaginal ultrasound-guided egg retrieval, the eggs are fertilized and the embryos cultured as they would be for traditional IVF.

Approximately 72 to 120 hours following egg retrieval, the embryos are transferred to the surrogate's uterus. She then lies perfectly still for approximately one hour to try to enhance the chances of implantation and is then discharged from the clinic.

Management and Follow-up after the Embryo Transfer

The surrogate will be given daily progesterone injections and biweekly estradiol valerate injections and/or suppositories in order to sustain an optimal environment for implantation, and approximately 10 days after the embryo transfer will undergo a pregnancy test. A positive test indicates that implantation is taking place. In such an event, the hormone injections will be continued for an additional four to six weeks. In the interim, an ultrasound examination will be performed to definitively diagnose a clinical pregnancy. If the test is negative, all hormonal treatment is discontinued, and menstruation will ensue within three to 10 days.

If the surrogate does not conceive, the aspiring mother may have her remaining embryos/blastocysts vitrified, to be thawed and transferred to the uterus of another woman at a later date. If in spite of both the initial attempt and subsequent transfer of thawed embryos the surrogate does not conceive, the infertile couple may schedule a new cycle of treatment.

Anticipated Success Rates with Gestational Surrogacy

In the event that a viable pregnancy is confirmed by ultrasound recognition of a fetal heartbeat, there is a better than 85 percent chance that the pregnancy will proceed normally to term. Once the pregnancy has progressed beyond the 12th week, the chance of a healthy baby being born is upward of 95 percent at SIRM. In our setting, we anticipate approximately a 50 percent birthrate every time two blastocysts are derived from the eggs of a woman under 35 years old. The birthrate declines as the age of the egg provider advances beyond 35. It is important to note that there is no convincing evidence to suggest an increase in the incidence of spontaneous miscarriage or birth defects as a direct result of IVF surrogacy.

The Bioethics of Gestational Surrogacy

The determination of ethical guidelines has not kept pace with the exploding growth and development in IVF. However, some leaders in the field are working together, sharing experiences and advice, in an attempt to formulate a code of ethics. We end this chapter with a suggestion made by Dr. William Andereck in a presentation called "Ethical Issues in the New Reproductive Technologies." He cited what he calls the "two-out-of-three rule" that he has applied to gestational surrogacy:

The genetic combination of the male and the female provide two of the essential elements which, along with gestation, are necessary to produce a human being. The two-out-of-three rule basically looks at these three elements: the egg, the sperm, and the gestational component. If at all possible, I recommend that at least two of these three components be contributed by the intended parents. If they can only contribute one, by all means please try not to get the other two contributed by the same person.

This is a good first step that can be applied to many of the situations discussed in this chapter.

In an earlier version of this book, which was published in 1988, we discussed the pros and cons of using fresh versus frozen sperm; the use of frozen sperm was considered cutting-edge technology at the time. In the edition published in 1995, we talked about such promising assisted-reproductive technology as fertilization/micromanipulation, including intracytoplasmic sperm injection (ICSI), and assisted hatching, including zona drilling. None of these techniques is discussed any longer in this chapter because, in many leading IVF centers, they have become standard procedures. This illustrates the short time span between ART development and practical implementation over the last two decades.

In previous editions we asked, "What would George Orwell have said about new fertility techniques such as cryopreserving eggs, sperm, and embryos for future use?" Now we ask, "What would George Orwell have said about gender selection and preimplantation genetic diagnosis?"

CHAPTER

16

MISCELLANEOUS CONSIDERATIONS

SAME-SEX COUPLES DESERVE AN EQUAL OPPORTUNITY TO HAVE A FAMILY

I have been treating infertile couples for more than thirty years and have had the great privilege of participating in the genesis of in vitro fertilization in the United States, virtually from its inception. During that time, my associates and I have helped hundreds of committed same sex couples go from infertility to family. With very few exceptions, the medical challenges faced by such couples, and the family relationships that emerged and evolved following the births of children have hardly differed from those experienced by other couples undergoing the same treatment. Many of these babies are now fully grown, thus providing me with a real-life opportunity to observe some of them as they have confronted life's challenges. Based on this experience, it is my opinion that the fact that they were born to same-sex couples did not disadvantage any of them.

In my experience, the commitment made by these same-sex parents to one another and to the raising of their offspring seems to me to have been no different than in the case of heterosexual parents. I have concluded that in spite of the enormous pressures imposed on same sex couples by an often bigoted society, they recognize their responsibility to maintain a cohesive relationship for the well being of their offspring.

Let's face it, while there are indeed many enlightened people who are willing to embrace same sex families, there is a segment of our society that is so caught up in religious and moral ideologies that they are not ready for this. Granted, the preservation of stable, monogamous relationships in same-sex couples is subject to more pressure and scrutiny. Yet, once cemented by a profound decision to have a child together, the chance of them falling apart appears to be no greater than for other partnerships.

Massachusetts was the first state to legalize same sex marriage. A few other states followed and it is probable that there will be more in the future. I believe that, in time, same sex marriage will be legalized throughout the United States. But even if I am wrong, what is indisputable is that marriage does not always provide a blueprint for enduring love and commitment. Nor is it an essential prerequisite for having a family. In fact, nowadays many couples are choosing to have children without first tying the legal knot. Some do so for financial reasons while others simply don't see the need for a legal contract to confirm their commitments to one another. Regardless of marital status or sexual preference, willfully creating a family together represents a profound expression of mutual love and commitment.

There are many options available to same sex couples seeking parenthood.

For Female Couples

In the case of female couples, the simplest approach is to undergo artificial insemination with donor sperm. However, in some cases the matter is complicated by the existence of infertility that cannot be adequately addressed through insemination with donor sperm . . . thus necessitating IVF. Regardless of the approach to treatment, stringent FDA guidelines require that all sperm donors—whether anonymous, known, recruited from a licensed sperm bank, or selected independently—be tested for potentially transmittable viral infections (e.g., HIV) at the time of producing the specimen, and that the sperm then be frozen/stored for several months, at which time the sperm provider be retested before using it for insemination or IVF.

In some cases, both female partners may wish to share in the biological contribution to a pregnancy. In such cases one partner will produce the eggs necessary to be fertilized with donor sperm and the embryos will be transferred to the prepared uterus of the other partner.

For Male Couples

Here, the available choices are insemination of sperm directly into the uterus of a surrogate (classic surrogacy) or IVF using an egg donor, fertilizing her eggs with sperm, and then transferring the embryo(s) to the uterus of a surrogate (gestational surrogacy). As with the use of donor sperm, the sperm provider needs to be tested for a variety of factors such as certain viral infections (including HIV). In addition, the specimen must be held in quarantine for several months before being used. Ever since the Baby M case about 3 decades ago (where a gestational carrier, who conceived after being inseminated with the sperm of the intended male partner, sued for custody and won), we have strongly advocated against the classic surrogacy approach, where the carrier is also the egg provider. In fact, at SIRM we confine the use of surrogacy to gestational surrogacy-situations where the carrier will have no genetic link to the offspring. This mandates the use of in vitro fertilization rather than artificial insemination.

In summary, aside from the effects of social and political pressures, same-sex couples experience similar concerns to those that occur in any other relationship. They wonder what the future holds and whether they will be able to fulfill their desire to have children and accomplish the dream of building a family. While at times this may all seem quite overwhelming, in today's age it is easier than ever for them to experience the joy of parenthood. There is no evidence that there is any harm to anybody from same sex couples having a child. Children need to be brought up in a loving, caring environment and it is the loving care that is most important, not the sexuality of the parent.

GAMETE/EMBRYO CRYOPRESERVATION

Embryo/Blastocyst Freezing (see Chapter 7)

Cryopreservation of human embryos has been a routine procedure since the early 1980s. Conventional techniques (which are still being widely used by most IVF centers) involve slow freezing which as previously stated unfortunately results in ice crystal formation inside the cell(s), damaging them and reducing embryo "competency," i.e. the subsequent ability upon thawing, to propagate a viable pregnancy. The relatively recent introduction of ultra-rapid freezing or vitrification changed all this.

Egg Freezing

It has been more than two and a half decades since Chen (1986) reported on the first birth following the transfer of an embryo derived from a frozen/thawed egg.

Hitherto, publications in the literature indicate that <25% of eggs cryopreserved actually survive in a condition where their subsequent fertilization could lead to the propagation of "competent embryos" (i.e., those that have the potential to propagate healthy pregnancies). This explains why the highest reported implantation rate per embryo (derived from frozen/thawed eggs) transferred is less than 10%. To put things in even greater perspective, based on previous reports in the literature, there is less than a 5% chance that any given frozen mature (MII) egg will survive the freeze/thaw and go on to propagate a live birth.

In spite of these relatively poor results, an increasing number of women, partly for medical reasons, but mostly because they feel trapped by the limitations of the "biological clock," are flocking to an ever-growing number of IVF programs in the U.S. that offer commercial egg freezing and banking. Presently, given the status of mainstream technology, any representation that egg freezing provides an assurance that women can presently preserve their fertility by banking their eggs for future use is both empty and misleading and will ultimately lead to major disappoint-ments with potential for public backlash.

Problems Associated with "Conventional" (Slow) Egg Freezing Techniques: Conventional "slow egg freezing" techniques cause ice crystal formation within the egg's cytoplasm, thereby compromising its survival. The intro-duction a few years ago of a freezing method known as *vitrification*, which freezes cells ultra-rapidly, avoids ice formation inside the cell(s), and, as such, largely precludes egg damage, yielding much improved survival rates.

Selecting Euploid, "Competent" Eggs for Selective Vitrification and Banking: We have reported on the use of full chromosomal assessment by CGH performed on the first polar body (PB-1) to test the DNA of mature eggs for their complete chromosomal integrity. We were able to demonstrate that 60% of eggs aspirated from the ovaries of women under 35 years have an irregular number of chromosomes (i.e., are aneuploid) and that the incidence of aneuploidy increases rapidly with advancing years.

Egg Freezing and Banking at SIRM: Against this background, we recently reported on a study where we selectively vitrified only "com-petent" chromosomally normal (euploid) eggs which upon thawing (warming) were fertilized by ICSI. Up to two blastocysts were then transferred to the uteri of designated recipients. Based on our experi-ence to date we are able to state that:

1. >95% of the vitrified euploid eggs survived the freeze/thaw and went on to be successfully fertilized.
2. About 60% of successfully fertilized eggs developed into expanded blastocysts.
3. The transfer of up to two such blastocysts results in about approximately a 50% implantation rate per transferred embryo and about a 60% birthrate per embryo transfer.
4. The baby rate per (warmed) egg was almost 30% (at least 7 times greater than ever reported).

All this clearly suggests that while pregnancy rates following egg freezing are profoundly affected by the freezing process itself, the pro-cess of selectively freezing and banking only "competent" (CGH-nor-mal) eggs represents the real breakthrough.

We believe that the ability, through PB-1 biopsy and CGH, to identify and thereupon selectively vitrify and cryobank only euploid, "competent" eggs for Fertility Preservation (FP) or for donor egg banking, will vastly improve the family planning options available to women and thereby will significantly impact the entire field of human reproduction. It has been estimated that the demand for FP-related IVF would be at least seven times greater than that which currently exists for infertility-related IVF.

FP-IVF could:

1. Allow women in the reproductive age to safely postpone having babies, without fear that the inevitable decline in egg quality which accompanies aging will deny them having a family they are ready.

2. Benefit women with existing medical conditions (such as breast cancer, leukemia, lymphoma, etc.) which preclude initiation of pregnancy until cured. In such cases treatment (e.g., by radiotherapy or chemotherapy) would otherwise often render these women permanently infertile. The successful cryopreservation and storage of their eggs could avoid denying such women the opportunity of parenthood with their own eggs.

3. Lead to the creation of better "egg banks" where donated eggs could be stored for subsequent dispensation (at comparatively low cost) to perimenopausal women and women with other causes of egg "incompetence" who wish to have babies (SIRM's egg bank will hopefully be in operation by 2014).

4. The creation of chromosomally normal (euploid) embryos could also serve as a much needed shot-in-the-arm for embryonic stem cell research and development.

5. With further advancement in egg freezing technology, it will no doubt ultimately prove to be far preferable to the use of embryos and become standard practice in the IVF setting.

Furthermore, there are several theoretical advantages to cryopreserving eggs rather than embryos:

An egg is a known quantity. It is likely to be healthy if it fertilizes and undergoes subsequent cleavage when thawed. In contrast, because the embryo is often transferred to the uterus immediately after thawing without undergoing further cleavage, one does not usually have the opportunity to observe whether it is indeed healthy at the time of transfer into the uterus. Because the embryo is further along the chain of evolution than an egg, the potential that an embryo damaged through freezing and thawing would produce an abnormal offspring is potentially greater than that which could be anticipated from an embryo derived from a previously thawed egg.

Egg freezing skirts the ethical dilemma as to whether life in its earliest form is being manipulated. Eggs, like sperm, are considered to be cells that do not have life potential on their own. However, some people believe that an embryo represents the earliest form of life and that any attrition of frozen-thawed embryos represents a form of abortion. However, the same argument cannot be applied to the freezing and thawing of eggs.

Ethics. If one were to argue that it is unethical to freeze an egg because its chances of survival and subsequent fertilization are questionable, then it should likewise be unethical to freeze semen because many of the sperm also die during cryopreservation. In this context it might also be argued that the practice of vaginal intercourse is wasteful because only one or two, and rarely three or four, sperm might be capable of fertilizing eggs and producing offspring—and the remaining sperm would die. Thus, most people who have a religious or moral aversion to embryo freezing would be unlikely to have the same objection to the freezing of eggs.

The role of egg donor agencies. The largest source of eggs for egg donation would be donors recruited through licensed agencies. This is already commonplace for the purpose of performing IVF with ovum donation. In addition, when more eggs are retrieved from a woman undergoing egg retrieval with IVF than are needed to optimize the likelihood that four to six embryos will be fertilized, the IVF couple might choose to donate or sell the surplus eggs to an egg bank or to other infertile women. We reject the sexist argument that it is immoral for women to sell their eggs while it is acceptable for men to sell their sperm.

It is indeed likely that the popularity of embryo freezing will in the long run be upstaged by egg freezing, but this will be some time in the future. However, embryo freezing will always have a place in the IVF setting because of the likelihood that when large numbers of eggs are fertilized in the laboratory, the couple will be left with more embryos than they or the IVF team would be willing to transfer into the woman's uterus. These excess embryos would either have to be allowed to die spontaneously or be frozen, stored, and kept available for a subsequent chance at conceiving should the initial IVF cycle be unsuccessful.

Nevertheless, we believe that, with few exceptions, egg cryopreservation is the better option for the future. As the technology continues to develop and be refined, we expect that egg cryopreservation will provide a variety of benefits to infertile couples.

IS BEING OVERWEIGHT DETRIMENTAL TO IVF OUTCOME?

There is little doubt that the prevalence of obesity in Western society is increasing at an alarming rate and that this is having a significant influence on the reproductive performance of women who are trying to have a baby. Recent evidence indicates that excessive weight in women of the reproductive age is associated with decreased birthrates, increased miscarriage rates, higher rates of premature delivery and a marked increase in pregnancy complications.

While being overweight clearly has an adverse affect on overall reproductive performance, the situation is less clear when it comes to its influence on women undergoing IVF. Several studies have been conducted and while the results vary and in some cases conflict, the general trend is in the direction of women who are moderately overweight (BMI of 25-30) and those who are obese (BMI greater than 30) having poorer IVF outcomes than those with a BMI under 25. It would appear that moderately overweight women, and more particularly those who are obese, exhibit a poorer ovarian response to fertility drugs (impaired follicle and embryo development with fewer blastocysts becoming available for transfer). They also might have a reduced ability to implant transferred embryos into their uterine linings (perhaps due to reduced endometrial receptivity).

It is of interest that many women with polycystic ovarian syndrome (PCOS) are also overweight. In such women, the hormonal environment in the ovaries is known to adversely affect follicle and egg development. Given that there is often no clear cut distinction between PCOS and overweight women, it is possible that many of the factors that are believed to affect egg/embryo quality in PCOS might similarly affect egg development and endometrial receptivity in overweight women. Such factors could include increased production of luteinizing hormone (LH), hyperinsulinemia and increased production of ovarian male hormones (androgens such as testosterone). The link between increased LH and resulting increased production of ovarian androgens (mainly testosterone) and poor follicle and egg development is well established. It is also well known that such hormonal changes can be transmitted to the adjacent uterus thereby adversely affecting endometrial development.

Clearly the question arises as to whether the negative effect of an elevated BMI (above 25) on general fertility potential and IVF outcome is due to compromised egg development, endometrial receptivity to the implanting embryo or both. In my opinion, while a direct ovarian influence probably predominates, there is also likely to be an adverse influence on endometrial development. This endometrial effect is commonly seen in PCOS women who, when they develop severe ovarian hyperstimulation (OHSS) often have a very thin endometrial lining.

Finally, it is important to emphasize that overweight women are at far greater risk during pregnancy than are women of normal body weight. As previously mentioned, the miscarriage rate is much higher. So is the incidence of diabetes, high blood pressure, preeclampsia, premature labor, surgically assisted deliveries, stillbirth, and neonatal death.

Maternal complications that occur after birth of the baby (i.e., infection, uterine post partum hemorrhage, etc.) are also much more common. Babies born to such mothers are also at great risk of developing respiratory distress syndrome (RDS). This condition which ordinarily only occurs in preterm babies can also occur in the absence of prematurity in such cases. RDS is the commonest reason for the newborn having to be admitted to a neonatal intensive care unit and also the commonest cause of death in the first week of life.

The clinical significance of a growing population of overweight women is enormous because not only can this compromise their overall reproductive performance but it also compounds the risk of chronic medical conditions such as diabetes and coronary/cerebral/peripheral vascular disease and thus compromises life expectancy as well as the quality of life. As such, being overweight represents an overall life hazard that should be addressed by the medical profession as well as by society as a whole. The answer is surely not a simple one but the solution does not lie in dieting alone (which rarely is of sustained benefit). Instead it requires an overall modification in lifestyle.

IN VITRO MATURATION (IVM) OF EGGS

In the mid-1990s a group at Monash University in Melbourne, Australia, reported the world's first baby born from an embryo derived from an immature egg that had been matured in the embryology laboratory, and then fertilized and transferred to the uterus. The process has come to be known as in vitro maturation (IVM) of eggs. In so doing these researchers in fact opened the door to retrieving numerous healthy eggs from women who had not received fertility drugs at all in advance of the egg retrieval and so potentially transforming the entire IVF arena. More recently, Sean Ling Tan, MD, from McGill University in Montreal, Canada reported impressive results using IVM, claiming success rates that are comparable to those being reported for conventional IVF.

How is the IVM process conducted? Within a few days of natural menstruation, an ultrasound examination is done to see how many early follicles have developed. A few days later, once the leading early follicles have reached about 10mm in diameter, 10,000 units of hCG is administered and a day and a half or so later, an egg retrieval is performed and eggs are aspirated from the follicles. These eggs are then allowed to mature in a special medium and under special conditions. Some develop into mature (M2) eggs and depending on the circumstances, these eggs may first be fertilized in vitro and thereupon the resulting embryos might either be transferred fresh as cleaved embryos or blastocysts (3-6 days after fertilization), or vitrified and cryobanked for subsequent dispensation.

But these findings need still to be substantiated by further studies. If that were to happen, it might become feasible to combine IVM with CGH testing of all M2 (matured) eggs. Doing so might improve results from embryo transfer post-IVM significantly.

What are the possible benefits and advantages of IVM? Immediate benefits of IVM would be seen in the arena of Fertility Preservation (FP) where women who for medical or personal reasons would bank their frozen eggs for future dispensation. This would be most needed in cases where women who have certain types of cancer need to undergo chemotherapy or radiotherapy that could damage their eggs and/or launch them into premature ovarian failure. IVM could also be used to access large numbers of donor eggs for dispensation to women who require egg donor-IVF. It would definitely simplify the entire process to the benefit of all.

No doubt, an ability to generate and acquire viable eggs and embryos without using fertility drugs to stimulate multiple follicle development would constitute a major breakthrough in the field of IVF. It would reduce cost dramatically (for IVF drugs often constitutes more than one-third of the total cost). It would eliminate side effects from and all risk of serious complications associated with use of fertility drugs, and it would expand the reproductive choices available to women.

Simply stated, IVM is a much needed approach in view of the potential hazards and the exorbitant cost associated with the administration of fertility drugs. Frankly, IVM, should it prove to be effective and practicable, could herald the end of an era where fertility drugs were indispensable to the removal of a sufficient number of eggs from a woman's ovaries....Wouldn't that be a blessing?

SHOULD NEW FERTILITY TECHNOLOGY BE REGULATED?

In addition to the questions raised by the cryopreservation issues, new ART technology raises a host of other moral and ethical issues that have yet to be resolved—and probably never will be answered to everyone's satisfaction. The basic question is: To what extent should technology be allowed to alter the normal course of nature? In other words, where does it all end?

The following three examples illustrate the kinds of moral and ethical questions the laboratory director of a major IVF program encounters:

A 28-year-old female medical student asked:

> *Is it possible for you to freeze two or three stimulated cycles of my eggs now? I'll be over 35 by the time I get out of medical school, and I'd like to begin my family at about age 40, but with age-28 eggs.*

When a graduate student received widespread publicity after the birth of identical twin calves from a cow embryo he had split, a couple inquired of the laboratory director:

> *Would you please split one of our embryos so we can have identical twins?*

And a terminally ill man asked:

> *My wife has agreed to bear me a large family after I'm gone. Would you freeze several samples of my sperm and artificially inseminate her over the years so she could have my family?*

The medical director and other key staffers of an IVF clinic should fully expect to be confronted with many such requests in the future. Although addressing these dilemmas is not within the scope of this book, the examples mentioned throughout this chapter illustrate but a few of the moral and ethical issues that arise with IVF and related technologies.

ARTIFICIALLY PRODUCED EMBRYOS

Another approach that is theoretically possible would be injecting one or more blastomeres into a zona whose contents had previously been removed or enveloping them with an artificial zona and then transferring the artificially produced embryos into a woman's uterus. It is also possible that human embryos potentially could be nurtured in the uterus of another species.

AUTISM AND IVF

Autism is a neurological, developmental disorder characterized by deficiencies in social interaction, verbal and nonverbal communication, and dysfunctional interests and behavior patterns.

At a meeting of International Society for Autism Research (INSAR) on May 20, 2010, a few papers were presented suggesting that in vitro fertilization is associated with an increased risk of autism in offspring. The worldwide alarm that this has evoked amongst infertile couples is understandable and is reminiscent of a similar "panic attack" that was sparked by a publication in the prestigious *New England Medical Journal* (NEMJ) in the '90s which suggested that the use of fertility drugs increased the risk of ovarian cancer. This study was seriously flawed in that it: a) was retrospective, b) failed to evaluate the effect of infertility itself on the incidence of ovarian cancer, c) did not adequately correct for the age of the women, d) failed to take into account a family history of cancer, e) did not carefully consider the clinical cause of infertility, and f) did not account for the effect of ethnic/racial influences. It was not until a decade or so later, following completion of several international studies in Australia, Europe, Israel, and the United States that the findings of the original study were finally negated. However, by that time the harm that had unnecessarily traumatized an already vulnerable infertile community and created pandemonium amongst medical care givers was done.

The data reported at the INSAR meeting on IVF and Autism and IVF is interesting, but anecdotal. As with the original study reporting an increase in ovarian cancer in women taking fertility drugs it was retrospective in design, which introduces recall and participation bias. The sample size was also small. The reported incidence of autism in IVF babies and the control group was also very small. Also the incidence of autism is more common in babies born to older mothers and also in low birth weight both of which are collectively and individually much more common in IVF. Thus the occurrence of autism in IVF babies most likely is related to the "type of woman who undergoes IVF" rather than to IVF treatment itself.

I am just waiting for the study that links breast cancer with IVF treatment, since overweight women are more likely to have conditions such as PCOS that increases the need for infertility treatment. Similarly, the average woman undergoing infertility treatment is also higher than the average age of women who conceive on their own spontaneously, and the incidence of breast cancer is more common in older women who are into the 2nd half of their reproductive careers. And women who do not breast-feed (as is the case with infertility induced delayed child bearing) are also at increased risk of ovarian cancer, since our patient population skews older. Thus it would come as no surprise if there were to be a slight increase in the risk of breast cancer in patients undergoing advanced fertility treatments such as IVF. However, that would not mean that IVF causes an increase in the incidence of breast cancer.

FRAGILE X SYNDROME AND IVF

Fragile X syndrome occurs in individuals who carry the gene FMR1 on an X-chromosome. The condition which occurs twice as frequently in males (1:1200) as compared to females (1:2500) is the commonest genetic cause of mental impairment which can range from learning disabilities to more severe cognitive or intellectual disabilities. *Fragile X syndrome* is the most common known cause of autism or "autistic-like" behaviors. Symptoms also can include characteristic physical and behavioral features and delays in speech and language development. Other manifestations include a variant known as Fragile X-associated tremor/ataxia syndrome, a condition characterized by loss of balance, tremor, and memory, which occurs in some older male carriers of the gene. Also, since some female carriers of the FMR1 gene may have associated diminished ovarian reserve, infertility, and early menopause, it is important to test women who present in this way for Fragile X.

Most males who have Fragile X syndrome are mentally compromised and usually have many of the physical and behavioral characteristics cited above. However, when Fragile X syndrome occurs in females it is often less severe. However, some gene carriers do not exhibit any of these features.

The severity of the manifestations of Fragile X syndrome varies, but most males with full blown clinical Fragile X syndrome are mentally retarded and exhibit physical and behavioral characteristics, while only about one-third of females are mentally retarded, another one-third are partially mentally challenged, while a third are unaffected.

The Fragile X gene, FMR1, can be passed on in a family by individuals who have no apparent signs of this genetic condition. In some families a number of family members appear to be affected, whereas in other families a newly diagnosed individual may be the first family member to exhibit symptoms.

Fragile X syndrome is diagnosed by DNA testing of cells using one of two methods: a) polymerase chain reaction (PCR) and b) Southern blot analysis. Both methods exhibit a high degree of interpersonal variability and thus when it comes to interpreting results, there are significant limitations. This is especially the case when diagnosing a "carrier state." Interpretation is further complicated by the presence of other fragile sites in the same region of the X chromosome.

The Fragile X gene (FMR1) contains a repeated sequence which is responsible for Fragile X syndrome. In a normal population, the number of repeated FMR1 genes varies from six to about 50. There are two types:

1. Where there are approximately 50 to 200 repeated premutations, and
2. Where there are more than approximately 200 repeats.

Individuals of Group A who carry a premutation are unaffected. Male carriers pass on the mutation to all their female offspring, who while themselves remain unaffected, are at risk of having affected offspring. There is no clear cut-off between the upper limit of normal and the lower limit of the premutation range. Accordingly, cases with 45-55 repeat copies fall into the so-called "gray zone," In some cases premutations expand from generation to generation such that over time they ultimately express as a fully fledged Fragile X syndrome. The larger the premutation in cases that fall in the "gray zone," the greater is the risk of subsequent expansion to a full mutation in the offspring.

It is recommended that in the following circumstances, patients undergoing assisted reproduction be tested for Fragile X:

1. All mentally challenged individuals, those who are autistic, and/or in cases of developmental delay,
2. Women with unexplained premature reduction in ovarian reserve or premature ovarian failure (menopause),
3. Individuals who have physical or behavioral characteristics of Fragile X syndrome,
4. A family history of Fragile X syndrome,
5. A family history of mentally challenged male or female relatives where no definitive cause has been ascertained,
6. Offspring of known carrier mothers.

Prenatal diagnosis can be made by 2nd trimester amniocentesis which yields definitive results. In contrast, results obtained from 1st trimester chorionic villus sampling (CVS) should be interpreted with caution because the status of the FMR1 gene often will not fully manifest in chorionic villi until the second trimester.

HUMAN CLONING

Following the successful cloning of an adult sheep in Scotland in 1997, scientists, theologians, physicians, legal experts, talk-show hosts, and editorial writers raised concerns about the prospect of cloning a human being. At the request of the President, the National Bioethics Advisory Commission (NBAC) held hearings and prepared a report on the religious, ethical, and legal issues surrounding human cloning. The report recommended a moratorium on efforts to clone human beings.

The term *cloning* refers to three procedures, each with very different objectives: reproductive, embryo, and biotherapeutic cloning.

Reproductive Cloning

The objective of reproductive cloning is to replicate an existing animal by removing the DNA of one of its cells and swapping it with the DNA in an egg from the same species. Following this process of "artificial fertilization," the resulting pre-embryo is either transferred directly to the uterus or is allowed to divide several times before being transferred to the uterus. This procedure has been used to clone sheep and other mammals. In the process, however, serious genetic developments have been noted in more than 30 percent of the offspring. It is likely that the same attrition rate would occur in humans; coupled with the belief that cloning disregards the sanctity of human life, reproductive cloning has caused many medical ethicists to find this procedure morally repugnant. There have been a few claims of successful cloning in humans, but none of these claims had been substantiated at the time of this writing.

Embryo Cloning

This experimental medical technique can also be referred to as "embryo splitting." It produces identical twins or triplets by replicating the process that nature uses to accomplish the same goal. In this process, the embryo is sliced in half or into thirds and allowed to develop further; the separate sections are transferred to the uterus. The procedure is unlikely to produce an increased risk of birth defects and has the potential to enhance the likelihood of pregnancy in infertile patients who have been classified as "poor responders." A possible advantage is the potential for achieving improved IVF success with one good-quality embryo. By increasing the number of transferable embryos derived per fertilization of each egg, there could be a potential to obtain acceptable IVF pregnancy/birthrates in women who because of age and/or poor response to fertility drugs are otherwise hard-pressed to produce even a single viable embryo with IVF.

Biotherapeutic Cloning

The first step in biotherapeutic cloning is the same as for reproductive cloning. The purpose of biotherapeutic cloning is to generate embryos for the purpose of research, mainly by harvesting the early embryonic stem cells that have the potential to develop into different tissue types, depending upon the environment into which they are delivered and the stimulus evoked. The production of a healthy replica of a diseased tissue or organ could be vastly superior to relying on organ transplants, and the supply would be unlimited. Theoretically, at least, there would be no risk of post-transplant organ rejection and therefore no need to use immunosuppressive drugs.

In 2004 a CNN poll found that 90 percent of Americans thought that cloning was bad, 67 percent felt that cloning animals was also a bad idea, 45 percent believed that humans will be cloned within a decade, and over half believed that human cloning is "against God's will," while 23 percent disagreed.

SOME ETHICAL CONSIDERATIONS

In the early 1980s, a plane crash cut short the lives of an infertile couple, leaving two frozen embryos orphaned. The ethical and legal questions that arose seemed endless. Did the embryos have a right to be born? If so, did they inherit the couple's estate? Who would have decision-making powers over the fate of the embryos?

Should we cryopreserve and store eggs from a young woman wishing to defer procreation until it becomes convenient? Would it be acceptable to eventually have a woman give birth to her own sister or aunt? Should we store viable ovarian tissue through generations? Should egg donation also become a future source of embryos generated for the purpose of providing stem cells to be used in the treatment of disease states or to "manufacture" fetuses as a source of spare body parts? If the answer to even some of these questions is yes, where are the checks and balances? Who will exercise control, and what form should such control take? Are we willing to engage this slippery slope where disregard for the dignity of the human embryo leads us to the point where the rights of a human being are more readily ignored? Personally, we hope not.

The answers to such questions must currently be formulated in the absence of clear ethical and legal guidelines to direct the use of IVF and related procedures. Because of this, leading professional organizations, such as the Ethics Advisory Board of the U.S. Department of Health, Education, and Welfare; the American Society for Reproductive Medicine (ASRM); the American College of Obstetricians and Gynecologists; and the Judicial Council of the American Medical Association (Ethics Advisory Board) are attempting to establish guidelines that would clarify the responsibilities of participants and set professional standards in the United States. All of the objectives dealt with by the various committees in this country and abroad are subject to a wide variety of interpretations. Furthermore, depending on demographics, geography, and the preponderance of different religious persuasions, ethical guidelines have to be modified to comply with acceptable standards within a particular community.

When one addresses the issues of morality and ethics in any particular IVF setting, it is imperative to examine not only the morality and ethics pertaining to sophisticated "Orwellian" developments in the field, such as embryo and gamete freezing, but also the "morality" of the entire technology. Examples of the kinds of questions one could ask in this regard are: Is the treatment of infertility itself justifiable? Where does one draw the line in implementing the various reproductive technologies?

In the absence of legally enforceable ethical standards of practice in the United States, each IVF program has virtually free rein with regard to the manner in which standards of ethics and morality will be applied. Largely for that reason, we work with an Ethics Advisory Board to review our ethical guidelines, to monitor our practical application of those guidelines, and to advise us in situations where difficult ethical decisions must be made.

The number of moral and ethical questions will only increase as new applications of assisted reproductive technology are introduced. Therefore, in order to answer those questions plus the ones that already confront us, we look forward to a day when clear ethical and legal guidelines directing the use of IVF and related procedures are available to everyone.

CHAPTER

17

THE NINE MOST COMMON QUESTIONS AND CONCERNS ABOUT IVF

QUESTION #1
Will IVF Increase My Risk of Cancer, Make Me Gain Weight, Affect My Emotional Stability, or Drive Me into an Early Menopause?

Risk of cancer: During the '80s and early '90s, articles appeared suggesting a link between fertility drugs and increased incidence of reproductive cancer. The fear was heightened by a retrospective (hindsight) study from Stanford University which suggested that the use of fertility drugs significantly increased the risk of ovarian cancer. This created such a degree of alarm that most IVF programs were compelled to include waivers in their consent forms and required their patients to sign these after full disclosure of potential risk. As stated elsewhere, prospective (forward looking) studies reported from Europe, Israel, the United States, and Australia completely discounted such a link and proved the original study from Stanford to be flawed.

Weight Gain: While the use of fertility drugs and corticosteroids such as dexamethasone, prednisolone, and prednisone can result in fluid retention and a temporary redistribution of body fat by altering the body's hormone and fluid balance, they are not a cause of permanent weight gain. The latter is far more likely to result from emotional stress associated with infertility and ART that often results in overeating. Besides, many women undergoing IVF are advised (often erroneously) to severely cut down on their activity thereby reducing their caloric expenditure.

Emotional Stability: Infertility is a condition of disempowerment. Most women feel very vulnerable and out of control. Those who go to an ART program simply because of its reported success rates and fail to take into consideration the people that will be controlling their everyday activities for a protracted period of time will, when confronted by insensitive individuals, often decompensate emotionally. Both information and human sensitivity are remedies to such problems. Information is empowerment and empathy and understanding are food for the soul.

There is no question that infertility as well as its treatment elicits an enormous emotional toll. This having been said, it is the ability to cope with this stress that differs widely from individual to individual. In my experience, those women who tend to "see the glass half empty" will usually find themselves extremely emotionally labile prior to, during, and after the IVF experience. Those that tend to "see the glass half full" tend to cope much better and in fact often are on an emotional high around the time of IVF treatment. Our responsibility as caregivers is to spot those that are under duress and counsel appropriately. When we are unable to make inroads with such patients they should be referred for professional counseling and on rare occasions will be candidates for psychiatric therapy. Clearly IVF performed in certain situations can be more stressful. For example, women who have failed IVF repeatedly, cases where older women and those with diminished ovarian reserve (using own eggs) feel that time is running out for them, patients who have or are running out of funds to support future IVF endeavors and those who have shaky relationships with their partners are more at risk of emotional consequences. They need special attention. It is usually not the hormones that trigger these emotional effects. Rather it is the circumstances surrounding the treatment being administered that are the cause.

Precipitating an Early Menopause: Menopause occurs when all the woman's eggs are used up. It is true that fertility drugs make more eggs available at retrieval. However, they do not increase utilization of existing eggs. In a natural menstrual cycle a varying number of eggs begin a developmental journey. Only one and sometimes two will ovulate but the remainder will absorb and never be available for use again. Fertility drugs simply allow those that would otherwise be lost to continue developing to the point that they become available for harvest. As such, the use of fertility drugs does not hasten the onset of menopause, and the number of ovarian stimulation cycles a woman undergoes will not reduce her overall egg population at a rate that is any greater than that which would occur under normal circumstances.

QUESTION #2
Will My Baby Be Normal?

One of the biggest concerns facing any pregnant woman is whether or not her baby will be normal. When it comes to IVF, that concern looms even greater because of the fear that the interjection of an "unnatural" component into the equation might increase the likelihood of an abnormal offspring. There have been several publications in the literature that have shown an increased risk of developmental abnormalities in IVF babies. Such reports have only served to heighten this concern. Some of these reports have suggested that because of an increased risk of chromosomal abnormalities in miscarriage specimens resulting from pregnancy loss with IVF, and because of an increased incidence in chromosomal defects such as Down syndrome (Trisomy 21), Edward's syndrome (Trisomy 18), and Turner's syndrome (XO monosomy) known to occur in IVF, there must clearly be a cause and effect relationship. However, a careful review of the growing IVF experience suggests that most of the above mentioned developmental defects are attributable to the fact that the average age of women having babies through IVF is significantly higher than the comparable fertile population at large, and chromosomal abnormalities definitely increase with advancing age. As an example, at the age of 30 years the chance, of a woman giving birth to a baby with Down syndrome is about 1 in 1000 whereas at 40 the risk is about 1 in 150 and at 45 it is 1 in 40. It is "wear and tear" over time of eggs that have been in the mother's ovaries ever since she was developing inside her own mother that is associated with an escalating risk of such chromosomal developmental abnormalities…whether the baby is born from spontaneous conception or IVF.

When it comes to non-chromosomal developmental abnormalities, it is possible that certain birth defects are indeed more common in the offspring of women undergoing IVF. Certain central nervous system disorders are increased in incidence in IVF babies but the increase is slight.

It is true that chromosomal deletions leading to early pregnancy loss are more common in men with male infertility and that infertile men are more likely to propagate IVF male offspring that likewise might turn out to have male infertility later in life. This is because some of the genes responsible for male infertility can be found on the Y chromosome. Some concern has been expressed about the possibility that Intracytoplasmic Sperm Injection (ICSI), a procedure used to procure successful fertilization (primarily in cases of male infertility) might increase the risk of developmental defects. If this is so then it is not the procedure of ICSI itself that is at fault, rather it is the male infertility for which ICSI is performed. In fact, when ICSI is performed using normal male sperm there is no reported increase in the incidence of developmental defects, thereby proving that the procedure itself is safe. In addition, without ICSI, the chance of successful IVF in cases of male infertility would otherwise be very low…so what choice is there other than to perform this procedure in such cases?

Because of the above, it is important for all women undergoing IVF to submit to careful evaluation in the first and early second trimester. At the very least, this should include a high level ultrasound examination. For women over 35 years of age, ultrasound and blood screening as well as chorionic villus sampling (in the first trimester) or amniocentesis (in the second trimester) is indicated to exclude chromosomal abnormalities. There are certain highly specialized centers where genetic testing of amniotic fluid using polymerase chain reaction (PCR) can be done. It all depends upon the identification of the involved DNA sequences.

Genetic defects are more common in certain couples. For example, Ashkenazi Jews are at an inordinate risk of genetically transmittable diseases (e.g., lipoidoses such as Tay-Sach's disease, Neimann-Pick disease, etc.), sickle-cell disease/trait is more common patients of African extraction and thalassemia is prevalent in individuals of Mediterranean extraction. Thus a careful directed pre-IVF genetic assessment should be done in such cases. The same applies in situations where cystic fibrosis is more likely to occur in the offspring (i.e., where there is a family history or the male has congenital blockage of the sperm ducts). Here again, pre-IVF genetic testing is essential. There are a whole host of additional genetically transmitted conditions and chromosomal balanced translocations where pre-IVF testing is likewise important.

Modern day access to chromosomal and genetic tests that can be performed on early embryos can minimize the risk of identifiable chromosomal and genetic abnormalities that can result in developmental defects. Tests such as Fluorescence In Situ Hybridization (FISH), Comparative Genomic Hybridization (CGH) and Polymerase Chain Reaction (PCR) can be performed on preimplantation embryos. It should be borne in mind however that such tests are not infallible. In fact, there is about a 5–7% diagnostic error rate. Accordingly, any pregnancy resulting after such preimplantation genetic tests suggest a normal pregnancy should be followed up with more detailed prenatal testing, including but not limited to ultrasounds, blood tests, and CVS/amniocentesis.

Conclusion: The risk of serious birth defects in the general population is 1-3% of all births. And, indeed, babies born from in vitro fertilization may also have birth defects. There are however a number of confounding factors that may lead to overstating the risk caused by the IVF process itself. First, birth defects occur more frequently in cases of multiple births, and the incidence of multiple births is much higher with IVF largely due to the purposeful transfer of multiple embryos rather than the technology itself. Second, the incidence of birth defects increase with advancing maternal age, and on average, women who conceive following IVF tend to be older than women who conceive naturally. Third, and perhaps most important of all, is the fact that couples who have infertility seem to have a higher rate of birth defects than the general population even if no fertility treatments are used. It follows that studies that use birth defect rates from the general population as a comparison to IVF probably over-estimate the risk from IVF.

This having been said, as with other medical technologies, IVF, while beneficial and highly effective, is not devoid of risk. Thus, all patients submitting to this treatment must be thoroughly, diligently, and empathetically counseled so that a decision to proceed is at all times a fully informed one.

Note: A multi-center study funded by the National Institutes of Health was performed in 2005. 36,000 pregnancies were analyzed. 95% were spontaneously conceived, 1222 (3.4%) conceived with ovulation-inducing drugs and 554 (1.5%) used IVF. This study found no causal association between fertility treatment and the incidence of serious birth defects.

QUESTION #3
Can I Afford IVF?

In most developed countries infertility is considered a "medical condition" and accordingly providers of health insurance will usually cover the costs. In contrast, in the United States insurance providers tend not to consider infertility as a "disease entity" and accordingly IVF is covered in less than 20% of cases.

A study reported in *Human Reproduction* in mid-2010 by the European Society of Human Reproduction and Embryology (ESRE) revealed that direct costs of fertility treatment vary considerably from country to country, with the United States topping the list. For example, the average price of IVF treatment was about $4,100 in Japan, $3,100 in Belgium,

$8,750 in Canada, and a whopping $13,800 in the U.S. It is even higher now. In addition, in the United States, approximately 25% of the estimated demand for fertility treatment was met. This underutilization appears to be most pronounced among minorities and the low-income population. Simply stated, when it comes to IVF in America, the size of the pocketbook usually determines the ability to have a family.

The above-mentioned study is really an understatement of the problem. The fact is that fewer than 100,000 women out of a pool of more than one million potential IVF candidates undergo IVF per year in the United States. About 150,000 fresh IVF cycles are conducted annually by more than 350 IVF programs. Thus, it is not simply a matter of modest underutilization. In reality, the number of IVF procedures performed annually in the United States barely scratches the surface of the demand. Furthermore more than one-half of all the IVF procedures are performed by fewer than 10% of the programs, with the remainder being divided among the rest of the clinics. Since large programs perform more than 600 procedures a year, it means that most others are performing fewer than 150. Since in most such programs more than one RE and more than one embryologist perform IVF, it follows that it is hard to gain the required experience. Simply stated, no one can gain optimal expertise doing so few procedures. In fact it is virtually impossible even to develop meaningful statistics with such small numbers, spread around several demographic and clinical categories of patients. Consumers should be attracted to an IVF program because of its reliability and quality. But merely interesting more consumers in the concept of IVF is not enough—the procedure must be made affordable,

This having been said, central to making IVF affordable is the need for widespread insurance coverage. However, the high cost of an IVF baby is linked to two factors. The first, is the fact that the absence of accurate data on IVF outcome statistics makes it difficult to actuarially determine costs, and the second is that the high incidence of IVF multiple births (largely due to the lack of control over the high number of embryos being transferred per IVF procedure) drives up cost per baby. Thus, before insurance companies are likely to cooperate and increase insurance reimbursement, IVF programs must become accountable when it comes to reporting their success rates, and the risk of IVF multiple pregnancies must be driven down. Unfortunately, as stated previously, annual outcome reporting by the Society for Assisted Reproduction (SART) and the Centers for Disease Control (CDC) does not demand any real validation or auditing of IVF outcome statistics by its member programs. In fact, presently these results are submitted without external oversight and are published as reported, in the annual SART/CDC report. Hopefully, this will change because until and unless it does, many insurance companies will, with some justification, remain reluctant to cover IVF. When it comes to the issue of reducing the number of IVF multiple births this cannot happen until the number of embryos permissible to be transferred per IVF procedure is regulated.

QUESTION #4
How likely am I to be successful and how many attempts might it take?

This is one of the commonest questions posed by patients undergoing IVF. It is also one of the most difficult to answer honestly. All too often a patient is glibly quoted a percentage as if it would apply to anyone in her age category. Nothing can be further from the truth, and any patient undergoing IVF should be cautioned that such a response should immediately raise a red flag and evoke skepticism.

IVF is a complex process whose success or failure depends upon the harmonious interaction of a multitude of variables that differ from patient to patient. In large part, a successful outcome, i.e., the birth of a healthy baby, requires a successful interplay of factors that are not dissimilar to those involved in the successful growth of a healthy plant in a garden. In both cases, success requires that a good quality seed be delicately planted in a receptive soil, only in the case of IVF the seed is the embryo, the soil is the uterine lining, and the gardeners are the RE and the IVF laboratory. You cannot expect a successful outcome when a poor "seed" is planted in a good soil, when a good "seed" is planted in a poor soil, or when the seed is planted in the wrong season or by a poor gardener. Accordingly, when it comes to IVF outcome, it is the factors that influence the quality of the embryo, the receptivity of the soil, and the competency of the IVF team that play a role.

Against this background let us analyze how these factors influence IVF outcome:

1. **Embryo quality**

    a) *Age of egg provider:* In the absence of severe sperm dysfunction, it is predominantly the chromosomal integrity of the egg that will determine embryo competency (the ability to propagate a viable pregnancy). Eggs with an irregular number of chromosomes (aneuploid), will either not fertilize or will propagate an incompetent (aneuploid) embryo, i.e., one that is incapable of attaching and/or developing into a healthy pregnancy. Since age of the woman is the main determinant of egg aneuploidy, it follows that ultimately the older the woman the lower will be the yield of competent embryos. When compared with other mammals, humans have the highest incidence of egg aneuploidy. Since most infertility and miscarriages (as well as chromosomal birth defects) are due to egg aneuploidy, and humans have the highest mammalian incidence of egg aneuploidy, it should come as no surprise that we as a species have the poorest reproductive performance of all mammals. In fact, at age 25-35 about 60% of human eggs are aneuploid and thus incompetent. This incidence increases rapidly with age such that by the early to mid-40s the incidence of aneuploidy is higher than 90%. In addition, with advancing age and encroachment of the menopause comes diminishing ovarian reserve. This translates into fewer eggs being available for processing and fertilization. The combination of declining egg competency and fewer eggs being available explains why above 35 years of age there is a profound decline in IVF success rates.

    b) *Sperm quality:* The advent of ICSI vastly enhanced the ability to force fertilize eggs. This dramatically improved IVF pregnancy rates which hitherto had been dismal when IVF was performed in moderate to severe of male infertility.

Notwithstanding this, it is a fact that the poorer the quality of the sperm, the lower the fertilization rate and the greater the likelihood of sperm aneuploidy contributing towards embryo incompetence. Therefore, male factor infertility does play a role in IVF outcome in spite of ICSI. In general, pregnancy rates are lower when the sperm is poorer, and miscarriage rates are higher. There is also an increase in certain developmental disorders and the subsequent incidence of infertility in the male offspring. The latter is probably due to the fact that a gene that is responsible for male factor infertility is carried on the Y chromosome (XY = male). While age can affect sperm function, it is rarely a significant factor when it comes to IVF outcome.

c) *Protocol for ovarian stimulation:* Patients with diminished ovarian reserve as well as those who are over the age of 39 years require a customized and individualized approach to controlled ovarian stimulation (COS). The ovarian follicles in such women are very sensitive to overexposure to the male hormones produced by surrounding tissue (theca) in the ovary. Unfortunately, these are the very women that either overproduce the hormone LH (which stimulates ovarian male hormone-testosterone production) or are hypersensitive to it. In addition, certain protocols of ovarian stimulation either do not protect the eggs from overexposure to testosterone in the early stage of COS (e.g., the use of antagonists such as Ganirelix or Cetrotide starting on day 6-8 of stimulation) or "flare protocols" which exacerbate the release of LH early in COS. There is compelling evidence to suggest that overexposure of developing eggs to testosterone and other male hormones can increase the likelihood of aneuploidy and thereby compromise IVF outcome.

d) *Laboratory expertise:* It goes without saying that in order to propagate a good quality embryo there must be a well-seasoned embryology team in place. It is also true that most IVF labs have such required expertise. One caveat is that the performance of certain technical procedures such as ICSI, egg/embryo biopsies (e.g., PGD), and assisted hatching (AH) require a lot of experience. No doubt, the longer the egg or the embryo is kept outside the incubator in order to perform such procedures, the poorer the results will be. This perhaps explains why smaller IVF programs where fewer such procedures are performed will often have lower success rates when it comes to the treatment of male infertility and the performance of egg/embryo microsurgical procedures such as PGD or AH.

2. **Uterine receptivity.** Approximately 30% of female attendees to the average IVF program will have a uterine impediment to embryo implantation. This can be due to a thin or inadequate lining or the presence of surface lesions (e.g., polyps, scar tissue, or fibroids) that can interfere with implantation. In addition, about 20% of women undergoing IVF have an immunologic implantation dysfunction (IID). In my personal practice, where more than 80% of the patients I treat have had 3 or more prior IVF failures, the incidence of undiagnosed IID is probably in the vicinity of 50%. Unfortunately, many IVF practitioners refuse to accept the concept of immunologic implantation dysfunction, and when their patients fail to conceive in spite of repeated embryo transfers, they recommend egg donation. The problem is that in the presence of an intractable implantation dysfunction, egg donation will also be unsuccessful. Failure to evaluate for and address such issues will inevitably reduce or eliminate the potential for successful IVF in such patients.

3. **The IVF Team.** Successful IVF demands that a rehearsed relationship exist between all members of the team (nurses, doctors, and laboratory staff). Without such a relationship outcomes will be poor regardless of individual expertise. The performance of the embryo transfer is a critical step in IVF and this demands a lot of experience as well as self-confidence on the part of the RE. Unfortunately, when it comes to this procedure there is a wide variation in expertise. Poor technique with regard to embryo transfer is one of the most significant variables affecting IVF

outcome. In my more than 30 years in the IVF arena, I've had the opportunity of observing scores of doctors performing embryo transfer and have witnessed good as well as atrocious technique when it comes to ET, and the results obtained by such practitioners was reflective thereof.

So, when you are glibly quoted an outcome statistic, you should demand of your doctor that he/she address how the above variables apply to your specific situation. Do not simply rely on verbal assurance. More importantly, do not rely solely on reported statistics by SART/ CDC where the results presented are based upon self-generated data presented by the IVF center and largely published as fact without any oversight, validation, or auditing.

At SIRM, we have developed a novel method of reporting IVF statistics known as the Outcome Based Reporting System (OBRS) which reports IVF statistics under age categories but subcategorizes the success rates on the basis of "categories of complexity" which attempt to analyze several other important variables (cited above) that can influence IVF outcome.

The decision as to how many attempts at IVF a patient/couple should undergo is a different matter altogether. IVF is expensive and since insurance reimbursements are available to less than 30% of those in need in the US, it follows that the pocketbook will determine access as well as the number of attempts at IVF that are feasible. From a pure medical standpoint however, the time to stop trying is when there is no remediable explanation for failure. This means that patients who fail to conceive, before deciding, need to take the necessary steps to try and identify the reason for failure, even if this requires getting a 2nd, 3rd or 4th opinion. In general, if IVF does not result in a baby after numerous embryos have been transferred over three attempts, it is probably time to move on. The good news is that for couples/patients who are willing and able to avail themselves of all IVF-related options, including but not limited to egg donation and/or gestational surrogacy as well as embryo adoption, more than 90% will ultimately be rewarded with a baby. Unfortunately, few can afford this luxury.

QUESTION #5

How Uncomfortable, Painful, and Risky Are the Injections of Fertility Drugs, the Egg Retrieval (ER), and the Embryo Transfer (ET)?

No one likes getting injections and with IVF there will inevitably be a lot of these. The good news is that most of the injections are water soluble and administered in small amounts via a short, thin needle subcutaneously, i.e., under the skin, and thus are less painful than others that are given deep in the muscle (intramuscular). Agonists such as Lupron and Buserelin, antagonists such as Ganirelix, Orgalutron, and Cetrotide, gonadotropins such as Follistim, Gonal F, and Puregon are all given subcutaneously and are thus usually well tolerated. In contrast, certain injections are oil based, are rather viscous, and thus do not disperse easily once injected, causing discomfort. The two notable examples are estradiol valerate in oil (Delestrogen) and progesterone in oil (PIO). Delestrogen is given twice weekly but in very small amounts and thus does not pose nearly as much of a problem as does PIO. This is administered starting with the egg retrieval (in conventional IVF cycles). In cases of embryo recipients (FET, egg donation, gestational surrogacy, and embryo donation) it is commenced at about five days prior to embryo transfer (ET) and, in both situations, is continued until near the end of the first trimester.

In some cases the woman will be allergic to the type of oil used in the injected medication. In the case of PIO there are several different types of oil used (e.g., sesame, peanut, ethyl oleate, and olive oil). When there is a local reaction to one type of oil, another can be tried. When Delestrogen oil causes a reaction it can be supplanted with estrogen skin patches, and in the case of PIO-reactions one can switch to a vaginal administration of progesterone (e.g., Endometrin, Crinone, etc.). While effective in non-hormone recipient cycles, it is, in my opinion, that vaginal preparations are less effective in the case of embryo recipients.

Severe, life-endangering anaphylactic reactions are very rare when any of these hormone preparations are administered.

In some cases, lack of sterile technique when administering fertility drugs will lead to infection at the site of injection and in some cases (very rarely) to abscess formation. Also, because the injection of PIO is given in the upper-outer quadrant of the buttock, there is a small risk of traumatizing the sciatic nerve. This can lead to pain radiating down the back of the leg, which goes away after several days. Sometimes the needle will inadvertently open a small blood vessel and this can lead to a hematoma and bruising. It will, however, rarely be severe enough to require medical intervention.

Obviously the use of any hormonal preparation can evoke side effects, and fertility drugs are no exception. The hormonal changes elicited by the gonadotropins can result in emotional liability. It is strange to say this but in my experience women who "see the glass half empty" tend to experience an exaggeration of their underlying demeanor and often become pessimistic, depressed, and emotional. On the other hand, women who "see the glass half full" and have a positive demeanor often feel upbeat, and at times even elated. Strange isn't it?

The side effects of the various medications used have been dealt with elsewhere in this book. One of the most serious of these is OHSS, which can be life endangering, but which only occurs after the administration of the hCG trigger. OHSS can be prevented through judicious treatment. Refer to Chapter 5 for more details on OHSS.

The Egg Retrieval

It should go without saying that any surgical procedure performed under conscious sedation carries with it certain anesthesia-related risks as well as surgical risks relating to infection, bleeding, and damage to surrounding structures. However, having performed thousands of egg retrievals, I can say with confidence that the risk of serious complications is very low indeed. In fact, I can count on 5 fingers the number of times over a period of approximately 30 years that I've had to admit a patient to the hospital because of a serious complication arising at the time of egg retrieval. The biggest danger occurs in women who have a bleeding tendency and go undetected. This is why it is so important to rule this out before proceeding to egg retrieval. One word of caution is that medications such as aspirin, and certain non-steroidal analgesics such as Motrin and Advil can prolong the bleeding time and increase the risk of hemorrhage. Accordingly, such medications should probably be avoided for approximately 5 days prior to the egg retrieval.

Clearly any procedure involving penetrating the nerve-rich capsule of the ovary (as with egg retrieval) will result in some discomfort. The bigger problem is that after extracting follicular fluid the follicle often fills and over-distends with blood, thereby stretching the ovarian capsule causing postoperative pain. This does not occur to the degree of causing severe discomfort in most cases but it can. In addition, the nerve reaction so evoked sometimes causes postoperative vomiting, sweating, and even diarrhea. However in most cases egg retrieval will result in some bleeding within the pelvic cavity (the blood usually collects behind the uterus, in the lowermost point in the abdominal cavity, i.e., the cul de sac). Most IVF physicians will aspirate as much of this blood as possible because it can be the source of pain.

It has been my practice to inject a dilution of a long-acting local anesthetic (bupivacaine) into the pelvic cavity at the conclusion of egg retrievals performed on women who for whatever reason are not planning to have an embryo transfer done in the same cycle. Examples include egg donors, women using a gestational surrogate, and those banking their eggs or embryos for future dispensation. This must be done cautiously, avoiding a direct injection of the local anesthetic into a blood vessel, because this can cause complications. However, if done carefully, the local anesthetic will numb the nerves on the membrane that envelopes the ovaries, uterus, tubes, bowel, and other pelvic structures, thereby reducing postoperative pain for at least 4-6 hours.

The Embryo Transfer

With rare exceptions, the embryo transfer is a painless procedure. However, sometimes the cervical canal, through which the ET catheter must traverse in order to deliver the embryos into the uterine cavity, is constricted (stenosed), tortuous, or has lesions growing in it that will obstruct the passage of the catheter. In some such cases, it is necessary to introduce a probe or a thin dilator through the cervical canal in order to create a clear passage into the uterus. This can cause pain and on rare occasions evoke a severe and even dangerous, abrupt autonomic (nerve related) response. When this happens, the woman's blood pressure will drop precipitously, she will have a slow and thready heartbeat, and she might even collapse or convulse. While this is very rare indeed, it is something that all IVF doctors must be on the lookout for. Accordingly, at times, when a prior clinical experience or ultrasound assessment suggests that the ET will be difficult, it is best to perform the procedure under conscious sedation with an anesthesiologist present.

Sometimes it is not possible to traverse the cervical canal with a catheter. In such cases (fortunately very rarely) the patient must undergo a transmyometrial embryo transfer procedure. Here with the woman under conscious sedation and using sterile technique a relatively wide bore needle is passed vaginally (under ultrasound guidance) through the uterine wall into the endometrial cavity. A thin catheter is passed through this needle and the embryos are so delivered. This transmyometrial procedure using a very special delivery system can be very effective but it requires significant expertise. I personally have performed about twenty-five such procedures over the years.

One of the most frequent complaints I encounter with the performance of embryo transfer results from the fact that in order to perform the procedure efficiently it is necessary that the bladder be filled in advance. This causes a varying degree of discomfort because some women's bladders fill quickly and overdistend while others take a longer period of time. As a result it is very difficult to time the ET procedure accurately so as to correspond with optimal but not overdistention of the bladder. In most cases, this can be accomplished through repeated abdominal ultrasound examinations but it is not always so. Very often, women complain that delaying the embryo transfer in order to ensure that the bladder is adequately filled was causing them undue discomfort. This is a tough problem to avoid but I wish to emphasize how important it is that the bladder be adequately filled so as to allow for proper visualization of the uterine lining, without which it is impossible to efficiently deliver the embryos into the uterus.

A varying degree of discomfort in the process of performing an IVF cycle of treatment is inevitable. For reasons cited above, some women experience more discomfort than others. I have found that proper disclosure and counseling in advance of performing a procedure prepares the woman and her partner for such a likelihood and goes a long way towards achieving compliance, tolerance, and appreciation. Furthermore, it enhances the doctor-patient relationship. Nothing is worse for any IVF physician to deal with than a disgruntled patient who does not get pregnant in the end. And of course no one can guarantee outcome. It follows that it is very important to try and establish the best possible doctor-patient relationship at all times.

QUESTION #6
Who Should I Believe When It Comes to Controversial Issues Such as the Value of Immunotherapy, PGD, ICSI, Assisted Hatching (AH), and Frozen ET (ET) versus Fresh ET?

Undoubtedly, for many couples planning to undergo in vitro fertilization this is a very perplexing issue. There are so many conflicting opinions out there, which are often presented with an equal amount of fervor and conviction, so as to truly confuse even the savviest patient. Who should be believed and who should not?

The problem is that IVF is as much an art as it is a science. Therefore, what may work best in the hands of one medical specialist might not be effective in the hands of another. A good analogy would be two different artists painting the same landscape. How likely is it that the two renditions would be the same? Very unlikely. It does not necessarily mean that the one rendition is better than the other, but rather that they express the independent experience and artistic interpretation of that particular artist. So it is with IVF; most of what we do is based upon our individual interpretation and expression of available scientific information.

Another issue is that more than 90% of published scientific data relating to IVF cannot be validated through gold standard statistical analyses, and thus lack reliability. I often say that if a textbook on IVF were to be confined to those things that have been proven through randomized statistical confirmation, it would probably be just a few pages in length. Why is this the case? Well, there are two important variables that influence the success or failure of IVF. The first is the "competence" of the embryo and the second is the receptivity of the uterine lining. I often compare this to the relationship between a seed and the soil in which it is planted. In order for a healthy plant to grow, a good seed must be planted in a receptive soil. In the case of human reproduction, for a healthy baby to result, a "competent" embryo (one that is chromosomally and genetically capable of making a baby) must find itself in a receptive uterus (one where the lining is both adequately prepared hormonally and is free of anatomical or immunologic impediments to implantation). The problem is that until recently there has been no reliable method for measuring embryo competence. Microscopic embryo grading and even preimplantation genetic diagnosis (PGD) using methods such as FISH are incapable of reliably defining the "competence" of an embryo. Consider the fact that a "pristine looking" top-grade day-3 embryo resulting from fertilization of a 31-year-old's eggs is approximately 10 times more likely to be genetically/chromosomally normal (competent) than an identical looking embryo derived from an egg of a 45-year-old. Since more than 70% of the time it is "embryo competence" rather than uterine receptivity that will determine the success or failure of an embryo to implant and successfully develop into a healthy baby, absence of knowledge regarding the "competence" of an embryo makes it virtually impossible to evaluate the success of any procedure or process involved in treatment, in terms of an outcome. If embryo competence cannot be determined with confidence, how then is it possible to assess the relative benefits of the various protocols, processes, and procedures in IVF? But, this all could change with the recent introduction of reliable genetic tests of embryo competence known as comparative genomic hybridization (CGH).

There can surely be no area of greater controversy in the field of IVF than that which relates to the value of selective immunotherapy for immunologic causes of implantation dysfunction. In fact, there are those that do not even accept that immunology plays a role in orderly implantation and placental development. Since both embryo competence and uterine receptivity together determine the success of implantation, and since it has been difficult until recently to assess embryo competency, it has accordingly not been possible to prove the potential value immunotherapy might have in terms of IVF outcome. Again, because of CGH, all this is likely to change in the near future. Now, for the first time, we are able to control for this variable and so confirm or refute the benefit of such immunotherapy in IVF.

It is a fact that about 70% of women who undergo IVF are at or below their mid-30s, have normally functioning ovaries, and have straightforward indications for undergoing the procedure. These women will usually respond well to standard "recipe" type protocols of ovarian stimulation, will produce an adequate number of mature eggs, and will readily conceive following one or two attempts.

However, for the remaining 30% who fall outside the bell-shaped curve of normal distribution, such a straightforward simplistic approach will often fail. These are the very women that might well be candidates for an approach that takes into consideration a thorough immunologic evaluation and the need for an individualized approach to ovarian stimulation that would optimize egg and embryo quality. Against this background, it is easy to see how IVF statistics that are simply based on the woman's age can be seriously flawed since they inevitably fail to take into consideration that there is a wide variation in patient clinical profiles, and that such variations often complicate matters severely.

So, when it comes to deciding whom to believe, the bottom line is that you need to a) be well informed by your physician as to what your options are and b) ask the right questions. To do so requires that you do your homework. This means communicating with others who have been treated by your physician for a similar problem, as well as speaking with other physicians. Many times, this can be facilitated through social networking channels such as blogs and discussion boards. Why go to such great lengths? Because it is against this background and ultimately, by your gut feeling, that you should make a final decision.

QUESTION #7
Which is Better, Day 2–3 ET or Day 5–6 (Blastocyst) ET?

The issue of whether it is better to transfer early cleaved embryos rather than blastocysts continues to rage. I wish to focus on the reasons why I strongly favor transferring blastocysts.

What we do know for sure (and reported on in 2008) is that cleaved embryos (day 2-4, post-fertilization) that fail to develop into blastocysts are with few exceptions "incompetent" (unable to propagate a viable pregnancy in a "receptive" uterine environment). So had they been transferred in the "cleaved" state, they almost certainly would not have developed to blastocysts and thus could not propagate a pregnancy anyway.

Simply stated, there is no difference in pregnancy potential by doing an earlier transfer of pre-blastocyst (cleaved) embryos versus forgoing an embryo transfer because none of the embryos developed into blastocysts. There is no validity to the often-stated opinion that an embryo would develop better and have a greater chance of propagating a baby by being inside the uterus earlier, than it would by being allowed to develop into a blastocyst in an incubator.

Don't get me wrong. I am not saying that there is no place for doing earlier pre-blastocyst transfers! Indeed, if it were possible to determine with confidence, by microscopic grading alone, which embryos would develop into blastocysts by day 5–6 post fertilization (and this is currently not possible), then in terms of outcome, it would not matter whether such embryos were transferred sooner or later. What we now do know for certain (and have reported on) is that if a day-3 embryo is found to have its full quota of 46 chromosomes (i.e., it is "euploid") as assessed by day-3 CGH, then, regardless of the age of the egg provider, more than 90% of such embryos will subsequently develop into a blastocysts by day 5–6 post fertilization.

By comparison, in the absence of CGH testing, about 40% of embryos derived from the fertilization of eggs extracted from a woman under 35 years, (and +/-10% in women in their mid-40s) will subsequently develop into blastocysts. Certainly, chromosomal integrity of the embryo is not the sole determinant of "competency" (epigenetic and metabolic factors also play a role), but it is by far the most important variable.

Keep in mind the following facts:

1. Embryos determined to be of a "High Grade," microscopically are not necessarily "competent" (i.e., euploid).
2. The likelihood of aneuploid (chromosomally abnormal) eggs increases as the age of the egg provider increases.

By waiting to day 5–6, many unworthy, aneuploid, and "incompetent" embryos can be culled out, thereby providing relative confidence that you will not end up with a high-order gestation. This allows for the transfer of fewer embryos, minimizing the risk of high-order multiple pregnancies.

Waiting until day 5–6 post-fertilization also affords important diagnostic benefits. Failure of the expected number of cleaved embryos to advance to this stage of development suggests either inherent embryo "incompetence" (which is usually a function of the age of the egg provider, the effect of the "biological clock"), and/or may be due to the wrong protocol of ovarian stimulation being applied.

Waiting facilitates the performance of CGH to identify and then selectively transfer only the most "competent" (euploid) blastocysts. In such cases, a single blastocyst transfer (SBT) should yield a 60–70% baby rate per embryo transferred to the uterus, provided there is no underlying uterine implantation dysfunction.

Of course, after everything IVF patients go through, it is much easier and far less stressful on the treating physician not to have to confront patient(s) with the heartbreaking news that they have no surviving embryos to transfer. Undoubtedly, this is one of the main reasons why IVF practitioners still prefer to transfer cleaved embryos rather than blastocysts. But as far as I am concerned, this is not justification to do what ultimately might not be in the patients' best interest. Rather, it is about doing what serves patients best and what they choose after being fully informed regarding associated risks and benefits.

QUESTION #8
How Do I Decide How Many Embryos I Should Have Transferred at a Time?

The decision as to how many embryos to transfer confronts most IVF physicians and their IVF patients. It is driven by a goal that both share in common, namely that of optimizing the chance of IVF treatment resulting in pregnancy. Clearly, the more embryos transferred, the greater the likelihood of success. Unfortunately however, there is a major downside to transferring multiple embryos, namely an inevitable increase in the rate of multiple pregnancies/births which in turn result in a marked increase in both maternal and neonatal (newborn) complications. Multiple pregnancies—especially high-order gestations (triplets and greater)—significantly increase the risk of pregnancy-induced complications such as miscarriage, pregnancy high blood pressure (preeclampsia), premature placenta separation (placental abruption), and placenta previa (front-lying placenta). It also markedly increases the likelihood of premature birth, low birth weight, perinatal death, and morbidity (including but not limited to severe neurologic complications).

Consider the fact that when comparing singleton with twin and triplet pregnancies:

1. Twins have three times, and triplets have six times, greater perinatal mortality rates.
2. Twins are six times, and triplets are eleven times, more likely to develop cerebral palsy.
3. Twins are 50%, and triplets are 80%, more likely to be born prematurely.
4. Mothers of twins are three times, and mothers of triplets are seven times, more likely to experience serious pregnancy-induced complications.

The anguish of losing one or more of your children at birth or watching them endure a lifelong disability is a situation no parent would wish to face, yet it is a frequent consequence of multiple births. Why then do so many IVF practitioners still insist on transferring multiple embryos at a time?

Most infertile patients simply do not perceive any great risk associated with multiple gestations, especially when it comes to twins. In fact most, consider multiple pregnancy to be a "bonus"...a favorable outcome. Faced with the high emotional and financial cost associated with IVF treatment, most couples prefer to complete their families in one attempt so as to "maximize the use of their resources." In fact, when asked, almost 90% of couples undergoing IVF in the United States are desirous of having twins. Some are even interested or covet having high-order multiples (triplets or beyond). Education is urgently needed to make IVF candidates fully aware of the risks associated with multiple gestations.

The inability to differentiate between embryos that will propagate a healthy pregnancy (i.e., "competent" embryos) and those that will not ("incompetent" embryos) is another possible reason. Most IVF patients erroneously believe that a "pretty" embryo (one given a high grade because it fulfills the microscopic criteria of "good quality") should invariably make a baby. This is simply not the case. Consider the fact that such a microscopically "good quality" embryo from a 30-year-old has about an 8-times greater chance of resulting in a normal birth than would an identical-looking embryo of a 45-year-old! This confronts IVF practitioners with a "damned if you do, damned if you don't" situation; driven by patient pressure to achieve a pregnancy and by competing market forces, they still too often choose to transfer multiple embryos, often with disastrous results. It is generally true that declining egg/embryo "competency" with advancing age justifies transferring more embryos in older women—especially in those over 40 years of age—but this still needs to be carefully measured against the risk of multiple gestations.

Not only is multiple gestation the most common complication of infertility treatment, it has also become the most costly in terms of its social impact. If all of the factors associated with multiple gestations

are considered, including the costs of antenatal maternal hospitalization, neonatal intensive care for premature infants, as well as the costs of
chronic medical care, rehabilitation, and special education, the projected
annual cost of IVF-associated multiple gestations in the United States is
approximately $1.5 billion as compared to about $550 million for all the
other IVF cycles performed.

Risk of Multiple Pregnancies

On the positive side is the fact that the last decade has seen a slight
but significant decline in the IVF twin pregnancy rate from about 25%
to about 22%, as well as a decline in the incidence of triplets from 5% to
about 3%. Still, IVF multiple birthrate are about ten times higher than
those associated with natural conception. Clearly, multiple pregnancy
(especially high-order multiples) represents a complex problem that can
no longer be justified as an acceptable outcome following IVF treatment.

Most in the IVF field are in agreement that it is probably best not to
transfer more than 2 embryos at a time in younger women. The reason is that embryos derived from the eggs of a young woman (under
35 years) are much more likely to lead to a pregnancy than are those
derived from older women. That is why most IVF programs in the
United States therefore recommend transferring up to 2 embryos at a
time in such cases. For women over 40, many still transfer 3 or even 4
embryos. For those between 35 and 40 years of age, 2–3.

Advances in IVF technology (see below) have brought the noble goal
of transferring a single embryo at a time without reducing the chance
of a successful IVF, well within reach. Numerous studies have demonstrated that the cumulative birthrate after single embryo transfer
(SET), followed by subsequent transfers of individually thawed leftover
embryos, is as effective in achieving pregnancy as implanting multiple
embryos at one time. And by this approach the risk of multiple births
can be virtually eliminated. Moreover, using the SET approach, more
than 80% of women under 40 years of age will deliver babies within the
first four single embryo transfers. At the same time, SETs would likely
cut the cost of healthcare per IVF baby by about $50,000 per livebirth.

A recent study found that, compared with singleton deliveries, the costs for twins, triplets, and higher-order deliveries are approximately four, 11, and 18 times greater, respectively—mostly due to maternal and neonatal complications.

In the past, the ability to select competent embryos for transfer has been thwarted by lack of reliability of microscopic morphologic (appearance) embryo grading and the inability of traditional preimplantation genetic diagnosis/sampling—and chromosomal evaluation (karyotyping) by conventional Fluorescence In-Situ Hybridization (FISH)—to be able to access all of the embryo's chromosomes.

The Hippocratic Oath decrees that the cardinal rule of medicine is *"primum non nocera"* ("foremost do no harm"). Since multiple pregnancies is the most serious complication of Assisted Reproductive Medicine, and IVF has been responsible for a virtual explosion in the incidence of twins and higher-order multiples, those of us that practice medicine in this arena have a solemn responsibility to educate our patients and then to restrict the number of embryos we transfer at one time. Central to achieving this goal is to optimize the ability to select the most "competent" embryos for transfer.

QUESTION #9
Do I Need to Use Donor Eggs?

Women are born with all the eggs they will ever have. After menarche (the earliest onset of menstruation) a monthly process commences whereby a number of eggs are used up each month. This process continues until the number of eggs remaining in the woman's ovaries falls below a certain threshold beyond which there is a progressive diminution in "ovarian reserve." Ovarian hormonal activity often becomes erratic and dysfunctional and the woman becomes progressively more resistant to ovarian stimulation with fertility drugs. In such cases the dosage of fertility drugs needed to achieve follicle/egg development progressively increases until the point is reached where she can no longer respond regardless of the dosage of FSH that is administered. This 6-8 year phase of the woman's reproductive life is referred to as the "climacteric."

The onset of the climacteric is heralded by gradually increasing blood concentrations of FSH on the 3rd day of a spontaneous menstrual cycle and a decline in AMH and inhibin B levels. This continues for a number of years until the vast majority of remaining eggs have been used up, at which time ovulation and menstruation both cease and "the menopause" has arrived. Symptoms such as hot flashes, mood changes, and vaginal dryness producing local discomfort with intercourse usually signal the imminence of menopause.

The timing of the onset and the duration of the climacteric both vary from person to person. Genetic factors, exposure to environmental toxins and radiation, disease, drugs, and pelvic disease associated with severe periovarian adhesions that compromise blood flow to the ovaries, can all influence the timing of the onset of both the climacteric and the menopause. Most American women will enter the climacteric in their early to mid-forties and go into menopause around 45-55 yrs. However, some women enter the climacteric much earlier on.

Reduced ovarian responsiveness to fertility drugs is usually the direct consequence of a decline in ovarian function brought about by the onset of the climacteric and pending menopause. Egg quality, on the other hand is directly related to the woman's age. It is the age of the woman rather than diminished ovarian reserve (DOR) that results in an increased incidence of embryo "incompetence" (failure to propagate a normal baby) and this is primarily attributable to egg aneuploidy.

Obviously, regardless of the age of the woman, the greater the number of eggs harvested at ER, the better the relative opportunity to find and select competent embryos for embryo transfer (ET).

As previously stated, the ovaries and developing eggs of women with DOR (regardless of age) are highly susceptible to the adverse influence of excessive LH-induced overproduction of male hormones (mainly testosterone).

While nothing can be done to lower the incidence of age-related egg aneuploidy, it is indeed possible to avoid a further increase in egg/embryo aneuploidy by individualizing the protocol of ovarian stimulation used.

In my opinion the following ovarian stimulation protocols should certainly be avoided by women with diminished ovarian reserve because they either contribute towards a higher LH/testosterone ovarian environment or do nothing to regulate these hormones prior to or during ovarian stimulation:

1. Microdose agonist (e.g., Lupron) "flare" protocols.
2. High doses of LH/hCG-containing fertility drugs such as Menopur.
3. Traditional GnRH antagonist protocols.
4. Clomiphene citrate or Letrozole.

Egg Donation

For women whose advancing age and/or ovarian resistance make having a baby with their own eggs unappealing or unlikely, ovum donation (using eggs from a young donor— usually compatible and anonymous) is a highly successful option. Here, outcome is unaffected by the age of the intended mother— assuming she is healthy.

Embryo Banking

Embryo banking allows older women and those with DOR to undergo several IVF procedures in relatively quick succession and in the process freeze/bank (vitrify) all blastocysts derived from CGH-normal (euploid) embryos for future dispensation, rather than having them transferred fresh to the uterus. Such embryo "stockpiling" can literally stop the biological clock in its tracks since it allows women who are running out of time to prolong their reproductive potential. As such Embryo Banking could help offset progressively declining egg/embryo "competency" over time.

CHAPTER

18

PUTTING THE IVF HOUSE IN ORDER

This book is based on the premise that IVF consumers (infertile couples and referring physicians) are at a great financial and informational disadvantage, and that the situation is not likely to change in the near future. If it is to improve at all, everyone who has an interest in IVF in the United States—physicians and others involved in IVF programs, insurance companies, fertility support groups, legislators, and IVF consumers—must work together in a concerted effort to help get the IVF house in order.

Many experts agree that there is a great need for the IVF community to deal with the consumer more openly. As far back as 1986, Dr. Gary Hodgen made the following statement at a medical conference:

> *I really believe that public trust is the single greatest factor that has allowed the miracles of medicine to evolve in the twentieth century. … The public has allowed us a great deal of latitude to decide where we are going to go and how we are going to get there. I don't believe we have in all cases returned that respect with an equal degree of explanation and understanding, speaking to the fears and concerns of the public in general. Certainly we are not of a single mind among ourselves as to the appropriate course or end-point in decision-making with regard to the ethics of in vitro fertilization therapy and research.*

We believe this statement to be as true today as it was then.

How can the IVF medical community respond to that public trust? We believe the first step would be to make IVF more accessible to all consumers. IVF programs could work toward this goal by (1) cooperatively standardizing procedures so consumers can expect about the same success rates wherever they go, (2) willingly providing reliable and understandable data to consumers, and (3) working with insurance companies and legislators to make the process affordable.

A proactive approach toward compiling and disseminating IVF information on the part of the medical community would go a long way toward educating members of the media, who all too often misunderstand and consequently misrepresent what IVF is all about. We are faced with too many contentious newspaper editorials and oversimplified TV news reports that paint an inaccurate and sometimes alarming picture about the success of IVF. Reversing the harmful trend of bad press by being openly accountable is one giant step that could be undertaken immediately.

CONSUMERS HAVE THE RIGHT TO EXPECT MINIMUM STANDARDS IN ALL PROGRAMS

Standards must be established for IVF programs in the United States, and consumers must have easy access to understandable data about success rates. In almost all other medical disciplines, consumers can safely assume that the physician who is going to perform a certain procedure has, or has access to, the required expertise. This should be true with IVF programs as well.

Consumers deserve to have similar outcomes from every IVF program in the United States. It is unacceptable that certain programs can promise a birthrate in excess of 50 percent per treatment cycle while others report less than half this success rate—or have no track record at all on which to base any statistical analysis. Is it right that a couple should pay such a huge amount when they don't know what their chances are?

One way in which IVF programs can meet minimum standards is by learning from and replicating proven programs. The general factors that contribute to a successful IVF program can be viewed as a triangle, with each side of the triangle representing a crucial ingredient: (1) technical expertise, (2) proven clinical and laboratory protocols and techniques, and (3) rigid quality assurance. The people who make an IVF program effective constitute the glue that holds the sides of the triangle together: commitment, teamwork, and determination are essential ingredients for the successful IVF program.

The structural integrity of this triangle might be compared to the interdependence between a lock and key. Once established (i.e., the IVF program functions effectively and the key opens the lock time after time), the winning combination should not be weakened through needless, ill-conceived tinkering. In the IVF program, as in the lock-and-key example, there is zero tolerance for deviation from a successful relationship. Just as it would be silly to file away at a key that fits a lock perfectly, it is also shortsighted to refuse to take advantage of state-of-the-art technical expertise, proven protocols and techniques, and unwavering quality assurance in the IVF setting. The technology exists. Lock-and-key IVF procedures can be replicated at many sites, enabling settings that adopt them to standardize their programs and, consequently, their success rates.

The difference between a poor and an excellent IVF program may have nothing to do with availability of expertise, equipment, or technical know-how. It simply may be the way in which the components are put together. In the case of a poor program, all the components may be in place, including technical expertise, but the program may be so poorly administered that there is no uniformity of outcome. An IVF program that doesn't have any set protocols and procedures might, with luck, come up with some good outcomes over a period of time—some good results in simple cases and worse results in difficult cases, with no consistency in success rates. A consistently successful IVF program will, depending on individual requirements determined beforehand, arrange the same components differently, but the components will be the same. A consistently successful IVF program can repeat the same strategies over and over and still adopt a reliable format for cases whose special circumstances require a special approach. The only time change would be called for would be in the introduction of new technology that improves the process.

We strongly believe that there should be a way to guarantee that the components of successful IVF programs can be replicated everywhere. Consumers should be able to have confidence that no matter where they live, they will have access to a program offering the same success rates as all others. The only way to accomplish this is by ensuring that all IVF programs use practiced and proven formulas for success, and that all results are validated and available to the public. Adoption of such techniques would be a giant step forward.

CONSUMERS HAVE THE RIGHT TO AFFORDABLE IVF

The high cost of IVF confronts consumer, physician, and insurance company with this chicken-and-egg situation: IVF is expensive because it is a high-tech procedure; however, a greater volume of IVF consumers could lower both fixed and variable costs; but, few customers can afford IVF because most insurance companies will not cover it; and, insurance companies are reluctant to reimburse for IVF because the success rates vary so widely and there is no accountability; therefore, IVF continues to be prohibitively expensive because . . . and the cycle continues.

The reluctance of most members of the insurance industry to cover IVF should be viewed from their perspective: They are unwilling to accept the current statistics on clinic success rates. There are many reliability problems with current statistics. There is no universal method for measuring success. Only with accurate data can insurers calculate their risk and decide on a fair premium for this kind of coverage. Then, and only then, will IVF be covered by insurance companies.

What Can Be Done to Reduce the Cost of IVF?

We believe that because fewer than 200,000 IVF procedures (out of the pool of more than 2 million potential IVF couples) are currently performed yearly in the United States, most of the approximately 400 programs in this country are grossly underutilized. The number of procedures performed barely scratches the surface of the demand. It is impossible even to develop statistics, let alone confidently report them, when they are based on such small samples.

Most importantly, consumers must be attracted to IVF because of its reliability and quality. But merely interesting more consumers in the concept of IVF is not enough—the procedure must be made affordable, which brings us back to the issue of medical insurance coverage.

Financial Risk-Sharing (FRS) with Patients

The absence of insurance coverage for IVF, with its high cost, makes it unaffordable to most that need it. Furthermore, given an approximate 35 percent national IVF birthrate, most women will require more than two attempts to have a baby. As such, when it comes to IVF, the traditional "fee for service" system of payment puts having a baby outside the reach of the majority of infertile couples. It is against this background that SIRM introduced a new concept in payment for IVF services: Financial Risk Sharing allows couples to undergo more than one cycle of IVF for a fee that is more than the usual cost for a single IVF treatment but substantially lower than the cumulative cost for undergoing more than one cycle at regular rates. Moreover, unlike with "refund plans" where there are almost always strict qualification criteria, there are virtually no restrictions to participate in FRPs. The arrangement simply ends with the live birth of a baby or with the completion of all fresh or frozen embryo transfers—whichever occurs first. Those patients/couples who have a baby with the first attempt pay a premium, and the center accepts an overall reduction in fees in order to make it affordable for women who are not successful in their first attempt to be able to try again. So, the infertile patient/couple and the IVF program are always on the same page throughout as both want the IVF to succeed, as quickly as possible.

Financial Risk Sharing plans have met with uniform acceptance on the part of consumers. At first, most IVF physicians opposed the concept of FRS, arguing that the value of medical care is inherent in the service itself and not in the outcome. Central to this argument was the fear that were FRS to be adopted universally for IVF services, the relatively low birthrates reported by many programs would threaten their economic survival. Consumer pressure coupled with a progressive improvement in IVF outcomes over the last 10–20 years has led to FRS garnering growing support in the IVF community.

Insurance Coverage Is the Key to IVF Affordability

Some years back, during an appearance on the *Oprah Winfrey Show*, I made the following observation about the double standard that exists today with regard to insurance reimbursement for certain fertility treatments in the United States:

> *When most insurance companies reimburse for procedures such as penile implants done in cases of male impotence and yet refuse to cover infertility, it makes one wonder how many directors and CEOs of these companies are older men who view male impotence as a life-endangering condition and the desire of a woman to have a baby as a vanity.*

This double standard also applies to reimbursement for tubal surgery (see "Tubal Surgery vs. IVF: An 'Apples to Oranges' Comparison," in Chapter 9). Until insurance companies change their outlook, this double standard will be perpetuated.

Before insurance companies are likely to cooperate, IVF programs must openly account for their success rates. All United States IVF programs should submit their statistics on quality of service for review by an impartial accrediting agency.

Why Insurance Companies Are Reluctant to Cover IVF—And What It Will Take to Fix It!

In the United States, one of the richest and most technically advanced nations on earth, millions of couples remain involuntarily childless. A conservative estimate places the number of U.S. couples that grapple with infertility annually at 4 million, yet less than 20 percent of those couples will undergo some form of definitive treatment. The high cost of infertility treatment, especially IVF, has resulted in reluctance on the part of most insurance companies to provide benefits for infertility and, therefore, has rendered such medical intervention financially inaccessible to the general infertile population. Although a few states have enacted legislation requiring health insurance providers to offer or provide infertility benefits, such coverage is often limited or absent altogether due to regulatory loopholes. The majority of employer groups as well as health insurance providers continue to avoid voluntarily including infertility benefits. They recognize that such benefits would spawn an increase in the demand for these specialized services. This fuels their fear of the spiraling costs that might be brought about by a disproportionate increase in the demand for IVF and the costly neonatal services required to deal with the potential influx of premature babies resulting from IVF-related multiple births.

Some Novel Approaches

The first step towards attaining the worthy objective of universal infertility coverage requires introduction of a method that will allow for reliable verification of clinic-specific outcome data (birthrates per embryo transferred) for every possible demographic and clinical category. A computerized data collection system could be placed in every participating ART program, with the requirement that only those procedures that are fully entered within 72 hours of completion would be eligible for insurance reimbursement. This would permit accurate and verifiable outcome reporting along with oversight relative to the number of eggs/embryos being transferred. All ART programs could be required to meet specific performance standards in order to qualify for insurance reimbursement and be rewarded with financial incentives if performance exceeded required standards. In this way, by shifting the focus from service to outcome, there would evolve a strong incentive to upgrade standards of care, improve outcomes, and minimize the number of treatment cycles necessary to achieve a live birth.

It is imperative that health insurance providers be embraced as part of the solution rather than being regarded as part of the problem. An all-inclusive multi-institutional "think tank," made up of physicians, consumers, and insurance providers, should be convened without delay to discuss the feasibility of introducing universal infertility insurance coverage in the United States. It is time to take the cause for optimal, safe, and affordable infertility care to the ones who need it the most—the consumers. The overriding goal must be to have the insurance industry join all interested parties in the immediate establishment and enforcement of a workable regulatory process.

Change is sometimes difficult to accept and implement. We anticipate that these novel approaches will create anxieties and objections from established, albeit outdated and inadequate, data-collection programs such as the ones currently in place and overseen by SART and the CDC. But we believe that the approaches outlined above would create necessary checks and balances to provide cost-effective, voluntary, universal insurance benefits for IVF, with widespread and far-reaching advantages for the employer, the pharmaceutical companies, the physicians, and—above all—prospective and existing patients.

We have to make a start and there is no time like the present.

IVF CONSUMERS HAVE AN OBLIGATION TO GET INVOLVED

Ultimately, consumers can control the debate. They may have to band together to make their voices heard against the forces of the marketplace, but they can bring about change. Now is the time for IVF consumers to be outspoken. If they do not participate in the campaign to put the IVF house in order, they have only themselves to blame if progress comes slowly. One of the most promising lobbying avenues would be to join one of the infertility support groups such as INCIID and Resolve, both to become more informed and to speak with a louder voice before the medical profession, legislative groups, and the insurance industry.

It is time for consumers to marshal their buying power to demand that the "big A's" in the field of high-tech infertility management, outlined in the previous section, are met:

1. Accreditation of IVF programs
2. Accountability by the medical profession with regard to providing validated and verifiable statistics or a track record, and instilling rational expectations in infertile couples who seek their advice
3. Availability and access to the consumer of state-of-the-art standards of care
4. Affordability

WHERE DO WE GO FROM HERE?

After an initial shakeout period following accreditation, the United States could ultimately have fewer IVF programs, but they will be programs validated by peer review and offering a uniformly reliable success rate. Just because there are fewer programs, however, does not mean that access to IVF will be more restricted than it is now for consumers who do not live in metropolitan areas. On the contrary, mobile units could bring IVF and related procedures to the couple's own area, where they are familiar with the doctor and feel most comfortable.

For example, instead of 25 small programs in one geographical area, all of which have relatively high costs because they cannot benefit from economies of scale, consolidation and regionalization might provide better service to the entire area. A few large, well-equipped centers could serve outlying communities as well as the metropolitan area, reducing overhead costs while maintaining an optimal level of technology and research.

THE BOTTOM LINE

Ultimately, society itself must determine whether technology should be allowed to run rampant or to progress in a controlled manner. We recognize the widespread concern of the medical community that regulation of one aspect of medicine may lead to creeping regulation of the entire profession. Nevertheless, we believe it would be socially responsible to adopt, at the national level, directives or requirements that would control this developing technology for the public good.

The social responsibility that confronts practitioners of IVF and related technologies was underscored by the late Dr. Gary Hodgen almost 3 decades ago twenty five ago at an IVF conference in Nevada when he asked:

> How can we in the area of in vitro fertilization do anything other than search and struggle together to find what this moral and ethical obligation is, define it, and attempt to refine it as we move forward with research results, technology, and new capabilities to help infertile couples? There is little difference of opinion in this pluralistic society about the needs of people to have well children. The issue that's at risk is how we get there.

The time has come to move from recommendations and guidelines, inconsistently applied, to strong directives that can be enforced. Loosely stated guidelines do not provide enough direction, and they leave the field wide open to abuse. All too often, guidelines have been adopted because decision makers are afraid to say, "This is what you will do," and thus settle for, "This is what we recommend you might do—if you want to."

Decisions about the future directions of fertility technology cannot be left to one interest group. In our pluralistic society, varying viewpoints and backgrounds must be represented in order to make the consensus process work: consumers, physicians and other practitioners of IVF, the clergy, fertility support groups, lawyers, insurance carriers, ethics specialists, the media, and legislators must all work together to bring about the national adoption of comprehensive, enforceable directives to guide the implementation of research and clinical care in the field of infertility.

Note: For the thousands of couples whose lives have been enriched by the gift of life through IVF and the other assisted reproductive technologies, for the many more infertile couples who have little hope of conceiving without the assistance of these procedures, and mindful of the sacred doctrine that obliges the medical profession to improve the human condition and alleviate suffering wherever possible, we challenge consumers, the medical/scientific communities, and the insurance industry to strive together to expand the technology, improve the quality, and promote the affordability and accessibility of IVF and related technologies.

Glossary

A/ACP   See agonist/antagonist conversion protocols.

acrosome   The protective structure around the head of the sperm. The acrosome contains enzymes that enable the sperm to penetrate the egg.

acrosome reaction   The second stage of capacitation, when a sperm sheds its outer membrane to expose receptors that interact with the egg's zona pellucida to initiate fertilization.

activated natural killer cells (NKa)   immune cells in the uterine lining that compromise embryo implantation.

adenomyosis   A condition in which the endometrial glands grow into the uterine wall, creating a sponge-like effect; can be associated with poor uterine linings. Women with this condition may experience heavy, painful periods and uterine enlargement.

adrenal glands   Small structures located at the top of each kidney that produce a number of hormones indispensable to proper growth, development, and a wide variety of physiologic functions.

AF   See assisted fertilization.

AFC   See antral follicle count.

agonist/antagonist conversion protocols (A/ACP)   Administration of GnRH agonist for approximately five days prior to menstruation, at which point the agonist is discontinued and a GnRH antagonist is administered daily until the hCG trigger. Simultaneous with GnRH antagonist administration, the woman receives gonadotropins daily until the hCG trigger.

AID   See artificial insemination by donor.

AIDS   Acquired immunodeficiency syndrome, sexually transmitted disease believed to be caused by one or a variety of viruses that are harbored in the nuclei of cells and attack the immune system. Infected individuals become highly susceptible to opportunistic infections; left untreated, AIDS ultimately leads to death.

alloimmunity   Immunity that develops against the proteins of another individual of the same species.

alpha fetoprotein   A chemical in the blood and amniotic fluid that if found might point toward a neurologic fetal malformation.

American Fertility Society   Former name of the American Society for Reproductive Medicine (ASRM).

American Society for Reproductive Medicine (ASRM)   A professional society that primarily includes physicians but also includes laboratory personnel, psychologists, nurses, and other paramedical personnel interested in infertility. Formerly known as the American Fertility Society.

androgens   Male hormones produced by excessive LH that directly stimulate the tissue surrounding the ovarian follicles; some of these androgens may filter into the surrounding follicles and adversely affect both follicle and egg development.

aneuploid   Numerical chromosomal abnormalities.

antibodies to sperm   Substances in the man's or woman's blood and in reproductive secretions (semen, uterine and tubal secretions, and cervical mucus) that reduce fertility by causing sperm to stick together, coating their surface or killing them.

antimullerian hormone (AMH)   A measure of ovarian reserve. (Also spelled *anti-Müllerian hormone.*)

antiphospholipid antibodies (APA)   Antibodies to some of the chemical substances that coat the root system of the placenta as it grows into the uterine wall. Women with high concentrations of these substances may have a higher incidence of miscarriages or may fail to conceive after repeated attempts.

antral follicle count (AFC)   An ultrasound examination of the ovaries during the first few days of the menstrual cycle that reveals the presence of small antral (fluid-filled) follicles, the number of which suggests the potential number of eggs that could become available for egg retrieval under optimal stimulation.

anus   Excretory opening of the intestinal tract.

ART   See assisted reproductive technology.

artificial insemination by donor (AID)   The most common form of insemination into the vagina or uterus; AID involves the use of donor semen or sperm in cases where the woman's partner is infertile or the woman chooses to conceive without having intercourse with the sperm provider.

ASRM   See American Society for Reproductive Medicine.

assisted hatching   A technique in which the zona pellucida (outer shell of the egg) is chemically or mechanically thinned prior to embryo transfer in order to improve the likelihood of subsequent hatching.

assisted reproductive technology (A.R.T.)   Procedures involving retrieval of eggs and the enhancement of eggs and sperm outside the body. Includes procedures such as gamete intrafallopian transfer (GIFT), in vitro fertilization (IVF), and zygote intrafallopian transfer (ZIFT)/tubal embryo transfer (TET).

autoantibodies   Antibodies that are formed against the proteins of the individual's own body.

basal body temperature (BBT) chart   A daily body temperature chart that provides a rough idea of when ovulation occurred. This is possible because body temperature rises when the corpus luteum produces progesterone (after ovulation) and drops at or just before the beginning of menstruation, when estrogen and progesterone levels fall (see also biphasic pattern of temperature on BBT chart).

BBT chart   See basal body temperature chart.

Billings Method of contraception   A method of predicting ovulation in which the woman examines the quality and quantity of her cervical mucus secretions. This method can be used to help the woman determine her most fertile period for the purpose of conceiving or for contraception.

biotherapeutic cloning   Replication of an existing animal by swapping its DNA with the DNA in an egg from the same species for the purpose of generating embryos for research purposes (e.g., stem cells).

biphasic pattern of temperature on BBT chart   Charting pattern that occurs because the woman's temperature is likely to be 0.5°F to 1°F lower during the first phase of her menstrual cycle than during the second half, when the progesterone produced by the corpus luteum raises her temperature slightly (see also basal body temperature chart).

bladder   The anatomical reservoir that receives urine produced by the kidneys.

blastocyst   An advanced stage of embryo development during which a cavity develops within the young embryo.

blastocyst transfer   The process of culturing embryos until they reach the blastocyst stage before transferring them to the uterus; the transfer of good-quality blastocysts is associated with a higher pregnancy rate than transfer of embryos on day 3 after fertilization.

blastomere   Cell within the developing embryo. Each blastomere is capable of developing into an identical embryo until the embryo reaches about the 30-cell stage, after which the cells begin to differentiate into specific tissues.

blastomere biopsy   Biopsy of a blastomere at the seven- to eight-cell stage of cleavage (day 3 after fertilization) for the purpose of diagnosing aneuploidies.

blood-hormone test (LH)   When this test is performed several times daily around the presumed time of ovulation, the detection of a rapidly rising blood LH (luteinizing hormone) concentration can accurately determine the time of probable ovulation. This test, which requires blood to be drawn several times and is therefore painful, time-consuming, and expensive, has been virtually supplanted by serial urine LH testing (see also urine ovulation test).

blood-hormone test (progesterone)   Measuring of the concentration of progesterone in the woman's blood during the second half of the menstrual cycle about one week prior to anticipated menstruation; indicates whether or not she is likely to have ovulated because progesterone is usually produced only by the corpus luteum, which develops after ovulation.

capacitation   The process by which sperm are prepared for fertilization as they pass through the woman's reproductive tract (in vivo capacitation); sperm may also be capacitated in the laboratory (in vitro capacitation).

CDC   Centers for Disease Control.

cervical canal   The connection between the outer cervical opening and the uterine cavity.

cervical mucus   Mucus produced by glands in the cervical canal; it plays an important role in transporting sperm into the uterus and in initiating capacitation.

cervical mucus insufficiency   A condition in which the ability of the cervical mucus to initiate the capacitation process is compromised through a deficiency in the amount of mucus produced, an abnormality in the physical-chemical components of the mucus, the presence of infection, an abnormal hormonal environment, or the secretion of antibodies to sperm in the mucus. Cervical mucus insufficiency is responsible for about 10 percent of all cases of infertility.

cervicitis   Inflammation of the cervix due to ureaplasma, chlamydia, or other organisms.

cervix   Lowermost part of the uterus, which protrudes like a bottleneck into the upper vagina; the cervix opens into the uterus through the narrow cervical canal.

CGH   A genetic test that identifies all the chromosomes in cells. It is used to identify those eggs and embryos that are euploid (have all their chromosomes) or aneuploid (have an irregular number of chromosomes).

chemical pregnancy   Biochemical evidence of a possible developing pregnancy based on a positive blood or urine pregnancy test; at this point, pregnancy is presumptive until confirmed by ultrasound (see also clinical pregnancy).

chlamydia   Bacteria responsible for a sexually transmitted infection that may damage the fallopian tubes and/or the male reproductive ducts, thereby causing infertility.

chromosomes   Structures in the nuclei of cells, such as the egg and sperm, on which the hereditary or genetic material is arrayed.

classic surrogacy   The use of a third party to conceive and carry a baby to term. In this form of surrogacy, the baby would bear the genetic imprint of the surrogate and of the sperm provider.

cleavage   The process of cell division.

climacteric The hormonal change that precedes the menopause by a number of years and is associated with a progressive loss of fertility, an increased incidence of abnormal or absent ovulation, hot flashes, irregular menstruation, a progressive rise in blood FSH levels, and mood changes. The climacteric usually represents an important stage in a woman's life.

clinical pregnancy A pregnancy that has been confirmed by ultrasonic examination or through pathologic assessment of a surgical specimen obtained either from a miscarriage or from an ectopic pregnancy. A clinical pregnancy should be distinguished from a chemical pregnancy, which through a positive blood pregnancy test merely suggests the possibility that a pregnancy has occurred (see also chemical pregnancy).

clitoris The small structure at the junction of the labia minora in front of the vulva. The clitoris, which is analogous to the penis in the male, undergoes erection during erotic stimulation and plays an important role in orgasm.

clomiphene citrate A synthetic hormone that is used alone or in combination with other fertility drugs to induce the ovulation of more than one egg. When marketed in the United States, clomiphene citrate is also known as Clomid or Serophene.

comparative genomic hybridization (CGH) A new technique that involves the simultaneous evaluation of all chromosomes.

conception Creation of a zygote by the fertilization of an egg by a sperm.

conceptus A term used to describe the developing implanted embryo and/or early fetus.

Controlled Ovarian Stimulation (COS) In response to the administration of fertility drugs, the maturation of several follicles simultaneously, which results in the production of an exaggerated hormonal response.

corona radiata See cumulus granulosa.

corpus luteum A term for a follicle after an egg has been extruded. After ovulation, the follicle collapses, turns yellow, and is transformed biochemically and hormonally. The corpus luteum produces progesterone and estrogen, and has a life span of about 10 to 14 days, after which it dies unless a pregnancy occurs. If the woman becomes pregnant, the life span of the corpus luteum is prolonged for many weeks. A synonym for the corpus luteum is the "yellow body."

COS   See Controlled Ovarian Stimulation.

Crinone   A vaginally applied progesterone supplement.

cryopreservation   The process of freezing (in liquid nitrogen) and storing eggs, sperm, and embryos for future use.

cul-de-sac   The area of the woman's abdominal cavity behind the lower part of the uterus.

cumulative birthrate   The overall chance of a woman having one or more babies per egg retrieval or per embryo transfer following several attempts.

cumulative pregnancy rate   The overall chance of a clinical pregnancy occurring per egg retrieval or per embryo transfer following several successive procedures.

cumulus granulosa   The group of ovarian cells resembling a sunburst that surrounds the zona pellucida of the human egg; also called the corona radiata. These cells nurture the egg while in the fallopian tube.

cytokines   Cell growth factors that play a role in embryo implantation

cytotoxic lymphocytes (CTL)   Immune cells that compromise embryo. Implantation.

DES (diethylstilbestrol)   A drug previously taken by women during pregnancy that may cause infertility and/or pathologic conditions in the reproductive tracts of both male and female offspring.

DFI   See DNA fragmentation index.

diagnostic hysteroscopy   A procedure that can be performed under anesthesia in the outpatient or hospital setting with minimal discomfort for the patient. A thin telescope-like instrument is inserted via the vagina and cervix into the uterine cavity, and carbon dioxide gas or a liquid is injected to distend the cavity and allow direct visualization of its structure.

diagnostic IVF   The performance of in vitro fertilization for the purpose of assessing the ability for fertilization to take place. It is an objective test of sperm/egg fertilization potential.

DNA fragmentation index (DFI) Numerical form in which DNA damage in sperm is expressed after the sperm chromatin structure assay (SCSA) or the sperm DNA integrity assay (SDIA).

dysmature Condition of an egg unlikely to develop into a viable embryo capable of initiating a healthy implantation and pregnancy.

E2 See estradiol.

ectopic pregnancy A pregnancy that occurs when the embryo implants in a location other than the uterus; the most likely site for such implantation is the fallopian tube (in which case the term *ectopic pregnancy* is used synonymously with the term *tubal pregnancy*). If undetected, an ectopic pregnancy may rupture and cause life-threatening internal bleeding. Ectopic pregnancies almost always require surgical intervention.

egg The female gamete, which develops in the ovary; also known as an ovum or oocyte. An egg is the largest cell in the human body.

egg banking Cryostorage of eggs to preserve fertility.

egg retrieval The retrieval of eggs from the ovarian follicles prior to ovulation; the eggs are sucked out of the follicles through a needle during ultrasound guidance or, rarely, laparoscopy.

ejaculation The emission of semen through the urethra and penis that follows erotic stimulation and accompanies male orgasm.

embryo The term for a fertilized egg from the time of initial cell division through the first six to eight weeks of gestation. Thereafter, the embryo begins to differentiate and take on a human organic form; at this point it is traditionally referred to as a fetus.

embryo adoption This occurs when a woman receives into her uterus an embryo to which neither she nor her partner has contributed a gamete.

embryo banking Stockpiling embryos over several IVF cycles so as to maximize availability for future dispensation.

embryo cloning An experimental medical technique that produces identical twins or triplets by slicing an embryo in half or into thirds and allowing them to develop further before transfer into the uterus; also known as "embryo splitting."

embryo co-culturing   The addition of cells derived from the growth of other tissue (from the lining of human or bovine fallopian tubes, or human follicular lining) to the culture medium in which the zygote is being nurtured in the laboratory. This is thought to enhance growth and promote the development of healthier embryos.

embryo splitting   See embryo cloning.

embryo transfer   The process whereby embryos that have been grown in the petri dish are transferred into the uterus.

endometrial biopsy   Surgical removal of a specimen of the endometrium, commonly performed to permit microscopic examination of the effect of estrogen and progesterone on the endometrium. When performed by an expert, it is usually possible to pinpoint almost to the day when ovulation is likely to have occurred.

endometrioma   A cystic collection of altered menstrual blood in the ovary that interferes with optimal follicle/egg development.

endometriosis   A condition in which the endometrium grows outside the uterus, causing scarring, pain, and heavy bleeding, and often damaging the fallopian tubes and ovaries in the process. Endometriosis is a common organic cause of infertility.

endometrium   The lining of the uterus, which grows during the menstrual cycle under the influence of estrogen and progesterone. The endometrium grows in anticipation of nurturing an implanting embryo in the event of a pregnancy; it sloughs off in the form of menstruation if implantation does not occur.

endosalpinx   Inner lining of the fallopian tubes.

epididymis   Tubular reservoir that contains and transfers sperm to the vas deferens and subsequently through the urethra and penis at the time of ejaculation.

estradiol (E2)   A female hormone produced by ovarian follicles. The concentration of estrogen in the woman's blood is often measured to determine the degree of her response to Controlled Ovarian Stimulation with fertility drugs. In general, the higher the estradiol response, the more follicles are likely to be developing and, accordingly, the more eggs are likely to be retrieved.

estradiol valerate   A preparation of natural estradiol taken orally or by injection.

estrogen   A primary female sex hormone, produced by the ovaries, placenta, and adrenal glands.

euploid   A cell that has its full quota (normal number) of chromosomes.

exit interview   An interview prior to the couple's release from an IVF program after the performance of embryo transfer, GIFT, artificial insemination, or related procedures. An exit interview prepares the couple for their return home and provides valuable feedback to the program.

extracorporeal fertilization   Synonym for IVF.

fallopian tubes   Narrow 4-inch-long structures that lead from either side of the uterus to the ovaries.

fertility drugs   Natural or synthetic hormones that are administered to a woman to stimulate her ovaries to produce as many mature eggs as possible, or to a man to enhance sperm function or production.

fertility preservation (FP)   Preserving fertility by cryostorage of eggs, sperm or embryos.

fertilization   The fusion of the sperm and egg to form a zygote (see also zygote, conception).

FET   See frozen embryo transfer.

fetus   Once the embryo differentiates and begins to take on identifiable humanlike organic form, it is termed a fetus; the fetal stage of development usually begins around the eighth week of pregnancy.

fibroid tumor   A benign tumor in the uterus, which may prevent the embryo from properly implanting into the endometrium or cause pain, bleeding, miscarriage, and symptomatic enlargement of the uterus.

fibrous bands   Scar tissue that may distort the interior of the uterus and prevent the embryo from implanting properly.

fimbriae   Finger-like protrusions from the ends of the fallopian tubes that retrieve the egg(s) at the time of ovulation.

financial risk sharing   A financial arrangement where patients undergo a pre-defined number of cycle of IVF for a single fee that allows IVF treatment to continue until the live birth of a baby or with the completion of all fresh or frozen embryo transfers—whichever occurs first.

fluid ultrasonography (FUS)   A simple and relatively painless procedure whereby a sterile solution of saline is injected via a catheter through the cervix and into the uterine cavity. The fluid-distended cavity is examined by vaginal ultrasound. FUS is highly effective in identifying even the smallest intrauterine lesions and can supplant diagnostic hysteroscopy in the preparation of women for IVF.

fluorescence in situ hybridization (FISH)   A chromosome-staining technique that allows for diagnosis of both egg- and sperm-induced embryo chromosomal abnormalities.

follicles   Blister-like structures within the ovary that contain eggs and that produce female sex hormones.

follicle-stimulating hormone (FSH)   A gonadotropin that is released by the pituitary gland to stimulate the ovaries or testicles.

follicular phase insufficiency or defect   An abnormal pattern of estrogen production during the first half of the menstrual cycle, which could result in infertility or recurrent miscarriages.

follicular phase of the menstrual cycle   See proliferative phase of the menstrual cycle.

folliculogenesis   The process of follicle growth and development.

fornix (pl. fornices)   Deep recesses in the upper vagina created by the protrusion of the cervix into the roof of the vagina.

fragile X syndrome   The commonest genetic cause of mental impairment which can range from learning disabilities to more severe cognitive or intellectual disabilities.

frozen embryo transfer (FET)   Process in which previously frozen embryos are thawed and cultured for a few days, and those that attain the blastocyst stage are transferred into the uterus.

FSH   See follicle-stimulating hormone.

FSHr   DNA recombinant, genetically engineered FSH.

gamete   The female egg and the male sperm.

gamete intrafallopian transfer (GIFT)   A therapeutic gamete-related technique that involves the injection of one or more eggs mixed with washed, capacitated, and incubated sperm directly into the fallopian tube(s) in the hope that fertilization will occur and that a healthy pregnancy will follow.

gamete micromanipulation   A special procedure performed on eggs to promote IVF in cases where there is severe sperm dysfunction.

gastrulation   The stage of embryonic development in which blastomeres are dedicated to the development of specific organs and structures.

GES   See Graduated Embryo Scoring.

gestation   The period from conception to delivery.

gestational surrogacy   The performance of IVF using the prospective parents' gametes and the subsequent transfer of the embryos into the uterus of a third party who thereon would carry the baby to term.

GIFT   See gamete intrafallopian transfer.

GnRH   See gonadotropin-releasing hormone.

GnRHa   See gonadotropin-releasing hormone agonists.

gonadotropin-releasing hormone agonists (GnRHa)   GnRH-like hormones that block the body's release of both FSH and LH.

gonadotropin-releasing hormone (GnRH)   A "messenger hormone" released by the hypothalamus to influence the production of gonadotropins by the pituitary gland.

gonadotropins   The gonad-stimulating hormones LH and FSH, which are released by the pituitary gland to stimulate the testicles in the man and the ovaries in the woman.

gonads   The ovaries and testicles.

gonococcus   A bacterium producing gonorrhea, a common venereal disease occurring in both men and women that may cause sterility.

gonorrhea   A common venereal disease that may cause sterility in both men and women.

Graduated Embryo Scoring (GES)   Method for assessing embryo quality by means of a series of microscopic assessments throughout a period of 72 hours following egg insemination.

growth medium   A physiological solution that promotes cleavage and development of the embryo.

Hashimoto's disease   An autoimmune disorder.

hatching   Opening of the zona (outer shell of the egg) due to expansion of the volume of the embryo through repeated cleavage. It occurs a few days after the embryo arrives or is deposited in the uterus and immediately precedes implantation (see also assisted hatching).

hCG   See human chorionic gonadotropin.

hemi-zona test   Used to determine whether sperm are able to attach to or penetrate the surface of human eggs.

heparin   A blood-thinning drug that does not cross the placenta and is safe for the baby.

heparinoids   Heparin-containing drugs.

heterotopic pregnancy   When implantation occurs in two sites simultaneously (i.e., in the fallopian tube as well as inside the uterine cavity).

high-order multiple pregnancy   The presence of three or more gestations within the woman's reproductive tract at the same time.

hindsight CGH   CGH evaluation of eggs/embryos performed only after the ET has been peformed.

HLA antigens   The imprints of the man's immunologic makeup.

hMG gonadotropins   See human menopausal gonadotropin.

hormonal insufficiency   A condition resulting in infertility and/or miscarriage; in the IVF setting, hormonal insufficiency may be produced by an abnormal response to fertility drugs and may lead to the failure of an embryo to implant because the amount of hormones produced and the timing of their production and release were not perfectly synchronized.

hormone (sex hormone)   Chemicals produced by the testicles, ovaries, and adrenal glands that play a major role in reproduction and sexual identity.

HSG   See hysterosalpingogram.

Hühner test   See postcoital test.

human chorionic gonadotropin (hCG)   A hormone, produced by the implanting embryo (and subsequently also by the placenta), whose presence in the woman's blood indicates a possible pregnancy; hCG may also be administered to women undergoing stimulation with gonadotropins alone or in combination with other fertility drugs in order to trigger ovulation. Injections of hCG may also be administered to encourage the production of progesterone by the corpus luteum in the hope of promoting implantation following embryo transfer and thereby reducing the incidence of spontaneous miscarriage in a pregnancy resulting from IVF. In such situations, the hormone hCG is derived from the urine of pregnant women.

human menopausal gonadotropin (hMG) A natural hormone that is administered either alone or in combination with other fertility drugs to induce ovulation of more than one egg. The hormone hMG is derived from the urine of menopausal women.

hydrosalpinx A condition in which the fallopian tubes are distended with fluid.

hypothalamus A small area in the midportion of the brain that, together with the pituitary gland, regulates the formation and release of many hormones in the body, including estrogen and progesterone by the ovaries and testosterone by the testes.

hysterosalpingogram (HSG) A procedure used to assess the shape of the uterine cavity and the patency of the fallopian tubes; it involves injecting a dye into the uterus via the vagina and cervix, and tracking the dye's pathway by a series of X-rays.

hysteroscope A lighted, telescope-like instrument that is passed through the cervix into the uterus, enabling the surgeon to examine the cervical canal and the inside of the uterus for defects or disease.

hysteroscopy Examination of the cervical canal and inside of the uterus for defects, by means of the hysteroscope. Surgery designed to correct such defects can be performed through the hysteroscope during this procedure, thereby often making more invasive abdominal surgery unnecessary.

ICSI See intracytoplasmic sperm injection.

immature oocyte (or egg) retrieval The retrieval of numerous healthy but immature eggs from women who had not received any fertility drugs in advance of the egg retrieval; these eggs are subjected to a complex process of maturation in the laboratory and are then fertilized using ICSI.

immunologic implant failure   Failure of the embryo to attach properly to the uterine wall, in the presence of antithyroid antibodies (ATA).

implantation   The process that occurs when the embryo burrows into the endometrium and eventually connects to the mother's circulatory system.

INCIID   International Council on Infertility Information Dissemination; A web-based fertility support group (www.INCIID.org) with its national office in Washington, D.C.

inclusive pregnancy rates   Pregnancy success reports that combine rates for both clinical and chemical pregnancies and do not distinguish between the two.

infertility   The inability to conceive after one full year of normal, regular heterosexual intercourse without the use of contraception.

inner cell mass (ICM)   The specialized cells on the inner surface of the morula that eventually develop into the fetus.

insemination   In the laboratory, the addition of a drop or two of the medium containing capacitated sperm to a petri dish containing the egg in order to achieve fertilization. Also refers to placement of sperm into the woman's reproductive tract.

insemination medium   A liquid that bathes and nourishes the eggs and embryos in the petri dish just as the mother's body fluids sustain them in nature.

intracytoplasmic sperm injection (ICSI)   A form of micromanipulation whereby a single sperm is captured in a thin glass needle and injected directly into the ooplasm of the egg. Usually used to assist fertilization in couples suffering from severe sperm dysfunction.

intralipid (IL)   a high caloric solution infused intravenously to down-regulate activated natural killer cells (NKa).

intrauterine insemination (IUI)   The injection of sperm, processed in the laboratory, into the uterus by means of a catheter directed through the cervix; enables sperm to reach and fertilize the egg more easily or to bypass hostile cervical mucus.

intravaginal insemination (IVI)   The injection of semen (usually donor semen) into the vagina in direct proximity to the cervix in the hope that pregnancy will occur.

intravenous immunoglobin-G (IVIg)   A sterile protein preparation derived from human blood that may offset or counter the anti-implantation effects associated with reproductive immunologic deficiencies.

invasive procedure   Any operative procedure, major or minor, that traverses body tissues. In the case of fertility-related treatments, a surgical procedure that requires that one or more punctures or incisions be made in the woman's abdomen.

in vitro fertilization (IVF or IVF/ET)   Literally "fertilization in glass," IVF is composed of several basic steps: the woman is given fertility drugs that stimulate her ovaries to produce a number of mature eggs; at the proper time, the eggs are retrieved by suction through a needle that has been inserted into her ovaries; the eggs are fertilized in a petri dish or in a test tube, in the laboratory with her partner's or donor sperm; subsequently the embryos are transferred into the body.

in vitro maturation(IVM)   Laboratory maturation of immature eggs.

in vivo fertilization   Fertilization inside the body.

isohormones   Similarly structured components that have different levels of biological activity; the influence of isohormones may be responsible for the variations in potency among different batches of gonadotropins such as hMG and purified FSH.

IUI   See intrauterine insemination.

IVF or IVF/ET   See in vitro fertilization.

IVF surrogacy   Synonym for gestational surrogacy.

IVF third-party parenting   A situation in which an individual other than one of the aspiring parents provides gametes (as with sperm or ovum donation) or a uterus, and the woman who will carry the baby to term undergoes embryo transfer.

IVI   See intravaginal insemination.

IVIg   See intravenous immunoglobin-G.

K-562 target cell test   A blood test that measures uterine natural killer cell activity.

labia majora   The hair-covered outer lips of the external portion of the female reproductive tract.

labia minora   The small inner lips of the outer female reproductive tract, partially hidden by the labia majora.

laparoscope   A long, thin telescope-like instrument containing a high-intensity light source and a system of lenses that enables the surgeon to examine the abdominal/pelvic cavity and to perform other diagnostic or surgical procedures under direct vision without necessitating major surgery.

laparoscopy   A surgical procedure using the laparoscope. Laparoscopy may be used for egg retrieval, diagnostic evaluation, reparative surgery, and various other fertility procedures. Because of its dual abilities to enable the physician to assess tubal patency and visualize the abdominal cavity, laparoscopy has largely replaced hysterosalpingography as the most popular method of assessing the anatomical integrity of the reproductive tract (see also augmented laparoscopy). Once the favored procedure for egg retrieval, laparoscopic egg retrieval has been supplanted by ultrasound-guided needle-aspiration egg retrieval.

laparotomy   A procedure in which an incision is made in the abdomen to expose the abdominal contents for diagnosis or surgery.

Letrozole   An oral ovulation-induction agent that inhibits aromatase, an enzyme that promotes estrogen production by the ovaries. This causes a rebound release of FSH and LH that promotes follicle growth followed by ovulation.

LH   See luteinizing hormone.

LHr   Genetically engineered luteinizing hormone (recombinant LH).

lithotomy (position)   Position that a woman is asked to assume in order to undergo a gynecological examination or other procedure, such as embryo transfer or vaginal ultrasound examination.

LUFS   See luteinized unruptured follicle syndrome.

luteal-phase insufficiency or defect   The inadequate production of hormones during the second phase of the menstrual cycle, which may result in infertility or miscarriage.

luteal phase of the menstrual cycle   See secretory phase of the menstrual cycle.

luteinized unruptured follicle syndrome (LUFS)   When hormonal changes associated with ovulation and a commensurate rise in the blood progesterone level take place but the egg is not released from the ovary. Also known as "trapped ovulation."

luteinizing hormone (LH)   A gonadotropin released by the pituitary gland to stimulate the ovaries and testicles.

macrophages   Cells of the immune system that destroy invading organisms or foreign proteins.

male subfertility   Less than optimal sperm quality, including configuration, motility, and count (number produced in a semen specimen), that reduces the chance of conception without completely preventing its spontaneous occurrence.

meiosis   The process of reducing and dividing the chromosomes in both the sperm and egg, which occurs immediately prior to and during fertilization.

menarche   The onset of a woman's menstruation.

menopause   The period of a woman's life that begins with the total cessation of menstruation, usually between the ages of 40 and 55.

menotropins   A treatment-preparation consisting of gonadotropins extracted from the female patient's urine containing follicle-stimulating hormone and luteinizing hormone.

menstrual cycle   The time that elapses between menstrual periods. The average cycle is 28 days, with ovulation usually occurring at the midpoint (around the 14th day).

menstruation   The monthly flow of blood when pregnancy does not occur; the flow is composed of about two-thirds of the endometrium and blood, often including the unfertilized egg or unimplanted embryo.

MESA   See microsurgical epididymal aspiration.

messenger hormones   See gonadotropin-releasing hormones (GnRH).

methotrexate (MTX)   A chemotherapeutic agent that can be used to treat ectopic pregnancies.

micromanipulation   A term used to describe a variety of mechanical procedures used to promote the entry of sperm into the egg. Also called assisted fertilization.

microorganelles   Tiny intracellular factories that provide energy and perform metabolic functions in the egg, where the microorganelles are located largely in the ooplasm.

microsurgical epididymal aspiration (MESA)   A procedure that involves aspirating sperm from sperm-collecting ducts on the surface of the testicles.

miscarriage   Spontaneous expulsion of the products of conception from the uterus in the first half of pregnancy.

mitosis   The identical replication of cells by cleavage; mitosis is the process responsible for the growth and development of all tissues.

mock embryo transfer   A trial procedure wherein a thin catheter is introduced via the cervix into the uterine cavity. It is intended to simulate embryo transfer and evaluate the potential for embryo transfer.

morphology (of sperm)   The percentage of sperm that have a normal vs. abnormal shape, structure, or configuration.

morula   An early phase during which the developing embryo, which contains a large number of blastomeres, resembles a mulberry.

motility   The ability of sperm to move and progress forward through the reproductive tract and fertilize the egg; sperm motility can be assessed microscopically.

multiple pregnancy   The presence of more than one gestation within the woman's reproductive tract at the same time.

myceles   Microfibers within the cervical mucus that sperm must swim through to reach the uterus; the woman's hormonal environment determines whether the arrangement of the myceles will facilitate or inhibit passage of the sperm. Around the time of ovulation the myceles are arranged in a parallel fashion so that sperm can swim between them in order to reach the uterus; it is believed that capacitation is promoted during that process.

natural cycle IVF   A situation in which one or two eggs are harvested from a woman's ovaries during the natural menstrual cycle and are then subjected to IVF and embryo transfer. Success rates are much lower than with conventional IVF.

natural killer (NK) cells   Immune cells that regulate embryo implantation.

neonatal   Period of life from the time of birth until 1 month thereafter

nonpigmented endometriosis   A condition in which endometriotic deposits in the pelvis cannot be seen at the time of laparoscopy or laparotomy because blood pigment has not been deposited in these lesions. The condition is believed to often precede the development of visible lesions.

nucleus   Structure in the cell that bears the chromosomes.

oocyte   See egg.

ooplasm   Nurturing material around the nucleus of the egg that contains micoorganelles and nurtures the zygote and embryo after fertilization.

operative laparoscope   A laparoscope that has been modified to allow passage of a double-bored needle or surgical instruments through a groove or sleeve adjacent to the instrument (see also laparoscope).

organic pelvic disease   The presence of structural damage in the pelvis due to trauma, inflammation, tumors, congenital defects, or degenerative disease.

ovarian stroma   The ovarian tissue surrounding the follicles that produces hormones.

ovaries   Two white, almond-sized structures, the female counterpart of the testicles, that are attached to each side of the pelvis adjacent to the ends of the fallopian tubes; the ovaries both release eggs and discharge sex hormones into the bloodstream.

ovulation   The process by which an ovary releases one or more eggs.

ovum   See egg.

partial zona dissection   A mechanical form of assisted hatching in which part of the zona (outer shell of the egg) is dissected away in order to promote hatching.

patency   Openness, freedom from blockage (particularly referring to the fallopian tubes).

PCR   See polymerase chain reaction.

PCT test   See postcoital test.

peeling   Removal of the corona radiata from the embryo by flushing the embryo through a syringe or pipette, or by microdissection using fine instruments. An embryo often must first be peeled before it is possible to determine whether fertilization and cleavage have occurred.

pelvic inflammatory disease (PID)   Results from infection of pelvic structures, especially the fallopian tubes, and which can inhibit the passage of eggs, sperm, and embryos in a timely manner to and from the uterine cavity, thus compromising fertility.

penis   The male external sex organ.

Percoll   A chemical substance through which sperm are passed to enhance fertilization potential.

perinatal   The period of time ranging from prior to birth and for 1 week thereafter.

perineum   The outer portion of the fibromuscular wall and skin that separate the anus and rectum from the vagina and vulva.

peristaltic movements of fallopian tubes   Mechanism by which the fallopian tubes contract in a purposeful and rhythmical way to transport sperm, eggs, and embryos in a timely manner so as to promote fertilization and, ultimately, implantation.

peritoneal cavity   The abdominal cavity that contains pelvic organs, bowel, stomach, liver, kidneys, adrenal glands, spleen, etc., and is lined by a membrane called the peritoneum.

perivitelline membrane   Membrane that separates the ooplasm and nuclear material from the zona pellucida in the human egg.

phrenic nerve   Nerve that may be irritated by trapped gas or blood during laparoscopy or following internal bleeding, resulting in subsequent pain in the shoulder, arm, and neck (most commonly on the right side).

PID   See pelvic inflammatory disease.

pituitary gland   A small, grapelike structure hanging from the base of the brain that, together with the hypothalamus, produces and regulates the release of many hormones in the body.

placenta The uterine factory that nourishes the fetus throughout pregnancy and is connected to the baby's navel via the umbilical cord.

placentation Formation and attachment of the placenta to the uterine wall.

plasma membrane Double-layered membrane that envelops the entire sperm.

polar body biopsy Biopsy of egg-derived chromosome populations within 36 hours of fertilization for the diagnosis of both egg- and sperm-induced embryo aneuploidies.

polycystic ovarian syndrome (PCOS) Condition in which the ovaries develop multiple small cysts; it is often associated with abnormal or absent ovulation and, accordingly, with infertility.

polymerase chain reaction (PCR) Technology involving identification and amplification of one or more gene loci on the chromosome.

polyploidy Situation in which more than two pronuclei (conglomerates of chromosomal material) are present; because of this, the zygote will not produce a viable embryo.

polyps (uterine) Outgrowths that protrude into the uterus and may cause pain and bleeding or prevent an embryo from implanting.

postcoital test (PCT) Assessment of the cervical mucus after intercourse to evaluate the quality of the mucus and mucus-sperm interaction; also known as the Hühner test.

preimplantation genetic diagnosis (PGD) A new diagnostic technology involving chromosome and genetic assessment of the embryo in order to determine its health and potential to develop into a healthy offspring. A procedure currently used to determine the sex of the embryo and to diagnose a variety of genetic disorders.

premature luteinization Often also referred to as a "premature LH surge." LH is released "prematurely," i.e., prior to the hCG trigger, and this results in compromised follicle and egg development. It is often characterized by a >20% drop in the blood estradiol level over a period of 24 hours.

progesterone A primary female sex hormone produced by the corpus luteum that induces secretory changes in the glands of the endometrium. Progesterone may also be given by injection or in the form of vaginal suppositories to enhance implantation and reduce the risk of miscarriage.

prolactin   A hormone produced by the brain that may influence the activity of FSH on the ovaries.

proliferative phase of the menstrual cycle   Usually, the first half of the menstrual cycle, when the endometrium grows under the influence of estrogen and the follicles develop; also known as the follicular phase.

prolonged coasting   The discontinuation of gonadotropin medication and deferring hCG administration for a number of days, while continuing GnRH agonist therapy in cases where severe ovarian hyperstimulation occurs following COS in preparation for IVF.

prostaglandins   Natural hormones contained in a multitude of cells in the body as well as in the seminal fluid. The placement of semen, which contains seminal fluid with prostaglandins, directly in the uterus in quantities greater than 0.2 ml can cause life-threatening shock.

prostate gland   Gland in the male reproductive tract that secretes a milky substance that nurtures and promotes survival of sperm. The combination of sperm and milky fluid that is ejaculated during erotic experiences is known as semen.

purified FSH   A fertility hormone derived by processing and purifying gonadotropins to eliminate the LH component.

quantitative beta hCG blood pregnancy test   Test that detects and measures the amount of hCG (produced by an implanting embryo) in the woman's blood. Measured about 11 and 13 days after embryo transfer, it can diagnose a possible pregnancy before the woman has missed a menstrual period.

rectum   Lower portion of the large intestine that connects to the anal canal.

recurrent pregnancy loss (RPL)   Repeated (>2) miscarriages occurring in the same individual.

reproductive cloning   Replication of an existing animal by swapping its DNA with the DNA in an egg from the same species; the resulting embryo is either transferred directly to the uterus or allowed to divide several times before being transferred; sheep and other mammals have been cloned with this procedure.

Resolve, Inc. Fertility support group in the United States; its national office is in Somerville, Mass.

retrograde ejaculation A condition, sometimes caused by a spinal cord injury or following removal of a diseased prostate gland, in which the man ejaculates backward into the bladder rather than outward through the penis. It may cause infertility but can be treated by inseminating the woman with sperm separated from urine the man would pass immediately following orgasm.

salpingoscopy A procedure involving the introduction of a thin fiber-optic instrument into the fallopian tube or tubes to promote visualization of the tubal lining. It is usually performed during laparoscopy but may also be performed through a hysteroscope.

salpingostomy A form of tubal surgery in which the end of the fallopian tube(s) is opened at the time of laparoscopy or laparotomy, using small surgical stitches or a laser.

salpingotomy An incision made in the wall of the fallopian tube to remove an ectopic (tubal) pregnancy, a tumor, or drain fluid from the tubal lumen.

SART See Society of Assisted Reproductive Technology.

sclerotherapy (for ovarian endometriomas) Needle aspiration of the liquid content of the endometriotic cyst, followed by the injection of 5 percent solution of tetracycline into the cyst cavity.

scrotum Pouch in which the male's testicles are suspended outside the body.

secretory phase of the menstrual cycle The second half of the menstrual cycle, which begins after ovulation under the influence of estrogen and progesterone produced by the corpus luteum; the term *secretory* is derived from the secretion by the endometrium of nutrients that will sustain an embryo; also known as the luteal phase.

selective reduction of pregnancy Prior to completion of the third month of pregnancy, reduction of the number of fetuses in a large multiple pregnancy by injecting a chemical substance under ultrasound guidance; the fetus or fetuses succumb almost immediately and are absorbed by the body. It may be considered a life-saving measure for the remaining fetuses in high-multiple pregnancies (triplets and greater) and reduces the risk to the mother.

semen   The combination of sperm, seminal fluid, and other male reproductive secretions.

seminal fluid   Milky fluid produced by the seminal vesicles that is ejaculated during erotic experiences (see also semen).

seminal vesicles   Glands in the male reproductive tract that secrete a milky substance that nurtures and promotes survival of sperm.

sHLA-G   See soluble human leukocyte antigen-G.

Society for Assisted Reproductive Technology (SART)   Affiliated with the American Society for Reproductive Medicine, SART provides information about IVF programs and compiles a registry of audited IVF results from participating programs.

soluble human leukocyte antigen-G   A genetic marker excreted into the growth medium of the petri dish and measured to identify those embryos most likely to produce a pregnancy.

sonohysterogram   See fluid ultrasonography.

sperm   The male gamete; spermatozoa.

sperm antibody test   Test that determines whether either partner's blood or the woman's cervical mucus contains antibodies to sperm.

Sperm Chromatin Structure Assay (SCSA)

sperm count   A basic fertility-assessment test of sperm function, primarily involving counting the number of sperm, assessing their motility and progression, and evaluating their overall structure and form.

spontaneous menstrual abortion   An early miscarriage occurring at the time of menstruation without the woman's menstrual period being delayed.

SP-I   See pregnancy-specific glycoprotein.

sterility   See infertility.

stimulation   Induction of the development of a number of follicles in response to the administration of fertility drugs (see also Controlled Ovarian Stimulation and superovulation).

subzonal insertion (SUZI) The direct injection of one or more sperm into the perivitelline space to promote fertilization. It is a form of micromanipulation.

superovulation The ovulation of more than one egg induced through the administration of fertility drugs (see also Controlled Ovarian Stimulation and stimulation).

surrogacy Situation in which an infertile woman uses someone else's uterus to carry a child to term. Surrogacy can be divided into (1) cases in which the surrogate mother contributes biologically to the offspring by providing her own eggs (classic surrogacy) and (2) cases in which the surrogate does not contribute biologically and therefore must undergo IVF (gestational surrogacy).

SUZI See subzonal insertion.

syphilis A life-endangering venereal disease that in its late stages attacks most systems in the body, including the cardiovascular and central nervous systems.

T-cells Immune cells that play a role in embryo implantation.

testes See testicles.

testicles The male counterparts of the female ovaries; located in the scrotum, the testicles produce sperm and male hormones such as testosterone.

testicular sperm aspiration (TESA) A procedure performed on an outpatient basis (usually under local anesthesia) where sperm are aspirated from the sperm duct for use in ICSI.

testicular sperm extraction (TESE) A procedure performed on an outpatient basis (usually under local anesthesia) where one or more hair-thin biopsy specimens are removed and delivered to the embryology laboratory for sperm to be removed for ICSI.

testosterone The predominant male sex hormone, which influences the production and maturation of sperm.

test yolk buffer A sperm-enhancement solution derived from the yolk of a chicken egg.

therapeutic gamete-related technologies Procedures involving the use of gametes to enhance the chance of conception through subsequent insemination, or transfer of eggs and/or sperm into the woman's uterus, fallopian tubes, or peritoneal cavity.

therapeutic hysteroscopy A procedure, usually performed under general anesthesia, in which a clear liquid is injected into the uterine cavity via the hysteroscope. This permits exposure of surface lesions inside the uterus or cervix via X-ray. These lesions can be treated surgically through excision, obliteration, transection, etc.

third-party parenting Any situation in which an individual other than the aspiring parents assists by providing gametes (as with sperm and ovum donation) or a uterus in order to help the couple have a baby.

thrombophilia The inherited tendency to develop blood clots too easily.

thyroid-stimulating hormone (TSH) A hormone produced by the pituitary gland that stimulates the release of thyroid hormone by the thyroid gland.

transabdominal egg retrieval An ultrasound-guided egg-retrieval procedure in which the needle is passed through the abdominal wall and a full bladder into the ovarian follicles; it has largely been supplanted by transvaginal egg retrieval.

transcervical Refers to the physiological or surgical pathway whereby secretions, organisms, sperm, or surgical instrumentation passes from the vagina into the uterus.

transmyometrial embryo transfer A procedure that transfers embryos to the uterus via a needle and/or catheter introduced through the uterine wall (myometrium) rather than through the cervix. It is used in situations where severe narrowing of the cervix negates the performance of conventional embryo transfer.

transperitoneal insemination (TPI) The injection of washed sperm through a syringe into the woman's pelvic cavity at the time of expected ovulation to promote conception; it may be combined with intrauterine insemination.

transurethral egg retrieval An ultrasound-guided egg retrieval procedure in which the needle is passed through the urethra and the bladder wall into the ovaries; it has largely been supplanted by transvaginal egg retrieval.

transvaginal egg retrieval An ultrasound-guided egg retrieval procedure in which a needle is passed through the back or side of the woman's vagina into her ovaries. It is the most commonly performed egg retrieval procedure today.

trapped ovulation See Luteinized Unruptured Follicle Syndrome (LUFS).

treatment cycle The menstrual cycle during which a particular fertility treatment, such as IVF, IUI, AID, GIFT, etc., was performed.

T-regulatory cells T-cells that help regulate the immune response involved in embryo implantation

trophoblast The root system of the conceptus, which subsequently develops into the placenta.

tubal abortion A pregnancy that gained early attachment to a fallopian tube's inner lining is absorbed before the woman even knows that she is pregnant.

tubal embryo transfer (TET) A procedure, usually performed via laparoscopy, in which one or more embryos are inserted in the fallopian tube(s) via a thin catheter a few days following egg retrieval; also known as zygote intrafallopian transfer (ZIFT).

tubal pregnancy See ectopic pregnancy.

tubal reanastomosis A surgical procedure in which the fallopian tubes are reconnected, reestablishing patency. Usually performed after a previous tubal ligation (sterilization).

tuboscopy A procedure in which a thin fiber-optic telescope is passed into the fallopian tube(s) to evaluate their inner structure.

UCFD See ultrasound color flow Doppler.

ultrasound A painless diagnostic procedure that transforms high-frequency sound waves as they travel through body tissue and fluid into images on a TV-like screen; it enables the physician to clearly identify structures within the body and to guide instruments during certain procedures. Ultrasound is also used to diagnose a clinical pregnancy.

ultrasound color flow Doppler (UCFD)   A means of measuring uterine blood flow.

unexplained infertility   Infertility whose cause cannot be readily determined by conventional diagnostic procedures; this occurs in about 10 percent of all infertile couples.

ureaplasma   A microorganism that occurs in the reproductive tracts of males and females; it may interfere with sperm transport and/or embryo implantation. It might also be responsible for early miscarriages.

urethra   The canal-like structure through which urine passes from the bladder and through which semen passes during ejaculation.

urine ovulation test   A simple test that can pinpoint the time of presumed ovulation; frequent charting of the test results detects the surge of LH that triggers ovulation.

uterus   A muscular organ that enlarges during pregnancy from its normal pearlike shape and size to accommodate a full-term pregnancy.

vagina   The narrow passage that leads from the vulva to the cervix. The vagina's elastic tissue, muscle, and skin have enormous ability to stretch so as to accommodate the penis during the sex act and the passage of a baby during childbirth.

varicocele   A collection of dilated veins around the testicles that hinders sperm function, possibly through increasing the temperature in the scrotum.

vas deferens   Tube that connects the epididymis with the urethra in the male reproductive tract.

vasectomy   Surgery to block the male's sperm ducts for the purpose of birth control.

vestibule   The cleft between the labia minora; the entrance to the vagina.

vitrification (ultrarapid freezing)   The process of very rapidly freezing eggs and embryos, so fast that ice does not form in the cells, thereby minimizing damage.

vulva   The external portion of the female reproductive tract.

warfarin   A blood-thinning drug.

washing (sperm washing)   The processing of a semen specimen in a centrifuge in order to separate the sperm from the semen specimen.

yellow body   See corpus luteum.

ZIFT   See zygote intrafallopian transfer.

zona-cumulus complex   The mass of cells (zona pellucida and cumulus mass) through which the sperm must pass to reach the egg.

zona drilling   A form of micromanipulation whereby a small hole is made in the zona pellucida to promote free entry of a sperm into the egg.

zygote intrafallopian transfer (ZIFT)   Another name for tubal embryo transfer.

INDEX

Italic page numbers indicate illustrations or captions.
Boldface page numbers indicate glossary terms.

D

E

Z

12/14 = Ø (5/14)
10/15
6/17 Ⓘ 4/17